COMMUNITY HEALTH
AND SANITATION

COMMUNITY HEALTH AND SANITATION

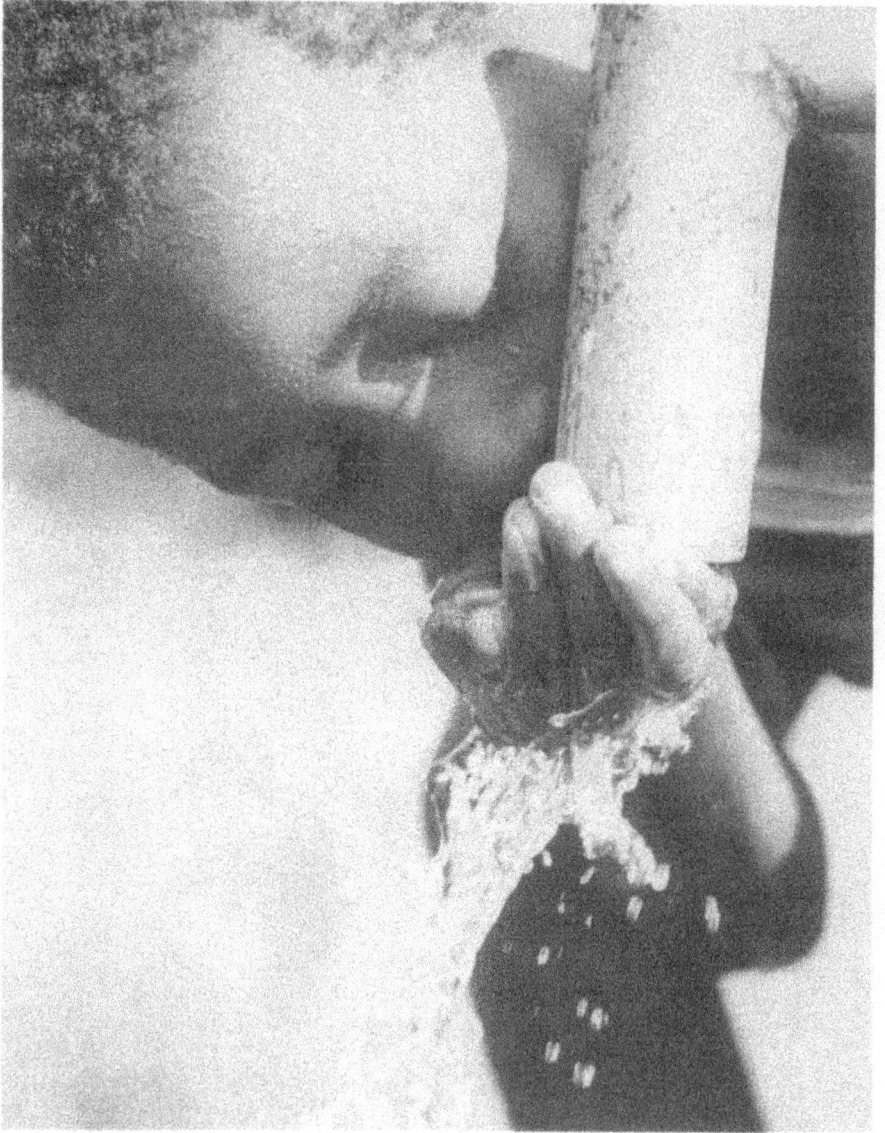

Community Health and Sanitation

Selectected and edited by
CHARLES KERR

**Practical
ACTION
PUBLISHING**

INTERMEDIATE TECHNOLOGY PUBLICATIONS 1990

Practical Action Publishing Ltd
27a Albert Street, Rugby, CV21 2SG, Warwickshire, UK
www.practicalactionpublishing.org

© Intermediate Technology Publications 1990

First published 1990\Digitised 2013

ISBN 10: 1 85339 018 6
ISBN 13: 9781853390180
ISBN Library Ebook: 9781780441856
Book DOI: http://dx.doi.org/10.3362/9781780441856

A catalogue record for this book is available from the British Library.

The authors, contributors and/or editors have asserted their rights under
the Copyright Designs and Patents Act 1988 to be identified as authors of
their respective contributions.

Since 1974, Practical Action Publishing has published and disseminated
books and information in support of international development work
throughout the world. Practical Action Publishing is a trading name
of Practical Action Publishing Ltd (Company Reg. No. 1159018), the
wholly owned publishing company of Practical Action. Practical Action
Publishing trades only in support of its parent charity objectives and any
profits are covenanted back to Practical Action (Charity Reg. No. 247257,
Group VAT Registration No. 880 9924 76).

Contents

A NOTE ON CURRENCIES

Although the articles in this book cover a number of different years in the 1980s, the following conversion rates from September 1990 will give the reader a general idea of the values involved.

	£ sterling	US $
Pakistan	38 P rupees	20.6
Sri Lanka	50 SL rupees	27.1
Thailand	47 Baht	25.5
Zimbabwe	6 Z dollars	3.3

ACRONYMS

ATA	Appropriate Technology Association
CUSO	Canadian Universities in Service Overseas
DANIDA	Danish International Development Agency
GTZ	German Technical Co-operation Agency
IRCWD	International Reference Centre for Waste Disposal
IDWSSD	International Drinking Water Supply and Sanitation Decade
IRC	International Reference Centre for Community Water Supply and Sanitation
ITDG	Intermediate Technology Development Group
NORAD	Norwegian Agency for Development
ODA	Overseas Development Administration
SATA	Swiss Association for Technical Assistance
SKAT	Swiss Centre for Alternative Technology
UNDP	United Nations Development Programme
UNEP	United Nations Environment Programme
UNHCR	United Nations High Commission for Refugees
UNICEF	United Nations Childrens Fund
USAID	United States Agency for International Development
VSO	Voluntary Service Overseas (UK)
WASH (E)	Water and Sanitation for Health (Education)
WHO	World Health Organization

Preface

Water and sanitation are essential for a healthy productive life. Over vast areas of developing countries, water is often remote and unsafe, while sanitation is at best primitive.

The poor suffer most, having neither the knowledge nor the means to improve their condition. Dehydration from diarrhoea alone kills over four million children each year in developing countries. The debilitating effect of endemic diseases together with malnutrition causes untold misery and suffering. Poverty is perpetuated by the adverse effects on productivity; a heart-breaking vicious circle. From the time of its foundation in 1965, ITDG has been all too aware of the problems associated with the lack of safe water and adequate sanitation facilities. Articles on water and sanitation have always been prominent in ITDG's quarterly journal, *Appropriate Technology*, established in 1973.

With the launch of IDWSSD in 1981, ITDG decided to make a contribution by starting a new journal featuring articles on appropriate technologies for safe water and improved sanitation. The first issue of *Waterlines* appeared in 1982, thanks to the financial support of Canada's International Research and Development Centre (IDRC), and has continued with the support of agencies which sponsor bulk subscriptions to fieldworkers, who would otherwise be unable to order the periodical. The main objective of the journal is to pass on practical, down-to-earth information to community planners and fieldworkers in developing countries who are tackling the problems day by day; a vital link in the chain along which information is disseminated for the Water Decade.

This is a companion book to the recently published *Community Water Development*, and, as with that volume, it was considered that publication of selected articles in book form would preserve the information as a valuable reference both for planners and workers in the field. Inevitably, although each volume could stand alone, several articles in each are relevant to the other: sanitation must progress simultaneously with water-supply improvements, as is emphasized in many articles.

This volume contains articles selected from the first seven volumes of *Waterlines* dating from July 1982 to April 1989, thereby covering much of the Water Decade. Again, because of the high standard of the articles and space constraints, a major problem has been to decide which articles to leave out. A secondary problem has been the question of whether to update the original articles. It was decided to minimize editing to retain the articles in their original context. Each has been dated and a further reading list has been included to replace the original references. An ancillary problem is that of changes in currency values; these have fluctuated widely and the conversion chart on page ix should give some guidance.

This volume has also been divided into 11 chapters, each preceded by a short introductory note for continuity and background. The first chapter establishes the theme that improved sanitation and hygiene, as well as improved water supplies, are necessary to achieve health benefits, and examines the methods to ensure successful projects. Chapter 2 shows how difficult it is to measure health benefits and gives examples of water health-hazards and their control. The next three chapters deal with measures to make water supplies more safe; in the home and for the community, and in particular through water-quality control.

Chapters 6 and 7 deal with sanitation: latrines in the former, and other aspects in the latter, including waste disposal and drainage. Training is covered in Chapter 8 and the related community education and participation programme (CEP) in Chapter 9. CEP is now recognized as an essential component of development programmes. Chapter 10 is directed to examples of programme planning, while Chapter 11 stresses the need for strategies for improvement. Articles include the evaluation of projects and an example of the introduction of CEP into a programme. It is considered that the adoption of the step procedure of Charles Chandler in Chapter 1, in conjunction with careful monitoring and evaluation, will achieve fuller health benefits and optimum resource use.

Water-quality control is an important component for the monitoring and evaluation of water-supply projects. The measurement of health benefits attributable to water and sanitation provide an essential foundation for community development programmes. As concluded in the final article, good health in the developing world can only come by the actions of the people themselves.

All credit for this volume also must go the the many authors who have contributed so much to *Waterlines*. My special thanks for their support and encouragement goes to the *Waterlines* editorial team, and to Robin Wiseman for undertaking all the real editing of this book.

These volumes have been dedicated by the publishers to Frances Stuart, editor of *Waterlines* from the first issue until April 1985. She died in a tragic accident in the course of her duties as a VSO in Nigeria.

Charles Kerr
1990

CHAPTER 1
Water and Sanitation

Health benefits cannot be achieved to any great extent through improved water supplies alone: improved sanitation must be implemented simultaneously. Even then, health benefits will only result with proper hygiene, and this demands education. Hence the equation:

$$\text{Health} = \text{Water} + \text{Sanitation} + \text{Hygiene Education.}$$

The articles in this introductory chapter emphasize various aspects of this now accepted wisdom. Martin Beyer, in his editorial article from the first issue of *Waterlines*, sets the keynote, employing the main points of the 1978 UNICEF/WHO recommendations from which the above equation was derived. Sumi Krishna stresses the basic components for significant health impact. As he says, the software component (education) is at least as important as the hardware. His quote, 'The simple practice of washing hands is the most important scientific and medical development of all time', warrants maximum publicity. Unfortunately, poor people may not be able to perceive that improved production and earning capacity is founded on their improved health and environment: 'Where sheer survival is the first priority, anything else, including health, comes second.' Technology will not produce results until community behaviour can be changed.

John Pickford, in his more recent article, discusses the importance of rural sanitation for health and well-being in the developing world with examples based on his experience. He also emphasizes the importance of software and concludes with a checklist for improved rural sanitation. Women as the key to success is the message from Mary Ellendorf and Raymond Isely. They underline the importance of understanding attitudes towards excreta in different cultures, and of latrine taboos and preferences. They quote a suggested checklist for guidelines relating user choice to national planning.

Development projects combining water supply and sanitation are often unsuccessful. Charles Chandler analyses some of the reasons for these failures and outlines methods to ensure success in a six-step procedure, involving people and planners in a joint search for the proper mix of hardware and software to meet community needs. He introduces a further factor in the equation for health, that of community participation. Chapter 9 is devoted to community education and participation (CEP), though this is a recurring theme throughout this book.

Pumps and pipes: do they really improve the quality of life?

MARTIN BEYER, UNICEF

Close to two billion people do not have sufficient access to safe water or to facilities for hygienic excreta-disposal to ensure the most elementary basis for decent living, together with adequate housing, food and nutrition. Overviews of the needs and the present situation in the world, especially of drinking-water supply and sanitation in the developing countries, have been compiled and presented by the World Health Organization as background to the work of the International Drinking Water Supply and Sanitation Decade, 1981-1990. They show tremendous discrepancies and outline the mammoth task ahead.

Governments, communities and their people around the world do take the Decade seriously. There is now concerted national planning in 60 major developing countries aimed at giving people the basic services and — in spite of the present tight economic situation — larger budget allocations.

Nevertheless, figures, even the most impressive ones, such as the numbers of water-supply schemes installed, latrines built and population covered, are one thing. It is another matter to look at the figures and see how many of these systems still function and are used properly by the population after one year, after 10 years and even longer.

The real measure of the effects of the physical improvements made for communities is the part played by water and sanitation in the improvement in health and well-being of their inhabitants. To ensure that health really is improved to the fullest extent, an effort is required by all the parties concerned — government, external co-operation agencies and the people of the communities themselves. This effort requires an awareness and knowledge of the highly complex factors involved. This need has only been properly realized and put into practice by government organizations throughout the world during the last 10 years.

In a way, this late recognition is understandable, taking into account that at first considerable time and experience was necessary to develop low-cost technologies that would permit more rapid provision of water supply and sanitation, particularly in dispersed rural populations. Especially since the 1960s, such technologies as high-speed water-well drilling, efficient submersible pumps, sturdier handpumps for community use, plastic pipes and lightweight PVC or glass-fibre latrine pans, have signalled quite a breakthrough.

After the first widespread implementation of community water-supply and sanitation schemes in rural areas of several developing countries, the results were not as encouraging as everybody had hoped. The examples are

manifold. Around the middle of the 1970s, there were still handpump installation schemes involving thousands of villages where over 80 per cent of
the handpumps were out of order after between three months and a year.
The same occurred with schemes for latrine construction. There were cases
of ceramic latrine pans being used as flower pots in public places in
villages, which may be more aesthetic but is less conducive to public health.

From an economic point of view, this means that enormous funds were
wasted in four continents. This does not include the human illness, suffering and death caused by the continued lack of appropriate facilities and
knowledge of sanitary practices.

All this has caused major rethinking in many quarters. It has stirred up
lively discussions both at international and national levels on the causes of
and remedies for what happened in the past. The conclusions are based on
worldwide experience and have been summarized in many documents. One
of the more discreet but effective ones was presented jointly by the World
Health Organization and UNICEF some years ago. It provides guidance to
both of these organizations and, by implication, to governments, on the
basic tenets for planning, programming and implementation of projects in
this field.

The main points of the WHO/UNICEF recommendations are:

O Water supply and sanitation should be regarded as integrated components of primary health care and community development.

O In order to combat diseases caused by contaminated water or related to
inadequate water supply and sanitation more efficiently, the installation of
sanitary excreta disposal facilities should be encouraged, with measures
taken to dispose of wastes and improve personal and food hygiene.

O Most important, it should be ensured that the communities and the individuals within them are not only fully aware of the relationships between
water, sanitation, hygiene and health, but also that they are motivated and
given the facilities and assistance to participate in all stages of improving
their own living conditions. In other words, work must be intensified in
providing encouragement to the communities to organize themselves for
self-help, and the necessary education to do this.

In this context, the exchange of ideas for practical, low-cost water and
sanitation projects is of paramount importance. Most of the work can —
and will have to — be done using simple methods and local resources.

The appearance of *Waterlines* signals the filling of a considerable gap in
communications. It has all the makings of an important tool for helping to
create the awareness and disseminate the knowledge necessary to improve
people's lives, largely by their own efforts.

Your part in *Waterlines* may not only be that of a subscriber and reader. It could be that of a contributor. You should also practice the ideas which appear in the magazine for the common benefit.

We are still far from reaching the goal of the Decade. To achieve this goal $40 billion would be needed each year instead of the $10 billion available. This would be less than 10 per cent of annual arms spending around the world, which totals about $600 billion. Even so, the Decade is becoming one of the most important factors in international development.

It will not only help alleviate human suffering and misery but contribute to a better economy by helping to liberate women from time-consuming labour and families from poverty and disease.[1]

(Waterlines Vol. 1 No. 1, July 1982)

Not by pumps alone

SUMI KRISHNA

The water pumped up from the depths of a tubewell is only as clean as the cupped hand of the person who drinks it. The simple installation of pumps, pipes and latrines will not automatically improve peoples' health. But the IDWSSD is based on this assumption. National governments have invested millions of dollars in the hardware, but almost no effort has gone into health and hygiene education — the software component of any water and sanitation programme. Diarrhoea, caused by dirty water, continues to kill four million children each year.

The Decade, pledged to providing 'clean water and adequate sanitation for all by 1990', has concentrated its attention on improving water supplies and building latrines. But, even before the start of the Decade, it had become clear to many specialists and planners that new water supply facilities, plus improved sanitation, plus complementary programmes of hygiene education, are all necessary for significant health impact. It was also recognized that water supply and sanitation schemes are most successful when integrated with other community development projects. In practice this rarely happens.

What will the impact be?

Worldwide, a multimillion dollar effort is going into the hardware — the pumps, pipes, taps and latrines. Although, globally, only a third of the funds required for the Decade have been raised, government allocations for water supply and sanitation are unprecedented. But several recent studies reflect that the technology of the Decade is not having the dramatic health impact that was initially expected.

The main anticipated health impact was a reduction in the incidence of diarrhoeal disease. The dehydration caused by diarrhoea, aggravated by malnutrition, is a major killer of poor children in poor countries. Diarrhoea also stunts the growth of infants and children. The new taps and latrines have not changed this noticeably.

Studies in the Philippines, Bangladesh, India and many other countries have failed to find significant, measureable health benefits produced by improved water supply and sanitation. Among the most rigourous of these studies is the one conducted by the International Centre for Diarrhoeal Disease Research, Bangladesh (ICDDR,B) in the remote Teknaf area, in the south-east of the country. Following an epidemic of dysentery in the area in 1973, a field laboratory was set up in Teknaf village to monitor the occurrence of diarrhoeal diseases. In 1975 a census was taken, and since then 500,000 people have been surveyed regularly for diarrhoea.

In July 1980, the Teknaf health impact study began in two clusters of villages. Health was measured by the incidence of diarrhoeal disease and the growth rate of children under five. In the project's first year, one village cluster was given handpumps; in the second year, they got pour-flush latrines, and in the third year they were given hygiene education. The control villages got no hardware or education, but could use the free treatment available at a small diarrhoea clinic nearby.

In the study villages, there was a tubewell for every six households; in the control villages, there was a tubewell for every 32 households. The percentage of households with access to tubewell water was about three times as high in the study villages as in the control villages.

The results of the weekly diarrhoeal surveys, and monitoring the growth of children every six months, showed that the study villagers were not markedly healthier — despite the hardware and the education. After four years, the project found that the new latrines had not significantly reduced the diarrhoeal diseases which are spread through poor sanitation, and that hygiene education had not improved health.

This is disappointing, says Dr William Greenough, Director of the ICDDR, B. But he points out that the lesson of the Teknaf project is that the software is at least as important as the hardware.

Studies often are incomplete

Many of the studies which do claim to show an improvement in one or more health indicators, such as the effect on children's diarrhoeal or parasitic diseases, or their nutritional condition, are unreliable or incomplete. After reviewing 50 studies published in English, Deborah Blum and Dr

Richard Feachem of the London School of Hygiene and Tropical Medicine, expressed 'serious doubts about them'.

For instance, one of the commonly used indicators is the occurrence of diarrhoea in young children. But information is notoriously difficult to collect. People do not remember, or they may be embarrassed or afraid to admit having diarrhoea.

Certainly new taps and latrines do produce some visible social benefits. In the Teknaf area for instance, villagers are pleased to be receiving so much attention. Some social attitudes have changed; for instance, many women no longer remain veiled in front of the male project staff. In areas such as Tamil Nadu state in South India, where the government has deliberately located new handpumps in the poorest low-caste section of a village, old patterns of segregation have begun to break down, as everyone has to share the same pump.

Moreover, in acutely water-scarce areas, as in sub-Saharan Africa, the time and labour that women save by having a nearby source of water may produce an indirect health impact, which may not be reflected by reduction in diarrhoea. Mothers may have more time for child care, for instance. In many parts of the world, for the people themselves, the convenience of the water supply and the quantity of water available may be much more important than the link between safe water and better health. Yet, if improved water supply and sanitation can produce some social benefits, and perhaps, even indirect health benefits, why have the new taps and latrines not resulted in a directly observable and measurable health impact?

Double standards

A film of daily life in a Bangladesh village, in the Teknaf area, showing 'what hands do all day' suggests one reason why all the technology is not producing results. The villagers have learnt the basic lessons of personal and household hygiene, and can repeat the lessons back to questioners. But in daily practice, they ignore these rules, as is clearly shown in the ICDDR,B film. Mothers clean infants who have defaecated, but do not wash their hands afterwards. The same hands are then used to clean other children's faces, and disease-carrying germs are passed from faeces to mouth, or to food and drink.

In a survey of two villages in Tamil Nadu, in India, we found that almost all the adults washed their hands, and feet too, before a meal. But the children did not. In the past, the ritual hand-washing emphasized by many religions may have helped control the spread of disease. Senior UNICEF official Tarzie Vittachi says, 'The simple practice of washing hands is the most important scientific and medical development of all time'.

Traditional sources safer

Dr Greenough says that in Bangladesh there is considerable evidence to show that water tanks belonging to zamindars (district governors under the Mogul empire), but used by other villagers, ensured a comparatively safe source of drinking-water during medieval cholera epidemics. The tanks may have helped check the spread of the disease, but, like the temple water tanks of South India, they are not used now.

Today, people are using the new hardware of pumps and pipes, but unhygienic individual and community behaviour is not changing. We know a lot about the technology of the village-level pump. The international aid agencies have put a lot of research, and funding, into evaluating the range of pumps on the market to discover which can be most effectively and easily operated and maintained in the village. But nothing like this effort has gone into discovering the best way to teach villagers why water that looks clean may not be safe, or how hand-washing and simple hygiene techniques can prevent the spread of disease.

Health education tends to use hit-and-miss methods. No one really knows how villagers can be helped to use their new hardware more effectively.

Providing the technology, the hardware of pumps, pipes and latrines, is necessary. But this alone cannot bring lasting changes to people's health, without changes in behaviour and behaviour changes slowly. Perhaps this is partly because poor, rural men and women believe they have no control over illness and death, particularly infant death, and must depend on a distant authority for emergency help. Such help comes too late for too many, reinforcing feelings of helplessness.

The software component of a programme cannot be shot like a bullet at a target audience. Health education requires a much greater receptivity to the villagers' own perceptions of their basic human needs, and of the benefits of improved water supply and sanitation. Behaviour changes rapidly when people perceive such changes as bringing immediate benefits.

Powerlessness

At present, poor men and women the world over do not see their own better health and environmental improvement in the community as a means to improve their own productive and earning capacity. In an acutely water-scarce situation, a convenient supply is important not just for drinking and domestic purposes but also for irrigation. However, when some water is available (regardless of its quality), other priorities — employment or land, more food for the family, a durable house — are more important. When sheer survival is the first priority, everything else, including health, comes second. In the health education field, there is also a great need to explore the different means of communicating information. In most parts of the world, health messages are mainly the responsibility of the community health worker. In some countries this works more effectively than in others. But for a single village worker, anywhere, the burden of responsibility is very great.

Changes in hygiene behaviour can, and do, occur in a variey of other ways than person-to-person contact. For instance, in parts of south India village boys have begun to use soap when they wash, imitating screen heroes.

Not just in the field of water and sanitation, but in the entire development field, the most prevalent mythology is still that the technology alone will produce results. This has not happened. Finally, the question is not whether water supplies can have an impact on health, but how to transform the potential impact into reality.

(Waterlines Vol.3 No.4, April 1985)

Rural sanitation and development

JOHN PICKFORD

Cities in many developing countries have an appearance of opulence. Modern airports and multi-storied offices and hotels bustle with well-heeled politicians, businessmen and international advisers. Those who become really rich usually live in the centre of things and share in the hurly-burly of city life.

Most people in developing countries know nothing of this wealth. They have few possessions and are often worried about what they will eat for their next meal. They sleep crowded together, children and parents sharing a tiny room. They are poor. Most poor people live and work in rural areas.

Much has been written and spoken about urban migration. It is often claimed that rural living conditions should be improved in order to reduce the flow of active young people from the countryside to the towns and cities. However, in most countries, the real problem is not just the drift of population, but the draining of all resources away from rural areas. The reward that should be given to those who labour on the land goes instead to providing cheap food for the towns or to foreign countries to repay debts or pay for imports which are largely enjoyed in the towns.

Consequently, rural sanitation often involves providing a service for people who are underprivileged in all respects. They have little cash. Their time is spent in their fields, or in walking long distances — for water in the dry season and for firewood throughout the year. They are subject to the vagaries of the weather — to floods and hurricanes and droughts. There are no hospitals or doctors nearby. Many people are ill for a large proportion of the time, suffering particularly from debilitating worm diseases and diarrhoea. Infant mortality is high.

Much of the sickness is caused by direct contact with excreta, or infection that is carried by flies from excreta. Many are sick because they eat food or drink water which has been polluted.

For this reason, the controlled disposal of excreta is terribly important for people living in rural areas. The whole question of rural sanitation demands considerable attention in development work.

Introducing new systems

Sanitation improvements in rural areas start from a low base. In many places, virtually no sanitation foundation exists on which to build. It is not a matter of extending an existing service as in towns, where there is usually already some kind of drainage system and some organization for sanitation.

In many rural areas, even the most rudimentary latrines are innovations, which may be resisted just because they are unfamiliar. When innovation is introduced from outside without consultation with community members, resistance may be so strong that the new ideas are positively rejected. There is nothing new about such rejection. In Nyasaland, before it became independent as Malawi, active opponents to colonial domination refused to use government-provided latrines.

Some idea of the state of rural sanitation can be gauged from the statistics published by the World Health Organization to show the 'progress' made in the early years of the International Drinking Water Supply and Sanitation Decade.[2] World-wide in developing countries, only 14 per cent of rural people had satisfactory sanitation in 1983. For the WHO regions of Africa, the Americas and the eastern Mediterranean, the proportion of the rural population with satisfactory sanitation actually fell between 1975 and 1983. Only the Western Pacific region reported a satisfactory level of provision, with just over half of the population served.

It is sometimes argued that sanitation is unnecessary for scattered rural communities. The fertility of fields in China for example, has been maintained for more than three thousand years largely because of the application of human excreta to the land.

A flight across low-density farmland in some comparatively barren parts of Africa shows fertile land near the farmers' dwellings because of open defecation there. As distance from the dwellings increases (and as the application of faeces to the land becomes less), the fertility decreases. However, the high incidence of excreta-derived diseases in such communities indicates that all is not well. In some places nearly all the children, and many adults too, are afflicted with intestinal worms. Roundworms and hookworms consume scarce food.

In order to reduce chronic and unnecessary faecal-derived illness it is important that human excreta be disposed of 'in a hygienic way so as not to endanger the health of individuals and the community as a whole'.[3] If the nutrients and the land-conditioning qualities of excreta are required to maintain the fertility of the soil, the types of latrine selected can be those which provide decomposed excreta for use as fertilizer.

The essential factor is time. If faeces are left in a safe place, organisms which transmit disease will die and so no longer present a problem. Bacteria and viruses die quite quickly. Even the longest-living pathogens, such as roundworm eggs, are totally inactivated within a year or so. With particularly unfavourable conditions for the disease-causing organisms (that is, favourable conditions for human health), the required period of storage for safety may be less than a year. These conditions apply in the alkaline environment of a carefully operated dry compost latrine in which users cover their faeces with wood ash. Latrines of this kind have long been used successfully in Vietnam.

Importance of health education

For health to improve because of improved sanitation, it is just as important for rural people to appreciate the dangers arising from excreta as it is for them to have good latrines. It is often rightly said that there are three equal elements for improving environmental health: safe drinking-water, good sanitation and health education. These three facets cannot be separated. Often drinking-water becomes unsafe because of poor sanitation. Health education — an understanding of the transmission of disease from excreta — can lead to a demand for good latrines. Equally, where good latrines have been provided without adequate health education or community involvement, there can follow such a degree of non-use or misuse that benefits are completely undermined.

From ancient times, people have practised simple sanitation by covering their faeces with soil. There is some truth in the old adage that 'out of sight is out of mind'. However, a shallow covering of earth is insufficient to prevent the spread of disease. The larvae of flies and worms have no difficulty in getting through a few millimetres of cover. Exceptionally, they have been known to emerge from faeces buried up to a metre deep, although a covering of 300mm to half a metre is usually enough to control them.

Perhaps the greatest need for excreta-related health education is concerned with children's faeces. It is commonly believed that they are harmless. In fact, the prevalence of diarrhoeas and worms amongst children of all ages, and the tendency of very young children to defecate whenever and wherever they happen to be, results in serious health dangers.

Costs and construction

Compared with other environmental improvements, sanitation can be improved with little external help. Latrines need cost little apart from labour. The essential feature of a simple latrine is a hole in the ground of sufficient size to contain the accumulated faeces for a year or more, with space on top for half a metre or so of soil. A pit a metre square and about a metre and a half deep should last a family of six people for between two and four years. If the owner of a latrine has plenty of space around his home, understands the importance of latrines and is willing to dig holes every few years, there is considerable advantage in small pits. Bananas are especially good for planting on a disused pit; they thrive on the rich nutrients available.

Squatting slabs can be made of locally available materials using techniques with which local people are familiar. Mud on a frame of sticks is common practice, but there is always a danger of the sticks being eaten by termites or attacked by rot. Collapse of a slab is not only dangerous — and thoroughly unpleasant — for anyone using the latrine at the time, but it also can prejudice neighbours against building their own latrines. Mud floors can be made hard and smooth. For example, in central Africa and other places, cow dung is soaked in water overnight, and the liquor is then mixed with local clay to produce a very good surface. Where wood is plentiful, it is often used for making floors or slabs for latrines.

Slabs are sometimes supported by a variety of scrap materials, including pieces of abandoned cars and lorries. Mud, boards, and old iron sheets can be used for the top surface. The crucial requirement is that it is smooth and hard so that it can be easily cleaned. The most satisfactory material for the surface will usually contain some cement. It may be plain concrete, reinforced concrete or terrazzo. The surface of terrazzo is made with marble chippings which can be polished to give a very smooth surface that gives the latrine an appearance of luxury.

One of the most common and useful ways to provide outside assistance for rural sanitation is to supply good floor slabs. These may be made centrally and sold to householders at the full market price. On the other hand, slabs are sometimes given free of charge to householders who have dug their own pits. Between these two extremes are a variety of strategies to encourage latrine builders to use good slabs.

A similar range of options can be used to supply other items for latrine construction where improved latrines are to be provided. These items include pans with water seals, pipes and material for lining the pits.

Where water is used for anal cleaning, pour-flush pans with a water seal provide an effective barrier between the pit and the user, reducing or eliminating nuisance from flies, mosquitoes and odours. The pit can be dug away from the latrine building and the pan connected to the pit with a short length of pipe or channel. Instead of digging a new pit when the old one becomes full, two more-or-less permanent pits may be used alternately. These twin-pit pour-flush latrines are becoming very popular in India.

In Africa and many other areas, it is customary to use solid material for anal cleaning. Materials in common use include hard paper (newspaper, old government forms and the like), leaves, stones, coconut husks, corn-cobs and grass. In some places, the used cleaning material is put in a basket and then burned. Elsewhere, it is put into the pit. A hole in the floor slab must then be provided through which excreta and cleaning material pass directly into the pit. Nuisance from flies and smells can be dramatically reduced by keeping the inside of the structure dark, and ventilating the pit by means of a pipe.

Lining of pits, at least near the top, is necessary in most soils, particularly if the pits are to be re-excavated for reuse. Linings may be of any locally available material, and should allow liquid in the pit to pass outward from the pit to the soil.

Any pit inevitably pollutes the soil around and beneath it. In many types of soil, the sideways movement of pollution is quite small — maybe as little as a metre or two. Nevertheless, it is sensible to locate the pits as far as possible from any wells which provide drinking-water, especially if the level of groundwater is close to the surface. Pollution may be due to microbes in excreta, or to dissolved chemicals derived from decomposition of excreta. From a public health point of view, pollution by microbes is most serious, since they can pass on diseases like the many different diarrhoeas and worms. Fortunately, the distance that micro-organisms are able to travel is fairly short, being limited to how far they can move in about 10 days.

The role of 'software'

Although many engineers and scientists are most concerned about the construction of latrines and the risk of pollution, the really important considerations in providing rural sanitation are those described as 'software'. Motivation of individual householders and communities must be very high on the list of priorities. To achieve this there is often a need for education. Sorting out financial aspects (whether all the cost is covered by beneficiaries or support is provided by governments or donors) is vitally important. So is the training of artisans, or the householders themselves, so that latrines are made in the best possible way to suit the local requirements.

Throughout the developing world there is ample evidence that rural sanitation can be improved where:
O there is determined leadership;
O local individuals and communities are aware of the benefits of improved

sanitation, and are fully involved in every stage of the programme;
O the types of sanitation offered are appropriate for local customs and can
   be provided within the resources available;
O training is provided in appropriate construction techniques.

(*Waterlines* Vol. 6 No.3, January 1988)

Women as the key to success

MARY L. ELMENDORF AND RAYMOND B. ISELY

It is primarily women who use new water-systems. Their role as household managers means that in food preparation, washing and bathing, women are the primary users and mediators between the water source and the household. Any planned change in water availability or excreta disposal should be based on information about their present knowledge, attitudes, and practices. Careful observation and discussion, not just standard surveys, are needed to get at perceptions and beliefs about water preferences and defecation behaviour.

The choice of water for drinking, cooking, laundry, bathing and other household functions is a result of women's careful decisions, based on what they have learned from their mothers and grandmothers, and on their observations of the costs and benefits of any change.

Qualitative criteria

Decisions about drinking-water are often based on colour, taste or smell rather than on technical purity. Decisions not to use improved drinking-water facilities such as tubewells or piped water are often related to unpleasant taste or smell such as that given by iron sulphide or chlorine. The processing of water also affects its perceived quality.

Many cultures hold beliefs about hot and cold food and drink which influence water use. For example, in some societies, cold boiled water is acceptable for daily use, but warm boiled water is just for invalids. Boiled water, even though cool, is considered hot unless specifically designated as cold boiled water after which it is no longer considered medicinal. Understanding these beliefs and practices is likely to lead to more successful attempts to introduce change.

The importance of understanding attitudes toward excreta cannot be overemphasized. The widespread perception that children's faeces are 'harmless'[4] can condition a continuous link in the chain of reinfection, whether the faeces are thrown on a nearby garbage heap or the diapers (nappies) are washed with dishes in an urban home with a newly installed piped connection. In many cultures infant faeces, even if not considered 'harmless', are not perceived as the harmful germ-laden carriers they so often are.[4,5,6] These factors should be understood, analysed and considered in the planning and preparation of educational approaches.

In some areas, women and children use the same latrines, but in many places the children defecate just outside the latrines, because they are afraid of falling through the large opening or because they are far away and the interiors are dark. These two problems have been solved in a very innovative way in Sri Lanka, where specially designed low-cost child-size water-seal latrines are available. These latrines are installed without any walls under the eaves of the home just outside the kitchen door. Mothers can thus easily train toddlers to use them and they double as an informal bathing area. Bath water is used to flush the latrines.

Many social and cultural variations in water-related beliefs and practices occur throughout the world. For instance it is a commonly held belief in Honduras that women might become pregnant if they use the same latrine as men. This limits the use of even household latrines to female members of the family.[7] In Nicaragua, women did not like to use new latrines because the metallic sides were 250mm off the ground, so that their feet were visible. On the other hand, some latrines were not used because the sides came to the ground and made a warm resting-place for snakes.[8]

Though these beliefs vary between country and country, and often between region and region within countries, there are a number of similarities. One, already referred to, is the idea that children's faeces are innocuous and therefore need no special handling.

Taboos are common regarding the mixing of the faeces of men and women, which is felt in many areas to make either one sterile. (In Tanzania for instance it is believed that the excreta of fathers and daughters should not be mixed.[9]) Latrines as a result are often only used by women. Streams and pools not infrequently are perceived to be the habitations of spirits and thus not to be disturbed. Other examples of fears and beliefs common to many cultures are numerous.

Such beliefs are very important for planning. They explain in part why a study of 120 villages in Bangladesh showed that latrines were used by only 12.8 per cent of children, while adult use (mostly women) was 59.9 per cent.[10] A similar study of 525 latrines in India showed that many more women used latrines than men, whereas children's faeces were thrown on garbage heaps.

Similarities in attitudes and perceptions surrounding water and excreta can often lead to ways of surveying attitudes and customs which can be used again and again within certain cultural and geographic areas, particularly those of similar size and environment. However, for effective project design, more detailed information concerning variations is needed at least on a regional basis. Failure to account for variation among populations may lead to inappropriate design and ultimate project failure.

Local pride

With respect to the introduction of excreta-disposal facilities, limited attention has been given to matters of local pride and aesthetics. A World Bank case-study of water supply and excreta disposal in Colombia revealed that the families preferred brightly coloured cement pedestals and slabs to drab grey facilities. [9,11] Similarly, in Yucatan, women expressed a preference for an aesthetically attractive latrine with a shiny porcelain seat or a brightly painted cement floor or pedestal, even if the cost and labour involved were much more. [12]

One other factor to be discussed with women in early planning is the reuse of grey water for flushing water-seal latrines. Even though more labour is involved in carrying water, such facilities may be preferred. Women are the key agents for acceptance, use and maintenance of new facilities in the home, and planners can benefit from incorporating their beliefs and wishes into programmes. As Feachem has noted, it is essential that planners when making 'designs' take account of user preferences and of the socio-economic setting of the project. [13]

This approach, which focuses on the product from the point of view of the consumer, has been described as 'user-choice' [14] and is elaborated on in relation to implications for planning delivery systems by Whyte and Burton. [15] Draft guidelines for relating the user choice to national planning for community education and participation have been suggested. [16,17] Whyte has developed a checklist system for:

O Identifying national experience in community participation;
O Assessing the social and economic potential for community participation;
O Anticipating problems in project implementation;
O Setting programme objectives and priorities;
O Project allocation and initiation;
O Project planning and design;
O Construction;
O Administration, operation, and maintenance;
O The education component;
O Performance evaluation and progress monitoring.

Alastair White[18] has elaborated the same concept into community participation options for different types of social systems and agencies. Although not enough emphasis is placed on the need to understand women's roles, careful analysis of social organization, formal and informal, is discussed with references to specific cases.

Sense of responsibility

If communities or households feel that new facilities really are theirs, they are much more likely to accept, use and maintain them. Simple adaptations at the local level increases the potential for adoption. Feachem noted and various studies verify[11] 'that in general, the design issues that will be improved through user participation are minor in their engineering or financial consequences, but major in the potential effect upon acceptance and correct use of the new facilities.'

In some instances effective community participation may slow down or stop a project. In Mexico, the Mazauwas in El Nopal would not accept a water installation connected only to some houses, nor wells accessible to clusters of huts. The community decided that everybody should have a household water supply at once or everybody would continue walking to the rather distant and poorly maintained well.[19]

A Maya community in Yucatan also delayed the construction of latrines until a model appropriate to their perceived needs and the specific environmental and geological requirements of their limestone soil could be designed and demonstrated.[12] Even though some may consider these cases failures, both communities were ready to work for what they felt they needed, and unwanted facilities were not installed to fall into disrepair.

Although the number of successful rural water and sanitation schemes is much smaller than the number that failed or achieved only limited success, there is increasing evidence that the user-preference approach combined with community participation is a viable strategy.[20,21,22] The hidden participant accepting or rejecting a new water supply or sanitation technology is most often a woman.

(*Waterlines* Vol 1. No. 2, October 1982)

Achieving success in community projects

CHARLES CHANDLER

There is no shortage of literature on what to do to provide water-supply and sanitation facilities in developing countries. Less in evidence is how to accomplish this aim in the real world, where social, political and environmental systems are complex, and problems abound.

Project planners face the task of designing projects that are not only technically correct and feasible, but also that continue to function for long periods of time, often under difficult conditions. Facilities may break down after a short time because of poor maintenance, and even those in good repair may be under-used if the people do not like the technology, or not used at all if people believe that traditional alternatives are more convenient. In the rural communities of developing countries, examples of past project failures are common: pumps in disrepair, taps broken or left unfitted, public latrines abandoned to nature, pipes and other materials damaged or diverted to unplanned uses.

If field results have been poor, current programmes must be held responsible — but why have they not always been effective? Three major problems are apparent:

O The conceptual gap between people and planners.
O The emphasis on coverage rather than on the continued functioning and use of facilities.
O The lack of effective back-up support to communities, particularly after completion of the project.

To overcome these problems, projects must follow a well-designed procedure, involving people and planners in a joint search for the proper mix of hardware and software to meet community needs. The six-step procedure presented here has been designed to accomplish this.

Step 1 Criteria, selection and training

Step 1 involves the planner selecting and using criteria to determine which communities to serve first, and recruiting and training project facilitators. Examples of criteria that might be applied include communities where:

O People are poor or disadvantaged, for example those with a per-capita income of less than the poverty level (as determined locally).
O Facilities are in need of rehabilitation.
O Traditional sources are highly polluted, such as village ponds, where farm animals also drink and wade.
O The incidence of diarrhoeal disease in children is expected to be high, for example, mortality in infants less than one year of age is greater than 50 per 1,000.
O Water is scarce, with an availability of less than 20 litres per person, per day.
O Bucket latrines are in use.
O Safe water is more than a 15-minute walk from most households.

Once measurable criteria have been established, communities are ranked into high-priority and low-priority groups, with the former selected for initial action.

Project facilitators may be chosen from primary health-care workers, teachers or other community-based workers. An approximately equal number of male and female facilitators will be required. Once chosen, facilitators are trained to observe the habits of the community in relation to water supply and sanitation, and to collect and analyse data. Interview techniques are emphasized during training, as well as methods for carrying out activities in the community. A particularly important aspect of training is communication with the disadvantaged groups through small group meetings.

Step 2 Involving the community

Community education and participation (CEP) helps to overcome any gap that may exist between people and planners as a result of their different perceptions of community needs. The objective of CEP is to improve communications so that planners can come to understand community problems, and people can participate in decisions on meeting community needs through development projects.

The first step is to meet the community. Contact must be established with village leaders and existing institutions, to inform them of the need for a base-line survey to verify the relevance of water-supply and sanitation improvements to overall community concerns. The permission of community leaders must be obtained prior to the design and construction of a water-supply and sanitation project.

Next, arrangements must be made for the facilitators to carry out the base-line survey in the community over a period of a few weeks (facilitators should live in the community through-out this period). The objectives of the survey are twofold:

O To determine the priority given to water-supply and sanitation improvement in relation to other priority needs within the community.

O To collect sufficient data to determine the existing habits of the community regarding water supply and waste disposal.

Communities where traditional sources are polluted can be given high priority for service

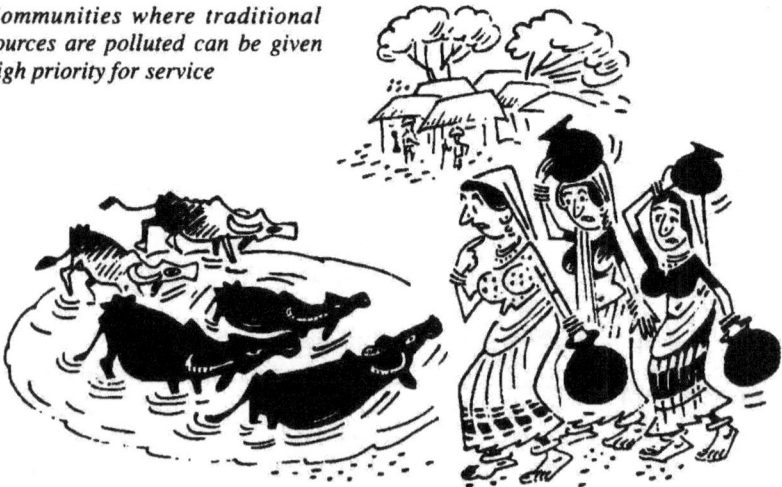

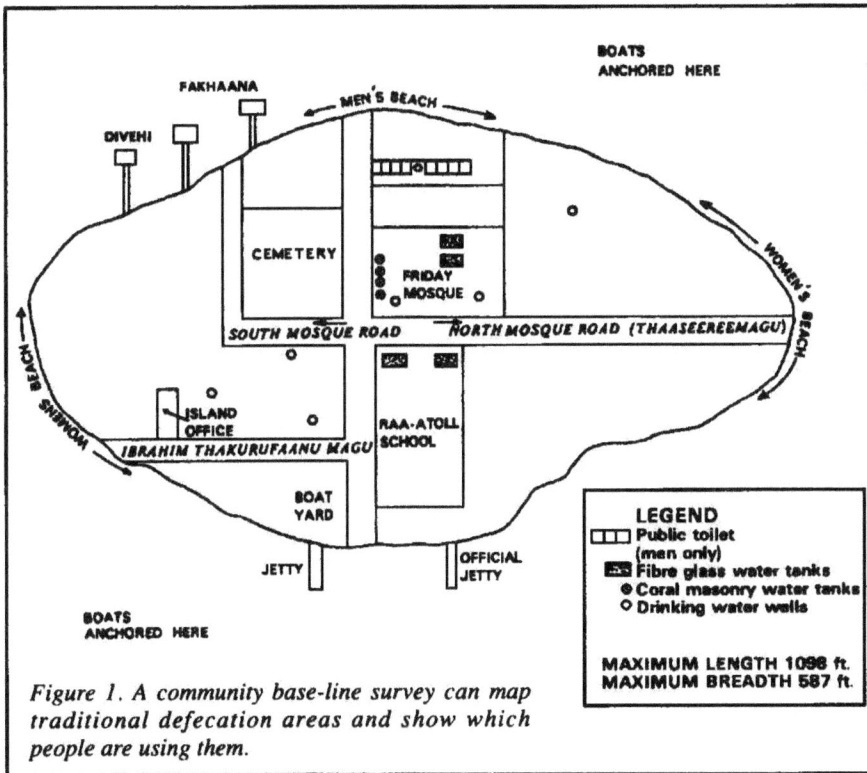

Figure 1. A community base-line survey can map traditional defecation areas and show which people are using them.

An important contribution of the base-line survey is a set of maps showing the existing sources of water supply for each household and the defecation sites in use (Figure 1). When the survey is completed a community meeting is held to discuss the results. If the community agrees that water supply and/or sanitation is a high priority need, the next step is to present the project resources that are available to meet these needs, the requirements to be met by the project and the responsibilities of the community during the process.

Step 3 Software and hardware

The planners' role in determining the most appropriate hardware/software mix to be used in the project is to work closely with the community, with the help of the facilitators, to develop alternative designs. Each alternative considered has both hardware (appropriate technology) and software (human resources and institutional development) components. Not all the alternatives are practical, feasible or even desirable. The challenge is to find the proper mix that will meet community needs and that will continue to function and be used within the existing social and economic environment.

Unless all the facilities to be constructed are to be owned by individual households, a local institution must take on the responsibility for the system's management, future operation and maintenance. This role may be designated to an existing institution such as a village council; alternatively, a new institution must be established. Institution leaders must then be selected and trained. Following training, their first job is to assist planners and people to draw up and consider a list of technological options.

Working closely with the people, the leaders must begin to formulate alternatives based upon suggestions received from the community. The planners' knowledge of technology and materials can be utilized in constructing and adapting new plans based on the ideas expressed in group meetings. Some alternatives may simply reflect the planners' own preferences, those of government officials or those adopted in other progammes. The emphasis must be on selecting alternatives that reflect all the diverse ideas of the community members. No effort is made at this point to eliminate or criticize alternatives, or to show why they may not be feasible. The local institution is acting as a facilitator to elicit different viewpoints, and to be sure that they are considered as a part of the planning process.

The next stage is to judge the feasibility of the alternatives. Only options that can be supported with spare parts, supplies and other necessary back-up through existing programme-support networks are considered. Where such networks do not exist, projects are as self-sufficient as possible, with no spare parts required other than those that can be purchased in the local market or made from indigenous materials using local skills.

At this stage, staffing patterns and the user fees required for each alternative are estimated. User fees are normally less than five per cent of the income of the heads of rural households. Where possible, consideration is given to maximizing the benefits to the community by choosing technologies and methods of implementation that are labour-intensive rather than capital-intensive.

A plan is then drawn up for presentation to the community in general, and to the disadvantaged groups in particular. The latter should be approached individually by the local institution, and small group meetings held, where required, to review the proposed plan and the method of implementation. If the disadvantaged groups are not satisfied, the local institution must work closely with the planners to incorporate the concerns expressed, where feasible.

Step 4 Involving everyone

The purpose of Step 4 is to develop a consensus and commitment within the community regarding the planned project. After agreement is reached with the disadvantaged groups, the planners and the local institution present the

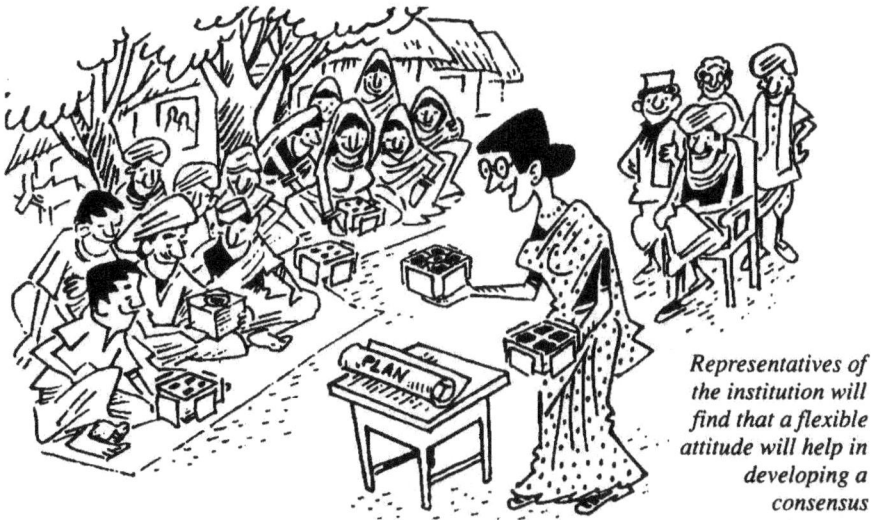

Representatives of the institution will find that a flexible attitude will help in developing a consensus

plan to a meeting of the entire community for discussion. The community then has the opportunity to introduce modifications to the plan as desired and where possible.

It is necessary for the community to demonstrate its commitment before construction starts. For example, the local institution may require a legal title to the land where facilities are to be constructed, or the community may first need to protect a spring catchment area. Users may be required to join a users' association, paying membership fees and additional monthly fees to make the system self-supporting as regards operation and maintenance. Construction should be delayed, if necessary, until these steps have been taken.

Step 5 Implementation

To implement the planned project, as agreed with the community, planners oversee project inputs and supervise construction while the local institution organizes community inputs of cash, manpower, and materials. The decisions remaining for individual users can be taken at this time, including the type of construction materials that will be used to ensure privacy in individual household latrines.

The on-the-job training of personnel for operation and maintenance should begin as soon as possible; some elements can start before construction is completed. Personnel from the local institution can assist in the construction process itself.

A follow-up survey is carried out after construction to determine whether the facilities have been completed as planned and are functioning and being used as intended. People's habits after the completion of the project are compared with habits observed during the base-line survey.

Health education efforts can be targeted to effect a change in those households that continue to use traditional water sources and defecation sites. This may be done in co-operation with primary health-care workers where appropriate. Training programmes may be planned through a programme support network, to teach the staff of the local institution how to carry out health education activities.

Step 6 Providing back-up

Step 6 is the establishment of links with a programme support network to ensure back-up assistance, where necessary. The role of the programme support network is to provide back-up to the communities and their institutions on request. Such support will require the provision of additional funds and manpower. Back-up support may be provided in conjunction with other programmes, such as hygiene education, which may be supported through primary health-care units.

Facilities may be required to train management or maintenance personnel under the supervision of the local institutions. Specific training needs should be identified and training curricula developed, such as curricula aimed at training accountants to serve the needs of local institutions. The programme support network may also include a unit to evaluate projects. This will make it possible to learn from past mistakes, and thus influence procedures in future projects.

Source

The procedural guide-lines described in this article were developed as the result of case studies carried out by local institutions in nine developing countries of the Asia and the Pacific Region (of the United Nations Development Programme) under the IDWSS Decade Advisory Service Project.

Suggested data to be obtained in the base-line survey

Community structure

An understanding of village organizational structures, official and unofficial.
Identification of different disadvantaged groups with respect to water and sanitation.
Key leaders and influential persons within the community.
Decision-making processes within the community, particularly the direct and indirect role of women.

Water usage, sanitation, management

Water rights and ownership and how they are obtained.
Seasonal variations in water source.
Preferred water source for each household for drinking/cooking/laundry/-bathing/animals/home and garden use (show desired source for each use on map).
Time taken or distance travelled for water collection (can be shown on map).
Household water-storage and use — practices for a sample of households, including quantity and source
Perception of community needs by the disadvantaged groups, women, children and the community as a whole.
Household practices for waste-water (sullage) disposal.
Household defecation habits (show on map separately for men, women and children).

Water and sanitation beliefs

General perceptions of community and personal illness; tolerance for disease.
Concept of 'clean' water and sanitation. Perceived relationship between water and health.
Credibility of official and indigenous medical personnel as opinion leaders.
Traditional beliefs concerning excreta and sanitation practices.
Personal hygiene habits and practices.

Community economic patterns

Means of subsistence.
Preferred spending patterns and ability to pay.
Co-operative and credit system.
Indirect measurement of average household income based on visual determination of housing type and evident amenities.

Education and communication behaviour

General formal and non-formal ways of communication with the outside world.
Effectiveness of different media for different tasks (entertainment, development education, traditional community events).
Audio-visual perceptions; literacy rates; language and dialect.

Technological alternatives

Data for deciding between technological alternatives including local technical skills, capabilities and traditional alternatives.

(*Waterlines* Vol. 5 No. 2, October 1986)

CHAPTER 2
Health Aspects

Sandy Cairncross co-ordinated the theme issue on 'Water and Health' in *Waterlines* (July 1988). In this, his introduction, he sets the four articles of that issue in the context of current debate about the impact of water and sanitation on health, and underlines the difficulties of measuring related changes in the health of a population. His remarks are most relevant for introducing this chapter, but the other four articles of the theme issue have all been included in the final chapter as each deals with different aspects of strategies for improvement, including evaluation.

The remaining articles of this chapter have been selected to give an overview of the problems of water health-hazards and their eradication. Annie Dufau brings out how, apart from the sheer hard work involved in carrying heavy loads of water, women are exposed to many health hazards, including skeletal problems which could lead to deformity and disability.

Denise Ayres discussed the massive effects of dehydration from diarrhoea, which kills over 4 million children each year in developing countries. She points out that, in the short-term, oral hydration therapy is a relatively easy and effective treatment for dehydration. But, in the long-term, there must be improved nutrition, more and better water supplies, improved sanitation, better personal and domestic hygiene and more health education.

George Davidson surveys the prevalence and eradication measures for malaria. Water management, with particular reference to small water supplies, is summarized. He concludes that success is only likely to be achieved where breeding grounds are few and well known, which is less probable in rural areas. An article on sanitation measures through drainage to beat mosquito breeding in India is included under chapter 7.

Finally, Kenneth Mott relates the current strategy for controlling schistosomiasis, which aims to reduce disease rather than attempt to eradicate it. The measure involves the use of more effective drugs in conjunction with health education, water supply and sanitation. Unfortunately, space precludes the inclusion of articles on Guinea worm and other water-related diseases, but these articles provide an inkling of the major problems experienced in developing countries.

Health aspects of water and sanitation
SANDY CAIRNCROSS

The health benefits of water and sanitation are often difficult to identify, and some studies which have tried to measure them have astonished and disappointed their authors by failing to detect any health improvements.

The first reason is that measuring changes in the health of a population is not a task for amateurs, and even experienced epidemiologists are sometimes defeated by the difficulty of doing so. Many past studies have had serious flaws, which meant that their results were not reliable. Some researchers did not even check that the water and sanitation facilities were being used, particularly by children, although children are often the chief sufferers from the diseases related to water and excreta-disposal. In other studies, the health of the users was not compared with that of people who lacked the facilities or, if it was, there were other differences between the groups of people studied which made the comparison invalid. For instance, a rich community is likely to be healthier than a poor one.

A more fundamental problem arises from the fact that a water supply serves a whole community. If one community is found to have more cases of disease than another at a particular time, this difference is not necessarily significant. People usually catch infectious diseases from their neighbours, so that an epidemic may sweep through one village, but miss another, simply because there is not enough contact between the two communities and not because of differences in their water supplies.

This does not mean that no attempt should be made to measure health. Rather, studies should only be carried out after careful planning, incorporating the lessons learned from health studies in the past.[23] and preferably with an epidemiologist in the team.

The second reason is that the health of a community is a complex issue, affected by many different factors. Anaemia, such as that described in the final chapter by Jamie Bartram and Warren Johns, may be caused by hookworm due to inadequate sanitation, but it can also result from malaria or malnutrition. Many cases of diarrhoea among children are caused, not by poor water supply, but as a side-effect of measles, even in a child which has apparently recovered from the disease.

Where other health problems play a major role, changes in water supply and sanitation may be necessary, but are not in themselves sufficient to bring about significant health improvements. Other measures, such as the measles immunization described in the final chapter by Mathew Onduru, may be needed, and the benefits may only become apparent after some time.

Thirdly, water supply and sanitation can affect the transmission of disease in several different ways and need to be considered separately.

Water supply and disease

Every water engineer has heard of the water-borne epidemics of diseases such as cholera and typhoid, which can occur when a community's water supply suffers from faecal contamination.

However, many epidemics which may recur in a poor community are only the tip of the iceberg of endemic disease, which is a familiar feature of everyday life and not necessarily water-borne. Even the classic 'water-borne' diseases such as cholera and typhoid can be transmitted from person to person in a host of other ways including the faecal contamination of hands, food or utensils. These other transmission routes are unlikely to be affected by improvements in water quality. More important are the improvements in hygiene which become possible when water is available in greater quantity for use in the house, to wash hands, plates, food and so on. This kind of disease transmission has been called 'water-washed', as it is not water-borne. It applies not only to diarrhoeal disease (including cholera and typhoid), but also to several other diseases of poor hygiene, such as trachoma and scabies.

An increase in the quantity of water used in the home is not an automatic consequence of a new water supply, even if it provides water closer to people's houses. Several studies in Africa have found a surprising relationship between the quantity of water carried home and the distance it must be carried (see Figure 1). Intuitively, one would expect that when the distance is reduced, the amount of water used would increase. Beyond a distance of about one kilometre, equivalent to a round-trip water-collection journey of 30 minutes, this does occur. At lesser distances, however, a plateau is reached beyond which water consumption only increases when water is supplied directly to individual houses. This means that if the traditional source of water is less than one kilometre away, the provision of a new water source closer to the home may not lead to an increase in water use, and this may not affect the water-washed transmission of disease. Significantly, many of the studies which failed to find a health impact from water supply were carried out in precisely those conditions, while many of

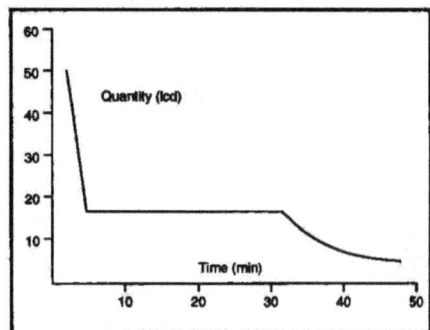

Figure 1. Schematic representation of how the time taken to collect a bucket of water affects the average quantity used for domestic purposes in litres per capita per day (lcd). Note the plateau for times less than 30 minutes. Although the exact height of the plateau depends on local circumstances, the general shape of the curve seems not to vary.

those which found a dramatic impact involved cases where water was piped to individual households, a level of service at which water consumption doubles or even trebles.

This illustration shows that the likely health impact of a water supply depends on the level of service which it provides, and also on the traditional water sources which it replaces. A baseline survey and community diagnosis, as described in the final chapter by Bartram and Johns, can help to clarify the existing situation and thus to assess the priority for water-supply improvements, as compared to sanitation or other public health measures.

Sanitation and disease

Excreta disposal can also affect disease transmission in quite complex ways. The infections most directly affected by sanitation improvements are probably the intestinal worms, mainly roundworm (*Ascaris*), hookworm (*Ancylostoma* and *Necator*), and whipworm (*Trichuris*). However, the effect of sanitation on these infections in a community is very different from the effect of treating the whole community with de-worming medicines.

To understand this, it is important to realize that these parasites cannot normally multiply inside the body in the way that bacteria and viruses do. Thus, for example, swallowing one microscopic *Ascaris* egg can only lead to infection with a single *Ascaris* worm. A person can be infected with one worm, or two or more. The intensity of infection (how many worms each person has) is at least as important as the prevalence (that is, the proportion of the population having at least one worm).

Generally, most people have only a few worms or none at all. Those who have a few are not likely to suffer serious symptoms, beyond a mild degree of tiredness or anaemia. The minority, infected by dozens or even hundreds of worms, is at much greater risk of serious illness such as stunted growth, intestinal obstruction or prolapse of the rectum. Typically, about 10 per cent of the population will have 50 per cent of the worms. Moreover, the faeces of this minority will contain much greater numbers of worm eggs and so be a more important source of infection for other members of the community. As a rule, children are more likely than adults to be among this minority. Contrary to most people's belief, therefore, children's faeces are more dangerous than adults' with regard to intestinal worm transmission. It follows that children's faeces must also be disposed of hygienically if latrines are to play a part in improving public health.

If everyone in a community is treated for intestinal worms, the result is that the prevalence of infection will immediately be reduced to zero. However, the environment will still be contaminated with worm eggs, some of which may survive for up to a year. The community will soon become reinfected, so that the situation will return to the status quo. On the other hand, if a sanitation programme succeeds in controlling transmission of the worms from one person to another its effect will be permanent. Its impact will only become apparent over a period of time, however, as the adult worms in people's bodies die off during the next year or so.

Controlling transmission by sanitation will have three effects. It may reduce the prevalence of infection to some degree. It is likely to have a more significant effect on the average intensity of infection — the average number of worms per person. Lastly, and perhaps most important of all, it should greatly reduce the number of people with very intense infections.

A simple analogy can illustrate this. Imagine a pile of 100 coins thrown into a crowd of 20 small children. Perhaps only the 10 children nearest to the place where they fall will manage to grab a coin — giving a 'prevalence' of 10/20, or 50 per cent. On average, these children will have 10 coins each — the 'intensity'. However, the strongest child may manage to get hold of as much as half of the pile — 50 coins. Now suppose that there were only 30 coins in the pile. Probably most of the same 10 children would manage to get at least one coin, so there would be little reduction in 'prevalence'. The average 'intensity', however, would fall from 10 to three coins per child. And the number of children with 30 coins or more would probably be reduced to zero.

Some of the studies of the impact of sanitation on intestinal worm infections have looked only at its effect on prevalence, and thus underestimated the full public health benefit. In particular, such studies cannot detect the degree to which it reduces the number of people with especially intense infections, who are most likely to become seriously ill and to pass on their infection to others.

The human factor

The role of hygiene in achieving health benefits from water supplies, and the need for children as well as adults to use latrines, are examples of the importance of human behaviour in the success or failure of water and sanitation schemes. To introduce a new water supply or latrine, or to improve domestic hygiene, requires a change to peoples' behaviour to some extent. They may need little persuasion to do so, but there can be little doubt that they are most likely to make the change in a satisfactory way if there is good communication between them and those who implement water and sanitation programmes. To incorporate a communication process within a technical programme is not easy, and is likely to require a smooth collaboration between several professions. There is plenty of room for the exercise of creativity here. Joanne Harmerijer's article is an excellent example of how it can be done.

Communication is important not only to achieve the full use of new water and sanitation facilities, but also to ensure their maintenance and even their construction. It is especially important for low-cost sanitation schemes, where households are usually expected to build their own. A latrine is part of a family's living space, and relates to some of their most intimate habits. People will not use a latrine, and certainly will not be willing to build one or contribute to its cost, unless they have been convinced of its advantages. The best people to convince them are not outsiders offering lectures, posters or even films, but their neighbours who already have a latrine of their own. This is why sanitation schemes usually take a long time to implement.

The process can be illustrated by a hypothetical example. Suppose an expert arrived in a village in Europe or North America, offering a new type of domestic central heating system which worked like a microwave oven and offered considerable savings in heating costs. Very few people would decide to install one immediately in their houses. Most would prefer to wait and see what happened when a few pioneers put them in, perhaps as a status

---

Quality vs quantity

Many infections can be accurately described as water-borne diseases, where the pathogenic organisms are carried passively in the water supplies, and they are prevented by attention to water quality.

There is another important group of diseases, however, which may be called water-washed infections as they result from lack of water for washing or personal hygiene. Clearly their prevention depends on the availability, access to, and quantity of domestic water supply rather than on its quality.

These two groups are shown as categories I and II in the table below. [15]

Category	Examples	Relevant water improvements
I Water-borne infections		
(a) Classical	Typhoid, cholera	Microbiological sterility
(b) Non-classical	Infectious hepatitis	Microbiological improvement
II Water-washed infections		
(a) Skin and eyes	Scabies, trachoma	Greater volume available
(b) Diarrhoeal diseases	Bacillary dysentery	Greater volume available
III Water-based infections		
(a) Penetrating skin	Schistosomiasis	Protection of user
(b) Ingested	Guinea worm	Protection of source
IV Infections with water-related insect vectors		
(a) Biting near water	Sleeping sickness	Water piped from source
(b) Breeding in water	Yellow fever	Water piped to site of use
V Infections primarily of defective sanitation		
	Hookworm	Sanitary faecal disposal

symbol. After some time, if the new systems proved to be worthwhile and to have no unpleasant side-effects, other residents might install them and their experience would subsequently convince their neighbours, one by one. Others again might wait until they had saved up the money to pay for the new system or until their houses needed other modifications or repairs. The whole process could easily take years. The extension of coverage with latrines, or with a new, more hygienic type of latrine, is likely to follow a similar pattern, as is illustrated very clearly by the graphs in Chris Smith's article in the final chapter. The lesson is that we should not be disappointed if sanitation programmes sometimes seem to advance rather slowly. Rather, we should look at the progress achieved so far and examine the factors which may have promoted it or held it back. This will help to identify ways to improve the programme, with a view to achieving the maximum possible benefit to health.

(Waterlines Vol. 7 No. 1, July 1988)

How carrying water affects women's health

ANNIE DUFAUT

Carrying water is one of the most arduous of tasks in the rural areas of developing countries; a task which is usually carried out by women and children. One of the aims of the Water Decade was to reduce the social. economic and health consequences of carrying water by providing a safe water supply within reasonable walking distance. Many projects have been developed, but few are concerned specifically with the health effects of carrying heavy loads of water over long distances.

Containers come in all shapes, sizes and materials, depending on local availability. Nowadays, women in many countries prefer buckets, tins or jerrycans to traditional containers such as calabashes and clay pots. The weight of an empty container varies between 500g and 4 to 5kg, depending on the material; plastic is the lightest. The average quantity of water held in a container ranges between about 12 and 25 litres.

The most common method of carrying water is on the head, particularly in Africa and the Middle East, though it is also used in Asia and Latin America. Carrying aids such as a simple ring of woven banana leaves may be used to increase the stability of the container and to free the women's hands; controlling the load is more difficult on steep or rough terrain.

Women sometimes carry several containers, increasing the weight of the load to 40 or 50kg. Carrying water on the head requires strength in the neck and considerable skill, a skill often acquired at around nine years old.

Carrying water on the back is also common throughout the world and

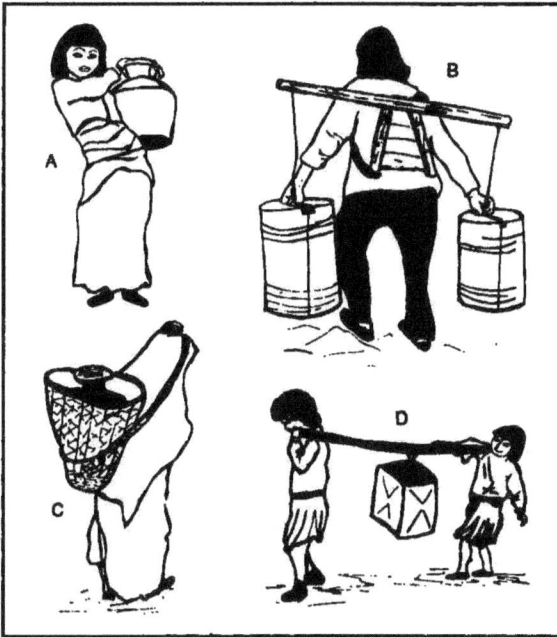

Different ways to carry water:
A. Bolivia
B. Korea's chee-geh.
C. Nepalese head strap.
D. Colombian shoulder pole.

different aids may be used to increase the stability of the load and allow it to be controlled more easily:

○ A head strap consisting of a loop of strong cloth or webbing in sisal or leather is used in Kenya, Tanzania and Sarawak. This aid requires very strong neck muscles.

○ In Ethiopia, a shoulder strap is made from a loop of strong cloth, webbing or rope.

○ Two strong forked branches with woven straw back-padding and shoulder straps make up the chee-geh from South Korea It allows some 50kg to be carried and is generally used by men.

○ The use of a wooden back-frame with extended arms allows the weight to be distributed evenly along the back.

Even with the use of these aids, women carrying water on their backs still walk in a stooped position.

Carrying water on the shoulder is much used in south-east Asia and Latin America. Because this method of water-carrying is asymmetrical, people's bodies tend to develop more on one side. A popular carrying aid is a shoulder pole or yoke which consists of two containers suspended by rope on a section of bamboo. It is easy to carry on flat ground where the bamboo acts as a shock absorber, but difficult to use on steep and rough terrain.

Water is carried on the hip in India, Bolivia and some African countries, often combined with other methods. The asymmetric position requires skill and muscular strength and, again, one side develops more than the other.

Carrying water on the hip may result in health problems such as pelvic damage, especially in children.

Carrying by hand is often used in conjunction with other ways of carrying water. It is more tiring than the other methods.

General health effects

The task of carrying heavy loads over long distances requires a great deal of energy, which comes from metabolized food. The longer the distance and the more difficult the terrain, the greater the quantity of food needed. Women carrying water are frequently exposed to malnutrition, anaemia and water-related diseases.

Women are most vulnerable to malnutrition at the end of the dry season when they have to travel even greater distances to fetch water. At this time of year, food is scarcer and work in the field may be very hard. Women and children suffering from malnutrition are also more susceptible to other diseases.

Some 230 million people are estimated to be anaemic, and pregnant women, in particular, are at risk. In Africa, 40 per cent of non-pregnant and 63 per cent of pregnant women are anaemic. During pregnancy, the arduous task of carrying water can cause problems with the growth of a foetus. Women have to resume fetching water soon after giving birth, which can affect the quantity and quality of breast milk, making the baby vulnerable to malnutrition.

Women collecting water from certain environments may by exposed to water-related diseases such as malaria, filariasis and schistosomiasis.

Energy consumption

The amount of energy used in walking with a heavy load can be expressed in terms of the consumption of calories and the consumption of oxygen. The quantity varies according to physical ability, the nature of the terrain, distances, the weight of the load and the method of carrying.

The International Labour Office recommends a maximum load — for women — of 25 to 30kg, but in practice this is often exceeded. The energy cost increases in steep and dry areas where women must walk further, such as the eastern side of Mount Kenya where the energy used by women to fetch water may represent 85 per cent of their total daily energy intake.

A study was carried out by the Medical Research Council of the UK to calculate the consumption of energy in terms of oxygen. This compared the efficiency of various methods of load-carrying, particularly the oxygen requirements for different weights and ways of carrying. Considering an average load of 25 to 40kg, it appears that the yoke is the most economic method, followed by bundles carried by hand and carrying on the hip, although neither of these methods is used alone. Carrying water on the back and head come next, with shoulder-carrying requiring the most energy, although it is used for shorter distances and on less rough terrain.

Effects on the skeleton

Carrying heavy loads over long periods of time can result in damage to the vertebral column (see Table 1). In normal physiological conditions, the vertebral column is resistant and can support great strains, but this changes as people age. A major problem arising from carrying water is the early ageing of the vertebral column. This may be influenced by several factors, the most important of which is overwork. A hereditary factor may also exist

Table 1. Pathology of skeleton according to way of carrying water

		Cervical column	Thoracic column	Lumbar column	L l
	On the head ⊕ Very strong muscles of neck +++ back +++ ⊕ Majestic, elegant posture ⊕ Symmetric position ⊖ No specific deformity but: ⊖ Limitation of flexion ⊖ Arthrosis ....▼	±	±	±	

	On the back
	⊕ Very strong muscles of neck (a)
	        back (a,b)
	⊕ Symmetric position
	⊖ Stooped posture (a,b)
	⊖ Cyphosis (a,b)
	⊖ Arthrosis ....▼(a)
	                  ▼(b)
	⊖ Hip and knee'arthrosis (a,b) ▼
		+++
		+
			+++
			+++
				+++
				+++	

	On the hip ⊖ Asymetric position ⊖ May lead to scoliosis attitude ⊖ and deformation of pelvic bone in children ⊖ Arthrosis ....▼	–	+	+	
	On the shoulder ⊖ Asymetric position ⊖ Muscles stronger on one side. back and shoulder ⊖ Arthrosis ....▼ ⊖ To children, scoliosis attitude	–	±	±	

Key
⊕ = positive aspects   ⊖ = negative aspects   ▼ = location of pain

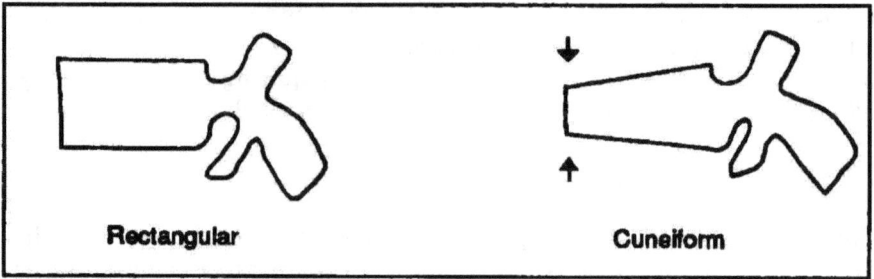

| Rectangular | Cuneiform |

Figure 1. Change of shape of vertebral bodies

in certain families, causing rheumatism; women are more susceptible to this problem. Ageing soon appears and arthrosis - a degenerative rheumatism - is common.

Problems occur in the organic tissue: the disc decreases and becomes thinner. The nucleus becomes fibrous and no longer acts as a shock absorber. The vertebral bodies become more fragile and tend to change shape from rectangular to cuneiform (Figure 1). This may lead to a deformity called cyphosis (Figure 2a).

At the same time, clinical symptoms appear in the form of pain, which increases with work, at the end of the day and in cold temperatures. It subsides with rest. Mobility often becomes limited: on waking up, considerable stretching is required before normal mobility can be achieved. As people move less because of pain, so their movements become more and more restricted until they may reach a stage where they cannot move at all. This is ankylosis, a condition most frequently found in people who carry

Figure 2.

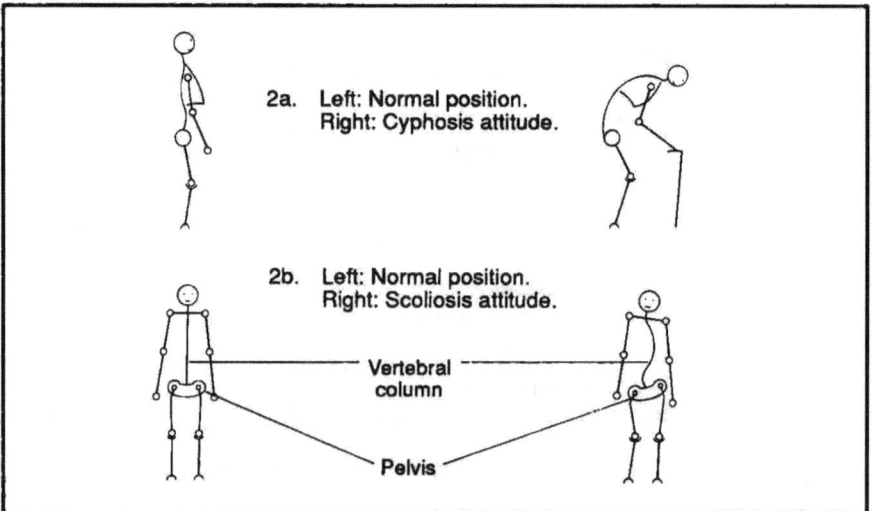

2a. Left: Normal position.
Right: Cyphosis attitude.

2b. Left: Normal position.
Right: Scoliosis attitude.

Vertebral column

Pelvis

water on the back. Because of modifications in physiological conditions, the vertebral column can no longer fulfil its functions.

Where children are concerned, the main problem associated with carrying heavy loads of water is the effect on the growth of bones. When children begin to carry water, they are still growing and a deformity known as scoliosis of the vertebral column may occur (Figure 2b), particularly when water is carried on the hip or shoulder. Carrying water on the hip may also cause deformed pelvic bones in children.

In Bangladesh, 50 per cent of the people treated for broken necks fell while carrying a heavy load on the head. A broken neck can have serious consequences and can even cause paralysis. People carrying water on their backs with a head strap exhibit a marked cranial depression, and many suffer from severe headaches. Also, because of the development of the neck muscles, they may have problems with the thyroid gland. Other problems include fractures, slipped discs and damage to the knees.

Improving the situation

Providing more appropriate means of transport and siting water supplies within a reasonable distance may lessen the health problems of women and children. Aids such as animals or wheelbarrows and handcarts may be introduced to decrease the muscular efforts required. The introduction and use of animal-drawn carts would be especially beneficial to women. Depending on the area, donkeys, buffalo or camels may be used, but, while they are well-suited to carrying water, they are expensive and can be difficult to obtain. The animals must also be trained, fed, watered and cared for, making it impossible for many poor families to use them. Also, women will not always benefit from such improvements unless the equipment is made directly available to them, as the animals are often claimed by the male head of the household.

Many designs of wheelbarrow and handcart exist all over the world, yet various obstacles restrict their use. The nature of the terrain, such as steep slopes, narrow paths, rocks, erosion gullies, fallen trees, roots, sand and mud can prevent the use of wheels or limit the use of handcarts.

Even on more favourable terrain, attempts to introduce these aids have met with little enthusiasm from women. Their muscles have been trained since early childhood for a particular way in which to carry water, and they find that the task of pushing carts requires greater effort. In fact, the muscles needed for pushing are different from those used in carrying; the latter requires very strong spinal muscles whatever method is used, whereas pushing uses the muscles of the upper limbs. Despite these negative factors, there are many advantages to these aids: they allow heavier loads to be carried, and so reduce the number of trips needed. With a wheelbarrow, the load is taken directly by the wheels, allowing 200kg to be carried. A container cart can take a weight of 72kg, and a water roller, 30kg.

The only way to shorten the distance over which water must be carried is to supply water near to or in the village. One of the aims of the Water Decade is to reduce health problems by providing safe water close to the houses. By reducing energy requirements, women will be less vulnerable to malnutrition; by providing safe water the incidence of water-related diseases will decrease; by reducing walking distances the skeleton will not suffer as much, and one of women's many carrying tasks will be considerably reduced.

Further reading

M. Carr, 'The long walk home', *Appropriate Technology*, Vol. 10, No. 1, 1983.

J. Castaing, J.J. Santine, *Le Rachis*, (Medicorama, Paris, 1971).

V. Curtis, *Women and the transport of water*, (Intermediate Technology Publications, London 1986).

G. Hathway, *Low-cost vehicles, options for moving people and goods*, (Intermediate Technology Publications, London 1985).

J. Kimondo, A. Agarwal, G. Moreno, J. Tinker, *Water, Sanitation, Health for All?* (Earthscan, London 1983).

R. Martinez, *Le Rachis*, (Masson, Paris, 1982).

R. Sohier, *La kinesitherapie analytique de la colonne vertebrale*, (La Hestre, 1970).

G.F. White, D. J. Bradley, A.U. White, *Drawers of Water*, (University of Chicago Press, 1972).

(*Waterlines* Vol.6 No. 3, January 1988)

Oral rehydration therapy: a cure but not a solution

DENISE AYRES

Dehydration from diarrhoea kills over four million children each year in developing countries. Most of these deaths are not only treatable but largely preventable.

Diarrhoea has diminished in the developed world through public health measures which ensure more and safer drinking-water, better sanitation and improved food-handling. Education has brought greater awareness of the dangers of poor hygiene — both personal and environmental. Such benefits have yet to reach many parts of the developing world.

In the long term, diarrhoeal disease-control programmes, which improve the quantity and quality of water supplies, excreta disposal and hygiene, are the only measures that will stop children being regularly reinfected. However, these measures take time to implement and to be accepted by communities. In the short term, there is a relatively easy and effective treatment for dehydration — 'oral rehydration therapy', replacing the lost fluid by giving the child a special solution to drink — which has already saved thousands of lives.

Dehydration from diarrhoea can kill a child within hours unless the vital salts and liquids lost from the body are replaced. Until relatively recently, the most common method of replacing them was by intravenous transfusion, introducing the fluid directly into a vein through the child's skin. This is costly and must be done in a hospital.

In the Bangladeshi refugee camps during the early 1970s, cholera and other diarrhoea-type diseases were a major problem. Obviously there were no facilites for intravenous therapy, so fluids were given by mouth and this method was found to be very effective. Since then, various groups and organizations, especially the Diarrhoeal Disease Control Programme of the World Health Organization (WHO), have been vigorously promoting the use of early oral rehydration therapy as a life-saver for children with diarrhoea.

Barriers to treatment

The treatment sounds simple enough, but putting theory into practice is not so easy.

In many communities, traditional attitudes to diarrhoea are barriers to using oral rehydration therapy. For example, diarrhoea is often seen not as an illness but a normal occurrence and, therefore, not something requiring any special kind of attention. It is rarely considered dangerous, as a child may suffer many episodes of diarrhoea and become very weak, but not actually die.

In many parts of the world mothers stop giving the child any food or liquid, including breast milk, with the start of a bout of diarrhoea. Breast milk is not only an easily digested food, but, if it is withheld, the amount of milk a mother can produce decreases rapidly. Breast milk also protects children against other infections. Mothers often do not feed their children for several days after the diarrhoea has ended.

This is particularly critical for the long-term health of the child as there is a dangerous link between malnutrition and diarrhoea. The badly-nourished child is more susceptible to diarrhoea, and diarrhoea sometimes impairs the stomach's ability to absorb nutrients for up to two weeks after the bout has ended. So the vicious circle continues.

Mothers' attitudes can only be changed through persuasive health education. What to drink and how to make it are of minor importance, until mothers firmly believe that their children should drink more when they have diarrhoea.[25] A change of attitude can often be achieved through demonstration. If one group of mothers in the community can be convinced about the value of early oral rehydration therapy and see it working for their children, others will soon be persuaded to use it.

Traditional attitudes do not, of course, exist only in villages. Senior doctors, paediatricians and all those involved in training health staff have to be convinced that oral rehydration therapy can play an important role in the management of diarrhoea, and that it has far more widespread application than intravenous therapy or often inappropriate drugs.

Once mothers have accepted that a child should drink when it has diarrhoea, it should be relatively easy to discuss what is the best drink under the circumstances. But again this is not as simple as it sounds. If mothers can be persuaded to encourage their children to drink as soon as an attack of diarrhoea begins, they can use any fluid that is available in the home to do this. For example, tea, milk, fruit juices or rice water. However, if rehydration therapy does not start quickly enough, and the child becomes dehydrated, he or she must drink sugar/salt solution. This can also be given at home at first, but the child must be taken to a hospital or clinic if there is no response and more fluid is lost. Mothers must be taught how to recognize the signs of dehydration.

Methods of measurement

The United Nations Children's Fund (UNICEF) and WHO are distributing sachets of oral rehydration salts (ORS) designed to be dissolved in one litre of clean drinking-water. Some countries are producing their own sachets of ORS.

One of the major problems with using the sachets is that it is often difficult to distribute them. Frequently, even where they are available, insufficient information is actually given to people about using them. This is unfortunate because if, for example, the ORS is mixed with too little fluid, the child will refuse to drink the over-concentrated solution, and treatment may be seen as unhelpful and discontinued.

There have been attempts in many places where sachets are not available to teach mothers and health workers how to make up simple sugar/salt solutions using locally available ingredients. The main problem here is to measure out even reasonably accurate amounts of unrefined sugar and salt. A simple formula for oral rehydration solution is to mix one level 5ml teaspoonful of salt plus eight level 5ml teaspoonsful of sugar in one litre of

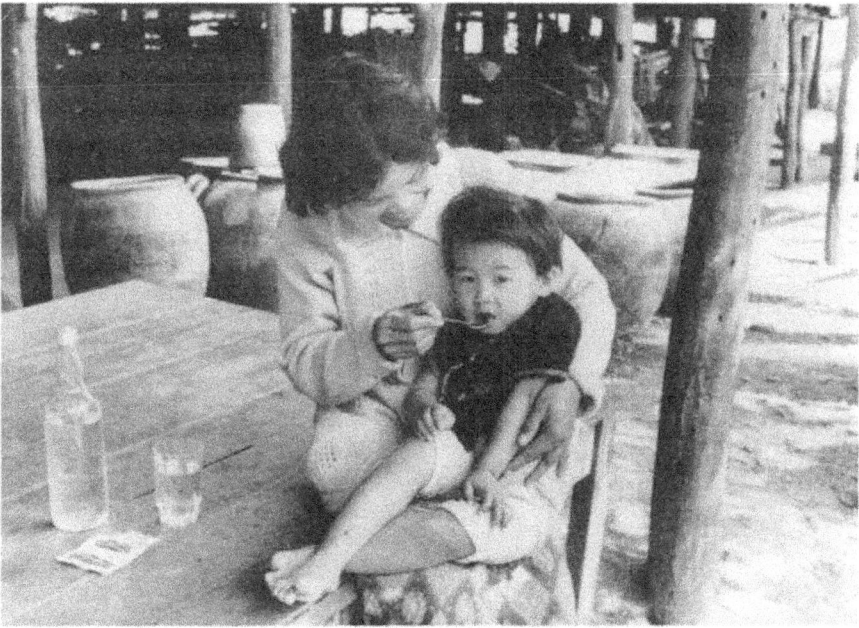

A primary health-care worker in Thailand gives a child oral rehydration salts to treat diarrhoea. (WHO)

Demonstration of oral rehydration at an open-air health centre near Dhaka. (WHO/A. Khan)

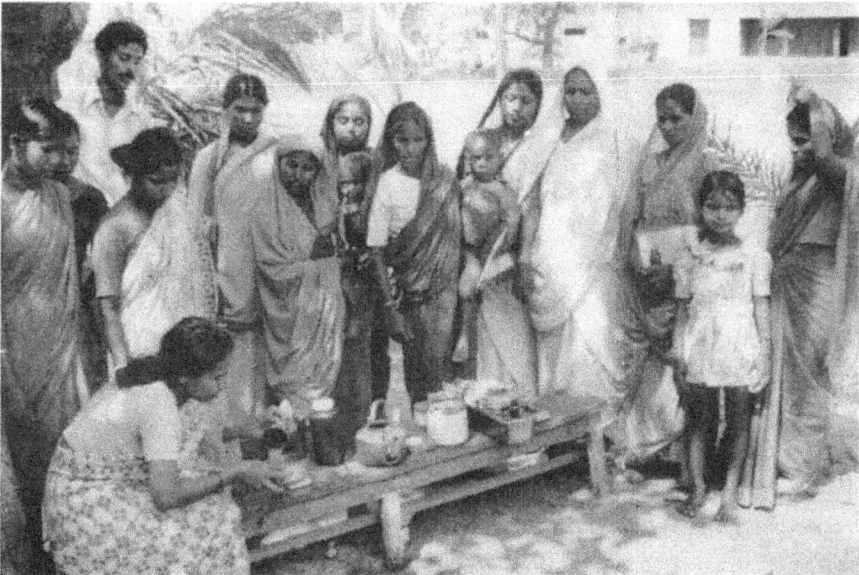

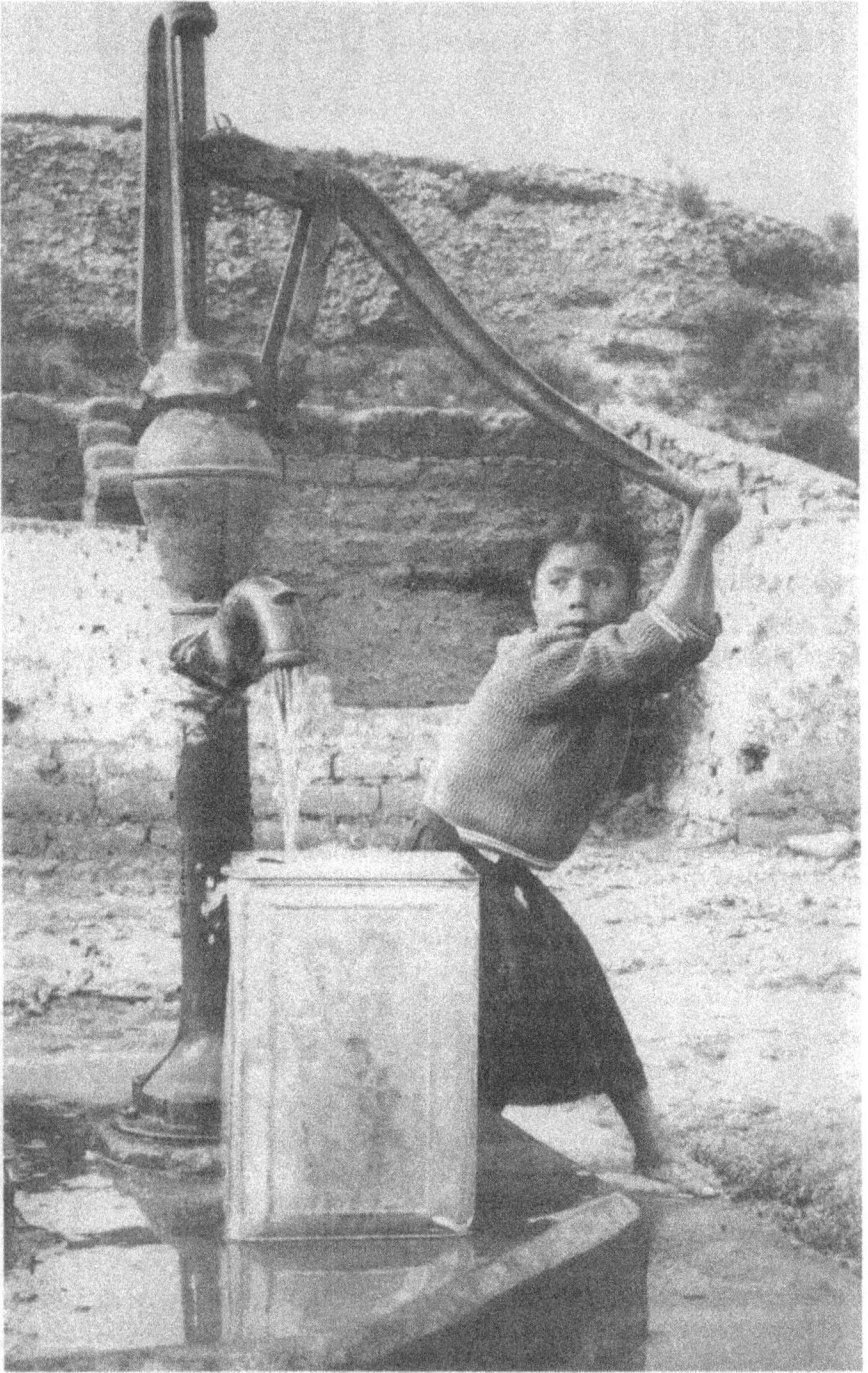

This well provides a little Peruvian girl with water that is good to drink.
(WHO/UNICEF/P. Almasy)

drinking water. A double-ended plastic spoon has been developed* to use for measuring out sugar with one end and salt with the other. The advantage of this spoon is that it measures out enough salt and sugar for a relatively small amount of water (200ml) so that the ORS is more likely to be drunk quickly and not be left standing for hours to become contaminated.

The main disadvantage associated with use of the plastic spoon is that mothers are often not given enough information on how to use it.

Sugar and salt can be measured out by hand, but measurement is often inaccurate. At least using this method people do not have to depend on supplies of equipment from outside. As with other measurement methods described, the success of this one depends on vigorous health education so that people understand not only how to prepare the fluid but why and when to give it.[26,27]

Health workers and mothers have to understand that they must be patient in giving oral rehydration fluid as the child may well vomit. Sparing time to give fluid is often a problem, especially for mothers, who have not only housework and cooking to do, but also have to work in the fields. This is one of the reasons why older brothers and sisters are being taught about oral rehydration therapy in many places so that they can help younger children.

In many places, it is unrealistic to expect mothers to have access to clean water or to be able to boil the water they have. Does it matter if dirty water is used to make up oral rehydration solution when clean water is unavailable?

Evidence indicates that the benefits of early replacement of water, sugar and salt during acute diarrhoea far outweigh the possible risk of using contaminated water.[28] A sound strategy is to advise mothers to use the cleanest water available, to boil it where possible and not to keep the rehydration fluid for more than 24 hours.

Oral rehydration therapy now forms an integral part of health-care programmes in many developing countries. Its value as a widely available, simple but effective life-saver is indisputable. There are few other treatments for childhood killer diseases that can be given as easily by anyone.

Nevertheless, if progress is to be made towards long-term diarrhoeal disease control rather than focusing exclusively on short-term treatment, there must be improved nutrition, more and better water supplies, improved sanitation, better personal and domestic hygiene, and more health education.[29]

---

*Plastic spoons are available from Teaching Aids at Low Cost (TALC), Institute of Child Health, 30 Guildford Street, London WCIN IEN, UK.

Water management and malaria control

GEORGE DAVIDSON

The disease malaria is carried from person to person by the bite of the female of certain species of mosquito. All mosquitoes spend part of their life in water. The female lays her eggs on water, and these hatch to release larvae, which live under the water surface, where they feed on microscopic food particles. They grow in size by a series of moults, eventually producing a non-feeding stage, the pupa, from which the adult mosquito emerges and flies away. This aquatic life-cycle occupies several days; at tropical temperatures about one week, but longer at lower temperatures. Thus water has to persist for at least a week to produce emergent adult mosquitoes.

The malaria parasite is a unicellular organism which invades certain cells and tissues of the body, in particular the red blood corpuscles, where it grows and multiplies, and eventually destroys the cells, releasing toxic substances causing fever and anaemia.

Some of the parasites are destined to become sexual forms, which only mature and fertilize in the stomach of the female mosquito if the right species takes them in with its blood meal. The product of union between male and female sexual forms then penetrates the stomach wall of the mosquito where it encysts. Within the resulting spherical cyst numerous divisions occur and the ripe cyst ultimately bursts to release large numbers of sickle-shaped sporozoites into the body cavity of the mosquito. These migrate to the head region and invade the insect's salivary glands.

When a female mosquito feeds, it inserts part of its proboscis into the skin in its search for blood capillaries. Having found one, it then injects its saliva, which contains an anticoagulant, thus ensuring that the blood, which is sucked up into its stomach, does not congeal and block its feeding tube. If the salivary glands contain sporozoites, these will enter the blood stream with the saliva, and thus the bitten person will receive an infection.

This cycle of the malaria parasite in the mosquito requires several days for its completion. The actual time depends on the species of malaria parasite involved (there are at least four species of human malaria parasites) and the prevailing temperature in the adult mosquito environment. At tropical temperatures, averaging something like 26°C (80°F), a malaria-carrying mosquito would have to live nearly two weeks after emerging from the water, taking its first feed on a person harbouring sexual forms of the two main species of malaria parasite, *Plasmodium falciparum and P. vivax*, within four days of its emergence and its second feed some 10 days later, before it could pass on the infection to a second person.

Factors limiting the disease

Temperature is the principal factor limiting the occurrence of the disease, which needs a warm climate. Its highest incidence is between the tropics of Cancer and Capricorn. What little infection occurs in subtropical and temperate zones is limited to the warmest weather.

In spite of intensive attempts to eradicate it in the 1950s and 1960s, malaria remains the most common of all the tropical diseases. The World Health Organization estimates that 107 countries are affected, and that about half the world's population is at risk. In addition to some 200 million people (mostly in Africa) chronically affected, something like 150 million new cases are occurring every year. Tropical Africa (where virtually no control is attempted) accounts for some 40 per cent of these cases, eastern Asia and Oceania some 30 per cent and the Indian subcontinent 20 per cent. The eastern Mediterranean and Central and South America produce the remainder.

Entomologists classify mosquitoes into two main groups on anatomical grounds: the culicines, which include the vectors of filariasis and yellow fever, and the anophelines, which include the malaria carriers. There are about 3,000 species of mosquitoes in all, and of these only 400 species are anophelines. Not all the latter are malaria vectors; in fact only 30 of them are of any great importance in carrying the disease. Whereas many species of culicines can breed in very small collections of water (tree-holes, artifical containers such as water pots, tin cans and the like) and polluted water, (sullage and excreta-contaminated water), most anophelines prefer larger and cleaner collections.

Worldwide distribution of malaria

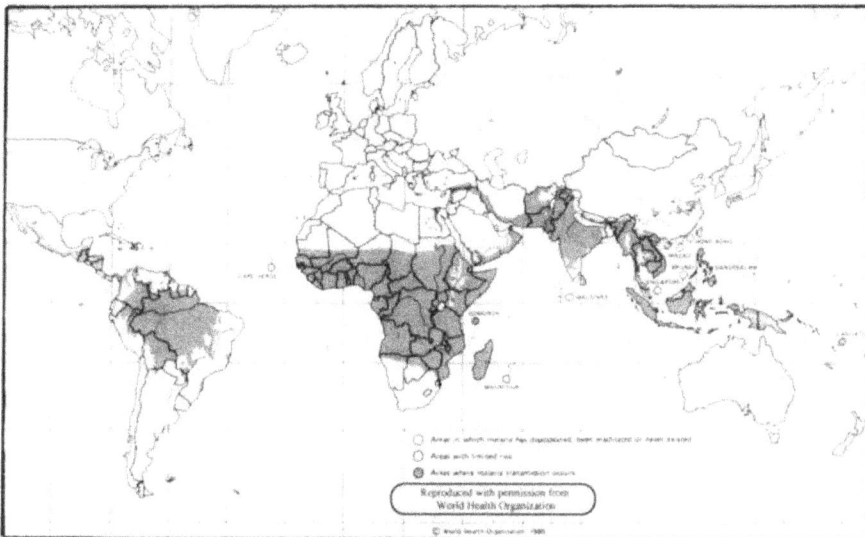

Reproduced with permission from
World Health Organization

Methods of disease control

Efforts to control malaria may be directed against the parasite or against the mosquito vector or at protecting humans from being bitten by the mosquito.

To kill the parasites, a number of efficient anti-malarial drugs exist, though resistance to them is fast becoming a major problem. As a major means of control of the disease, these drugs present problems of mass distribution and acceptance, however.

A single-shot medical treatment or long-lasting prophylactic (preventative) has not yet been discovered. Nor has a suitable vaccine, though certain recent developments give hope in this direction. The protection of humans from being bitten largely centres on health education and the provision of house-screening and mosquito nets at a price low enough for the predominantly poor countries in which the disease is usually found. Finally, the attack on the vector may be directed against the adult or against the aquatic stages.

The most noticeable progress in the fight against malaria has come from the spraying of long-lasting chemicals on the insides of walls and roofs of human habitations. Most malaria vectors spend part of their adult life resting indoors before or after feeding on the occupants and are thus vulnerable.

A single spraying of a uniform, adequate dosage of chemicals such as DDT, BHC, malathion, fenitrothion, permiphos-methyl, propoxur, bendiocarb, or permethirin may remain lethal to resting mosquitoes for several weeks and lead to such a reduction in life expectancy that the chances of any single female mosquito living long enough to complete the cycle of the parasite from sexual stages to the production of sporozoites becomes extremely remote.

The aim is not to eliminate the mosquito population altogether (this would be extremely difficult to do) but rather to intercept transmission of the disease. The principle of malaria eradication (which was arrived at in more than 40 countries between 1957 and 1969) was to maintain this interception for as long as it takes the human infection to die out (some two or three years in the case of *P. vivax* and one year in the case of *P. falciparum*). Then mosquitoes would no longer have a parasite to carry.

Successful eradication was largely restricted to peripheral areas of the disease's distribution: southern Europe for example. The reasons for failure in other parts of the world are numerous, complex and controversial. Resistance to the insecticides certainly played a part, but so did organizational and financial difficulties as well as changes in human motivation.[30]

Before the advent of residual insecticides, larval control formed the main method of vector containment. Chemicals used then included mixtures of unwanted fractions from oil-refining processes designed to produce continuous films on the water surface to prevent aerial respiration by the aquatic stages of the mosquito and, later, a compound of copper and arsenic known as Paris Green. The larva-eating fish Gambusia was also used and is still in vogue today in the now-favoured biological control approach.

Nowadays, bacterial larvicides as well as fungal, protozoan and nematode parasites are also being advocated as biological methods.

Water management methods

Water management methods aimed at rendering water collections unfavourable for vector breeding have been employed for many years, and the older textbooks[31] on malaria control elaborate on numerous mechanical and naturalistic modifications of existing or potential breeding places. A manual produced by the World Health Organization[32] reiterates most of these, which were first put into practice before World War II, and even before World War I in limited areas.

The most suitable type of water management method will depend largely on the type and size of the water collection involved. The WHO manual referred to classifies them as follows:

1. Large bodies of water such as lakes, reservoirs, marshes and swamps. Control of the more open water collections may involve straightening the shore-line and removing or filling in side-pockets. Water-level fluctuations leading to alternating inundation and drying of marginal vegetation may also help. Breeding tends to be restricted to this marginal vegetation. The draining and filling in of swamps and marshes may be necessary if they are the source of malaria-carrying mosquitoes. Very often, large water bodies are not. Exact knowledge of what is breeding where is an essential requisite for any larval-control method. 'Species sanitation' is the phrase in use signifying the practical application of this knowledge.

2. Small collections of water such as temporary rainwater pools, hoofprints and wheel-ruts. These are best dealt with by grading and filling-in.

3. Ricefields. Here, intermittent irrigation is the favoured means of preventing mosquito emergence, only allowing surface water to remain for less time than the aquatic cycle of the mosquito.

4. Saltwater marshes, lagoons and coastal fishponds. In such situations, the salt content of the water is critical as far as the mosquito is concerned, and altering it, either by admitting the sea, or in some cases excluding it by tidal gates, can make it unsuitable.

5. Partially or heavily shaded situations such as forested areas. Here removal of the shade by clearing vegetation may discourage breeding of some species. However, this might encourage equally or more dangerous light-loving species to invade. The addition of drainage to clearing would, of course, prevent this.

6. Running water. Here breeding is confined to grassy margins and quieter

backwaters. The straightening and clearing of edges in a general process of canalization helps in such situations. Various automatic means of alternating draining and flushing have also been designed to flush out marginal breeding.

7. Springs and seepages from streams, irrigation channels and the like. Drainage, filling-in and repairs of leaks in embankments are called for.
8. Plant hollows and cavities are best dealt with by the destruction of the plants.
9. Man-made containers such as wells, cisterns and tanks can be either covered to prevent access by egg-laying female mosquitoes or emptied at frequent intervals.

Dealing with any of these water management methods in detail is beyond the scope of this article, but it would seem appropriate to say a little about these.

Man-made problems

Much of the malaria present in the world today is man-made. Dam construction leading to the formation of lakes, and major agricultural irrigation schemes are obvious examples of man's creation of new and extensive breeding places. Removing earth to construct roads and railways leads to the ubiquitous 'borrow-pit' which soon becomes filled with water and forms a breeding ground.

Less obvious are the smaller-scale activities of individual people or small groups, which lead to the persistence of often quite small but nonetheless dangerous and often unnecessary accumulations of surface water. Depressions associated with the cultivation of certain crops, holes deliberately dug in search of precious stones ('gem-pits') for making bricks or sand or merely to reach the water-table are all liable to become breeding places.

Inadequate maintenance of drains and ditches often leads to blockages and the accumulation of still water, which, even if they are slightly polluted, can encourage certain species of malaria vectors. Water points, be they wells, handpumps or stand-pipes, are a continuous source of risk and will become an increasing problem unless provision is made to prevent the formation of puddles around them. Ideally, concrete aprons with a drain pipe should remove the waste water effectively. Where a drain or ditch is not available to receive and carry away the water, a suitable soakage arrangement should be provided.

Limitations to control

In conclusion, it must be pointed out that larval control in general and water-management methods in particular, have their limitations as far as the control of malaria is concerned. Unless a very high proportion of breeding places can be dealt with, they are unlikely to have sufficient effect on vector density to produce a major change in transmission. Success is only likely to be achieved where breeding grounds are few and well-known. This may be the case in townships, but is less likely to be so in rural areas — and malaria is primarily a rural disease.

Large-scale water management schemes are also likely to be prohibitively expensive for developing countries. They have considerable advantages, however, because they offer more permanent solutions than the repetitive use of insecticides and can be more acceptable to the population, involving less interference with individual householders. Ideally, they should be looked upon as ultimate objectives and in the meantime used in any way feasible to supplement short-term methods of control such as the use of anti-malarial drugs and house-spraying.

At the village level, community participation in small-scale work aimed at keeping the environment clear of unnecessary water collections and rendering those that cannot be removed unsuitable for vector breeding should be encouraged. At the same time, all the authorities concerned with managing water supplies in malarious countries should constantly be made aware of the possible dangers and implication of their work on the transmission of the disease.

(Waterlines Vol. 1 No. 4, April 1983)

A lesson about water: schistosomiasis

KENNETH MOTT

Schistosomiasis or bilharziasis has up to now been considered an inevitable plague in 74 developing countries. It is usually referred to as 'that disease caused by snails'.

It is not the snails that cause schistosomiasis, however, it is people themselves. Widespread acceptance of this fact now forms the basis of the new concept of schistosomiasis control. People cause schistosomiasis by defecating and urinating in ponds, streams and rivers, which can then re-infect them when they bathe there. So a person can be the sole source of his own increasingly heavy infection as well as that of neighbours, family and friends. The details of the life-cycle of the schistosome, a parasitic flatworm, are as fascinating as they are complex. But it is easier to understand how people cause schistosomiasis than to understand how the intermediate stages of the parasite enter and leave the snail host before reaching a human.

Heavy infections with large numbers of schistosome parasites, occurring

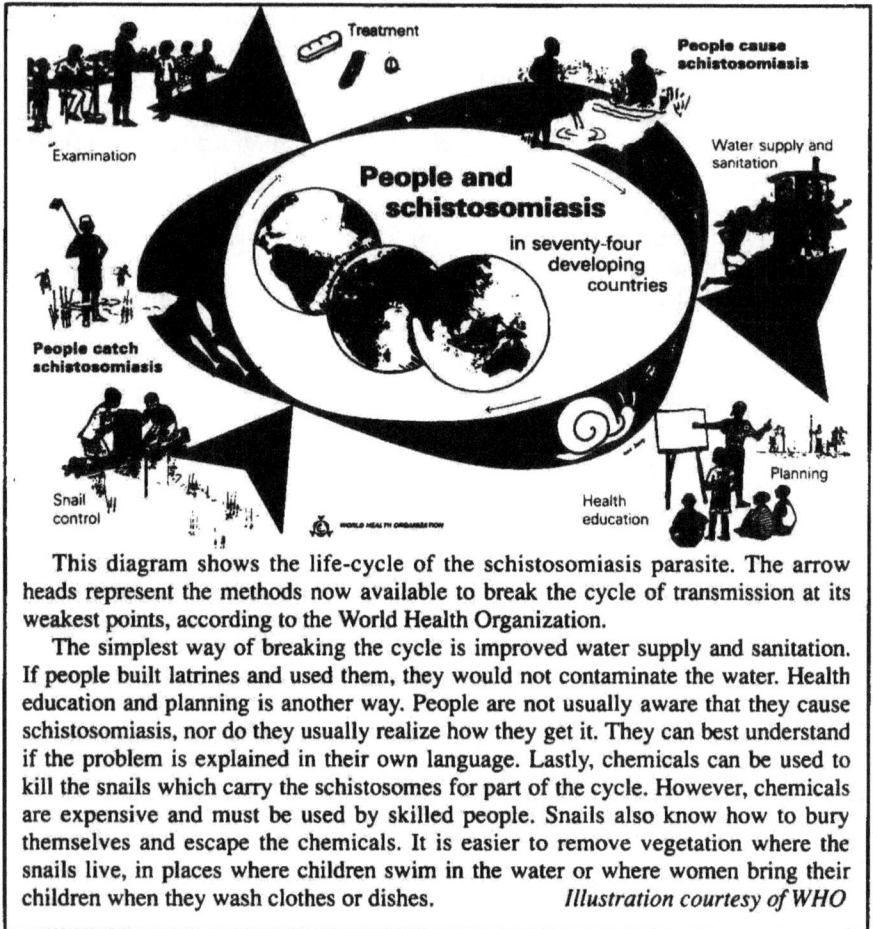

This diagram shows the life-cycle of the schistosomiasis parasite. The arrow heads represent the methods now available to break the cycle of transmission at its weakest points, according to the World Health Organization.

The simplest way of breaking the cycle is improved water supply and sanitation. If people built latrines and used them, they would not contaminate the water. Health education and planning is another way. People are not usually aware that they cause schistosomiasis, nor do they usually realize how they get it. They can best understand if the problem is explained in their own language. Lastly, chemicals can be used to kill the snails which carry the schistosomes for part of the cycle. However, chemicals are expensive and must be used by skilled people. Snails also know how to bury themselves and escape the chemicals. It is easier to remove vegetation where the snails live, in places where children swim in the water or where women bring their children when they wash clothes or dishes. *Illustration courtesy of WHO*

mainly in children, cause the actual disease. The eggs laid by the female — not the flatworms themselves — damage the bladder, intestines and other organs.

The symptoms of schistosomiasis include rash, coughing and chest pains, cramps, diarrhoea, fever, blood in the urine, and enlargement of the spleen and liver. With re-infections over a period of years, it can become a very debilitating and sometimes fatal disease. A specific form of bladder cancer occurring in endemic areas is also linked with long-term schistosomiasis infection.

If a child has many schistosome parasites, many eggs will be found in the urine (urinary schistosomiasis due to *Schistosoma haematobium*) or in the faeces (intestinal schistosomiasis caused by *S. mansone, S. japonicum* or *S. Mekongi*). The eggs may now be detected by simple low-cost diagnostic tehniques. The test to detect intestinal forms of schistosomiasis has been simplified. A small amount of faeces is pressed through a fine nylon or steel screen to remove large debris, which can be quickly examined for eggs under a piece of cellophane soaked in glycerine. Various simple techniques for filtering schistosome eggs out of urine have made diagnosis much easier.

WHO's strategy for reduction

The current strategy for controlling schistosomiasis is aimed at reducing the disease rather than attempting to eradicate it. The immediate and dramatic impact of this strategy depends on safe, effective drugs, which can be taken by mouth. All of these — metrifonate, oxamniquine and praziquantel — are included in the WHO Model List of Essential Drugs.

A high proportion of infected people are cured after a single treatment — the latter two drugs are given in a single dose. Many doctors feared that re-infection would eliminate any benefit from treatment, but these fears have not been confirmed by experience. In most areas, a reduction in the overall number of cases is maintained for one-and-a-half to two years without repeat treatment. In any event, the re-infections recorded are not as severe as before. In Brazil, over 5 million doses of oxamniquine have been given for intestinal schistosomiasis since 1975. The prevalence of infection has dropped remarkably in the north-east of Brazil, and the reduction in the rate of liver and spleen enlargement among children confirms that treatment with oxamniquine has been successful. Hundreds of thousands of people are now being treated with praziquantel in Egypt and Sudan.

The long-term impact of this strategy will depend on health education, water supply and sanitation. If people could be educated as quickly and as efficiently as they could swallow the drugs, it would be feasible to consider eradicating schistosomiasis. But health education has not yet been produced in pill form! Nevertheless, an approach emphasizing the use of chemotherapy affords a sound basis for educating the community in how they spread and cause schistosomiasis.

It would be short-sighted to assume that chemotherapy alone will provide a long-term solution. Under a bilateral programme between the governments of Mali and the Federal Republic of Germany through the German Technical Co-operation Agency (GTZ), communities are encouraged to build central standpipes before treatment programmes begin. An intensive health education programme reinforces these preventative efforts.

In the past, the high cost of installing new supplies, the difficulties of maintaining them and the traditional beliefs and customs which encouraged people to use ponds and streams for drinking-water, limited their effectiveness as a method to control schistosomiasis. Nowadays, fortunately, water supply is considered a fundamental element of development for the general well-being of the community.

Examples of successful programmes

Experiences in Egypt, Zanzibar, Zimbabwe, Brazil, St Lucia and elsewhere have confirmed that a safe water-supply reduces contact with water, where transmission of schistosomiasis occurs.

Providing washing and water-supply facilities is a realistic option in some countries where schistosomiasis is endemic. In St Lucia, combined stand-pipe systems with laundry, showers and toilets were built by the national control programme supported by the Rockefeller Foundation and the UK Medical Research Council. These have become permanent community institutions. At first, community volunteers supervised the facilities in half-day shifts. Now the same people receive a stipend from the Ministry of Health. This close supervision is essential to keep the showers and toilets in good condition.

In Zanzibar, the personnel involved in a pilot control programme undertaken by the UNDP/World Bank/WHO Special Programme for Research & Training in Tropical Diseases succeeded in motivating the community to build wells with their own resources. Additional funds from the Ministry of Health have now induced residents to build more wells. In this programme, the role of the 'schistosomiasis agent', a person selected by the community to liaise with the programme staff, has been crucial to promoting the control activities.

The most remarkable large-scale change in the role of water supply in schistosomiasis has occurred in Brazil. Illness due to schistosomiasis in the north-east of Brazil has been reduced in general, but localized areas are still heavily infected. The Ministry of Health has identified the areas which would benefit from improved water supply, and allocation of water supplies in the region is now carried out according to criteria established in co-operation with the Ministry of Health.

Schistosomiasis represents a human paradox. In their desire to be clean, people may wash in water where they, their neighbours or children have defecated or urinated. This vicious circle can only be broken by people themselves. They will only make the link between contamination and schistosomiasis after intensive health education. The success of sanitation programmes will be proportional to the health education efforts reinforcing them. We have much experience on how not to undertake such programmes. To help in the control of schistosomiasis, it is now time to associate our technology with the educational process.

(*Waterlines* Vol. 4 No. 1, July 1985)

CHAPTER 3

Safer Water in the Home

A safe water-supply source such as a protected spring or well does not guarantee safe water in the home. Contamination often occurs from handling,
dirty containers, or the introduction of extraneous matter during collection
and transportation. Similarly, storage in the home represents a major health
risk.

An important source of safer water in the home is rainwater harvesting
from roofing. The article by John Gould in Chapter 4 of *Community Water
Development* discussed the feasibility of water collection for domestic
purposes in Botswana. The thatching of the rondavels there is generally
unsuitable for this purpose, but corrugated-iron sheeting on permanent
buildings with gutters is eminently suitable.

Nick Hall discusses the difficult question of collecting water from thatch
and concludes that it is feasible, with suitable gutters and thatch. It is apparent, though, that a high standard of thatching is required, preferably with
tile substitution at the eaves' edge. Where thatching cannot be used, temporary catchments can be constructed by suspending lengths of cloth from
poles adjacent to houses, so that run-off can be discharged into receptacles
for drinking water. This important source of safe drinking-water supplies
warrants fuller investigation and encouragement.

The next two articles deal with the construction of water jars for domestic storage. The first, by Samia Jahn and Abdallah Omar, outlines the provision in the Sudan of elevated iron holders for traditional clay water-jars
incorporating a water tap. The second article, by Brian Latham, describes
the construction of reinforced cement water-jars in Thailand using a brick
form with capacities above $1.5m^3$. This is an extension of the work by
Simon Watt on ferrocement tanks.

The article by Dian Desa, the Indonesian non-governmental organization
working for rural development, discusses the use of a species of Moringa
seeds to precipitate solids together with some bacteria from dirty pond-
water. Villagers from a test village were quite enthusiastic about using it,
after health education, so Dian Desa proposes to disseminate the technology
further.

The boiling of drinking water is often advocated where water resources
are unsafe, particularly when there are outbreaks of enteric disease.
DeWolfe Miller provides evidence that this approach may have drawbacks
and limitations. He suggests that a closer look at the benefits could well
demonstrate that these disadvantages are understated.

Laurie Childers drew the pictures and Frans Claasen wrote the text for
the article on UNICEF's upward-flow water filter, an inexpensive device

which provides clean water for about 10 people. In Zimbabwe, the same principle using graded gravel and sand layers within a steel 44-gallon (200 litre) petrol drum has been used as a rapid gravity filter served by elevated storage for farming households. Plumbing provides for flow-reversal for backwashing.

Water collection from thatched roofs

NICK HALL

Thatch is still the most common roofing material in the world — on the Indian sub-continent for example, census returns indicate that well over 50 per cent of the population live under thatch.[33, 34]

Thatch, whether grass, palm leaves or some other plant material is most commonly used in rural areas, and it is in these same areas that adequate, planned, domestic water-supplies are generally lacking. This article describes some traditional ways of collecting water off roofs, particularly thatched roofs, and also suggests some practical, cheap and simple ways of taking advantage of this source of rainwater.

Thatched roofs made of grasses, reeds or palms are almost invariably constructed with wide, overhanging eaves. In England, reed thatched roofs, which have been known to last up to 100 years, are built so that they extend at least 40cm beyond the walls. In many other countries, this overhang may be considerably wider. The eave depth is usually a function of the length and stiffness of the thatching material and the local thatcher's technique, but it is often deliberately constructed to protect the walls, especially if they are made of unfired earth. It may also provide valuable shade from fierce overhead sunshine in tropical climates.

The eave is the most vulnerable part of a thatched roof, being exposed to wind, rain and other damage on both its upper and lower surfaces. Within a few years, the edge becomes ragged. Attempts at rainwater collection off thatched roofs are therefore usually very hit-and-miss, although collection at both eave and ground level can be improved.

Some societies have arranged their domestic building patterns to take advantage of dripping eaves. The Romans, who were very keen on plumbing, constructed impluvium* courtyards for water collection as well as for privacy and coolness.

Similarly, in Yorubaland, Benin and parts of Iboland in West Africa,

---

* An impluvium is a depression which collects rainwater in the middle of an open-air hall or courtyard.

rooms of houses were built adjoining four sides of a courtyard[35] (Figure 1). Rainwater was then either collected in large pots placed below the ends of the roof valleys, where the water flow was greatest, or in the courtyard itself. It was drained from the courtyard into storage. It is reported that every family compound in the Benin Republic town of Ketou (which was some way from a river) possessed several artificial subterranean storage tanks beneath an impluvium courtyard.[36]

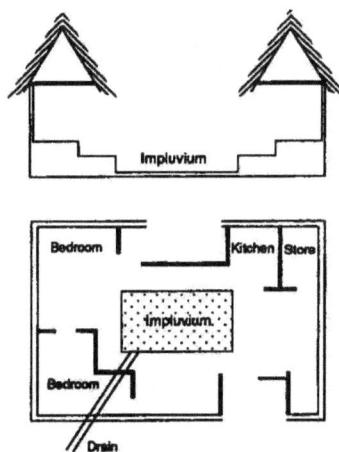

This simple and direct form of water catchment is especially suited to climatic zones with long rainy seasons or particularly heavy cloud-bursts, but the courtyards need regular cleaning and maintenance. Courtyard construction usually involves building several roofs that join each other at an angle; the resulting roof valleys carry a concentrated water flow, and are thus subject to more rapid weathering than adjacent slopes.

Figure. 1. Cross-section and plan of an Ibo house. Redrawn from African Traditional Architecture[35]

For this reason, when low construction and maintenance costs are a priority, valleys and other changes of roof pitch are not recommended. This would be the case whatever the roofing material.

It is possible to collect rainwater discharged from roofs through 'French drains', which are gravel-filled trenches dug immediately below the eaves. Water could then drain into a tank in the same way as from an impluvium.

Eaves level collection

Rainwater will generally be purer for drinking if it can be collected before it reaches the ground.

If rainwater is to be collected from thatched eaves, guttering has to be very wide - 30cm minimum - in order to catch all the water from the ragged edge. This means that it must be custom made, and thus rather expensive.

Wide guttering tends to be heavy, requiring specially robust, wall-mounted support brackets. These must also be very large to support guttering, which may be more than half a metre from the wall. Thatched roofs, therefore, rarely have gutters attached, and are said to have 'dripping eaves'.

To simplify water collection at eaves level, the first course of thatch can be replaced with a course of tiles or even corrugated roofing sheet

(Figure 2). This idea of mixing thatch with other roofing materials is not entirely new. In the Netherlands, for example, it is common to see buildings where two materials have been deliberately placed alongside each other. This is not done for collecting rainwater, but simply because thatch is only used on the part of the building where it is most needed for its excellent insulation qualities. For instance, 300 mm-thick reed thatch has a 'U' value of 0.3W/m²/°C.

The author has designed and tested a method called 'tile substitution' to make collection at eaves more efficient. Incorporating a hard, straight eave in an otherwise thatched roof allows the builder to fit a lightweight, narrow-diameter gutter, which in turn means that the supporting brackets do not need to be so robust. The brackets can then be fixed to the ends of the rafters instead of needing the added security of wall-mounting.

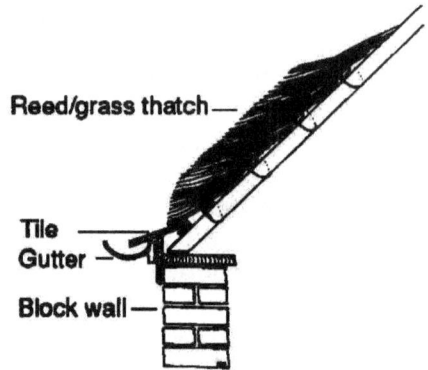

Figure. 2. Schematic diagram of water collection off thatch

Advantages of substitution

Substituting tiles for thatch on the first course has several advantages. Firstly, the eaves will be significantly strengthened, so increasing the life of the roof, and secondly the fire risk so closely associated with all thatched roofs is considerably reduced.

It will obviously be necessary to take into account local thatching methods and materials when substituting tiles for thatch. Although the details of thatching method vary from one region to another, certain common principles do apply to all good quality thatching.

Where stiff grasses, reeds or cereal crop stems are used, the thatcher can take advantage of this rigidity by fixing them to the roof structure under tension.[37] This tensioning of the thatch is achieved by tying down the course of thatch nearest the eave to the first batten, which is nailed to the rafters just behind the 'tilting board'. Figure 3

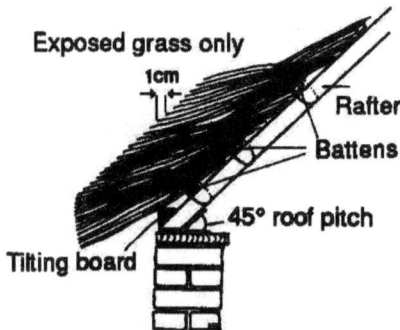

Figure. 3. Fixing thatch to the roof under tension with a tilting board

shows this tilting board and the effect it has on the first and subsequent courses of thatch. Only a centimetre or two of each reed is thus exposed on the outside face of the roof; the remaining metre or more of reed is isolated from the weather within the bulk of the thatch.

A tiled or corrugated eave course can replace the tilting board, but perform the same function. This is possible if the tiles are laid at a relatively low pitch: 30° for a roof that is built at 45°.

The first thatch course is then tied to a batten placed close to the top of the tiles. Failure to pitch the tile correctly will cause a gap to open between the tile and the thatch overlap once the thatch is securely tightened down; this gap will be particularly vulnerable to wind damage.

When flexible materials such as palm leaves or pliable grasses are used, this problem will not arise - this type of thatch will naturally lie flat onto the tile which can then be laid at the same pitch as the roof structure.

The wide eave overhang traditional in some regions can be retained whatever thatching material is used on the rest of the roof, using tile substitution.

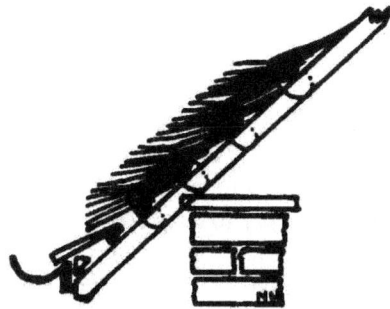

Figure. 4. Extending the rafters to produce an overhanging eave.

This method could well improve protection and shading of the wall-material. Protection of the wall now becomes a constructional, rather than a thatching detail, and involves extending the rafters (Figure 4).

Gutters

Semi-circular, 10cm-diameter gutter-piping is cheaply and readily available in the industrialized countries, where it is mass-produced in a number of different materials. Plastic and aluminium are currently the most economic gutters; they are sold as part of a complete package with suitable supporting brackets, downpipes and ancilliary fittings.

In regions where these are not available, or are very expensive, substitutes can be made locally. Split bamboo is one material that will serve the purpose admirably. Figure 5 shows one method of attaching

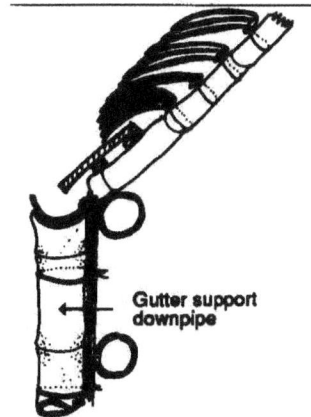

Gutter support
downpipe

Figure 5. Using split bamboo guttering with palm thatch.

bamboo gutters.[38] They are tied to the wall, or the rafter feet when a wide overhang is needed, and are additionally supported by bamboo posts, which may also act as downpipes to channel the water into storage. Different supports could be used with bamboo and other gutters — the details of local eave construction will determine precisely what fixing is suitable.

Water quality

The most important question now concerns the quality of water collected from thatched roofs.

Water collected off any roof will inevitably contain some debris, whether the roof is covered thatch or hard inorganic materials.

The upper surface of thatch does erode away, however, exposing previously uncovered reeds to the elements. Some of this old, weathered material will be washed off the roof and may find its way into rainwater storage tanks. Some of it will be blown away, especially during dry weather. Local climatic conditions will cause thatched roofs to weather at different rates, so no rules apply to calculations about the weight of thatch debris.

Nevertheless, it is possible to make a rough estimate of the weight of debris which will part company with the roof. In England, a new 30cm-thick water reed thatch has a dry weight of about $40kg/m^2$,[39] and will last on average 80 years. At the end of this time, the roof is reduced to approximately half its original thickness, with the fixing ties exposed on the surface, and needs stripping and rethatching. Thus, for each year of its life, about 20kg of dry matter will be eroded off a roof with a surface area of

Figure 6. Two designs for mechanisms to separate debris from rainwater collected from thatch. On the left is an Australian design. As funnel A fills it tilts slowly towards the ground, and after the first flush of debris-laden water has been discharged to the ground, funnel B is tilted into place above the downpipe and the remainder of the rainwater is directed into storage. On the right is a slightly simpler manually operated idea. The moveable deflector would be operated by a lever.

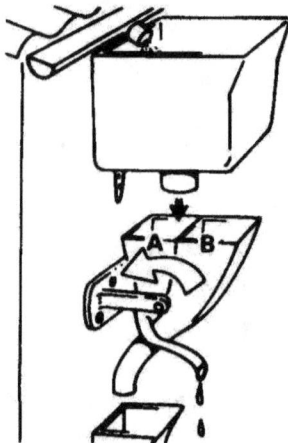

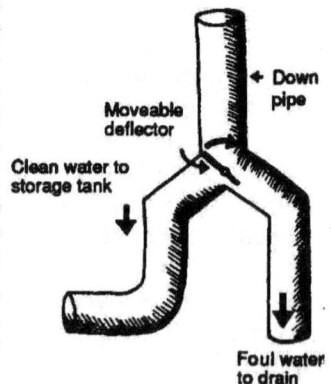

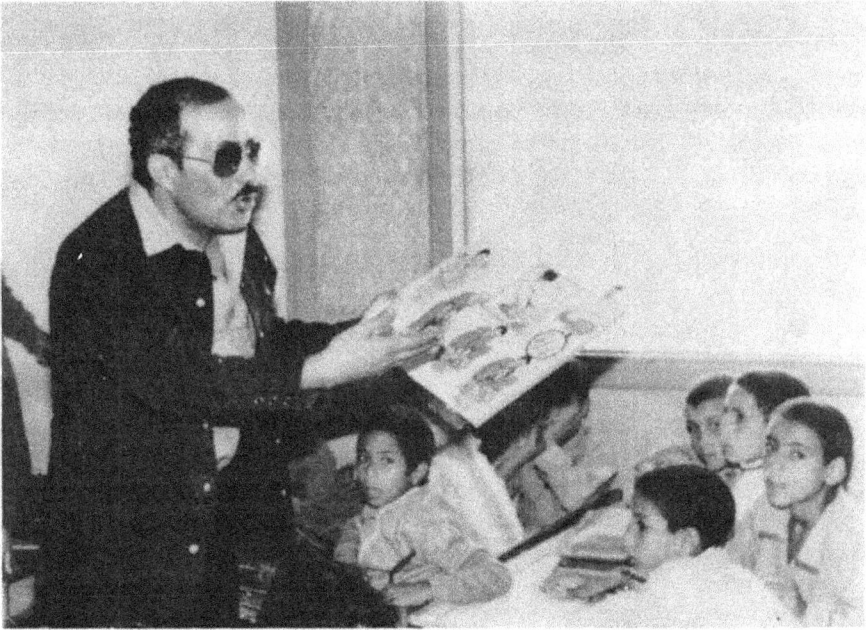

This Egyptian medical officer tells children about schistosomiasis.
(WHO/UNICEF/A. El Matawy)

The nurse is illustrating the difference between clean and dirty water in a Ghanaian village health education discussion. (WaterAid)

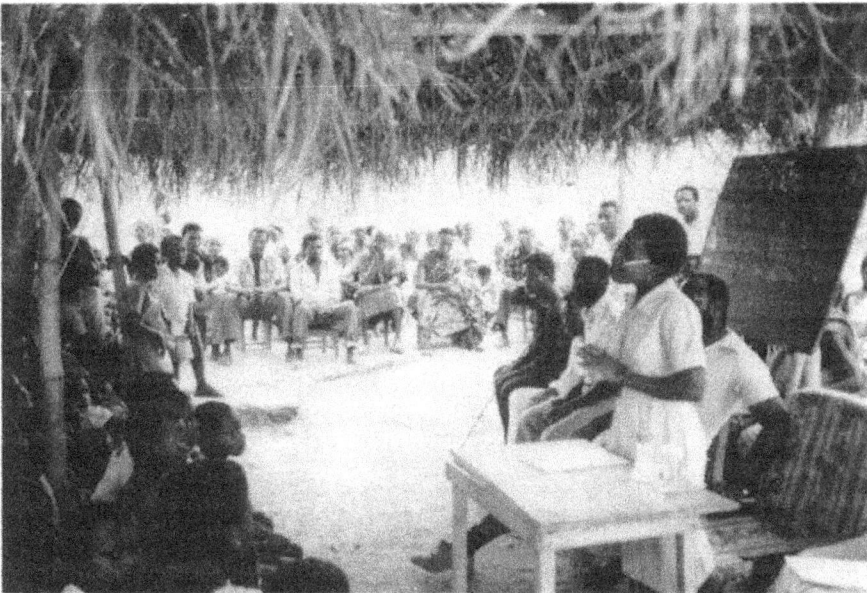

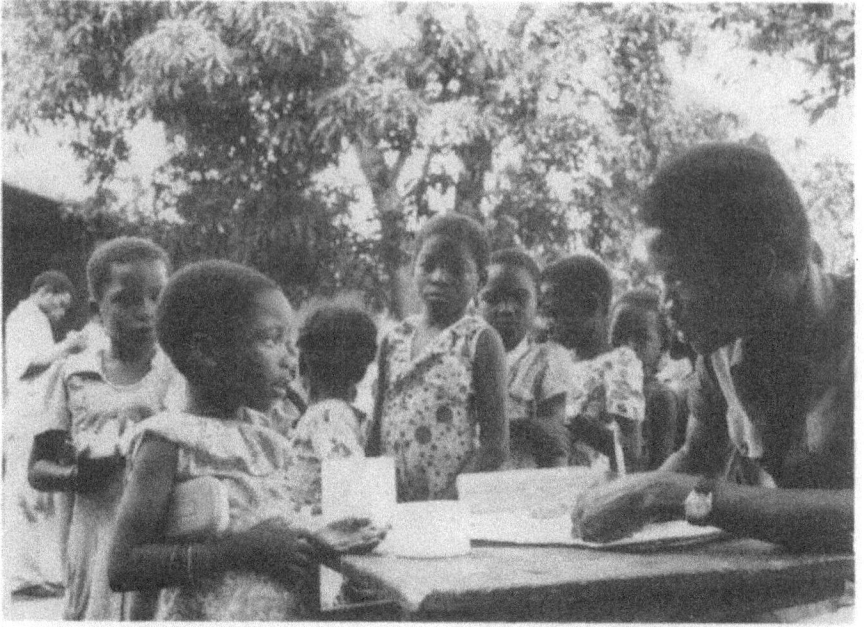

School children in Zanzibar being tested for schistosomiasis
(WHO/Kenneth E. Mott)

Primary health worker checking children's samples for schistosomiasis.
(WHO/Kenneth E. Mott)

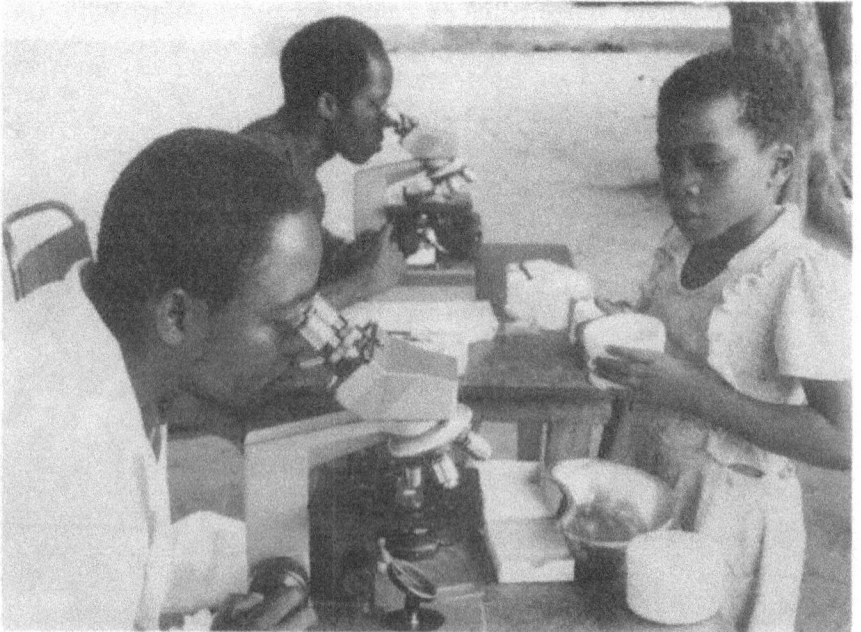

80m². An 80m² roof will cover a gabled building 5m wide by 11.5m long. Of the total 20kg per year lost, perhaps half will find its way into the gutters. Reed thatch is the heaviest thatching material, so it is unlikely that other roofs, especially if they are well thatched, will shed more debris.

Other debris would include dust, leaves, bird and small animal droppings, and both live and dead insects. There are several ideas for mechanisms to separate rubbish from collected rainwater. Figure 6 shows an Australian device to do this automatically, and a simpler baffle tank design. Information on how this device performs in the field, however, is sparse.

Roof-collected rainwater should be filtered, boiled or disinfected to improve its suitability for drinking. Storing it allows settling and permits disease-causing agents to die off.

Conclusion

It is feasible to retain the good qualities of thatch — low cost, high insulation value, and generation of labour intensive employment - and also to collect nearly all the rainwater that falls on the roof. This is particularly valuable for people not served by mains water supplies. Tile substitution need not involve total rebuilding of the roof or the wholesale replacement of thatch with mass-produced industrial roofing materials, except at the eaves edge.

Unfortunately tile substitution does not lend itself to use with circular buildings, unless bamboo can be trained to fit a curve.

(Waterlines, July 1982)

Improved traditional clay water jars

SAMIA AL AZHARIA JAHN AND
ABDALLAH HUSSAIN OMAR

To provide safe water is one of the key aims of Water Decade activities in developing countries, but most projects are not designed to include follow-up measures to make sure that the water is still safe when it reaches the stomach of the person who drinks it.

Even when households in Omdurman (Sudan) had their own piped supplies of chlorinated water from the public water works, this alone proved to be no protection against water-related diseases. Small children still died of diarrhoea.[40]

Water is seldom consumed as it comes from the tap. In hot weather, it is not perceived as pleasant unless it is cool, and so it is transferred to storage and cooling vessels. Only a few wealthy urban households in the Sudan can afford automatic electrical coolers and refrigerators are usually over-loaded with food and only used for making ice-cubes.

The most important storage and cooling vessels in towns and rural areas are the traditional spherical or amphora-shaped clay jars which have capaci-- ties of between 25 and 40 litres. This is very similar to other African coun- tries.

Poor maintenance and storage

Unfortunately, many clay jars are not well maintained. They are neither placed on elevated holders nor regularly cleaned inside and out. Often the jar is left completely open or the covering is inadequate. Hands can come into contact with the water whenever it is removed. When stored water is taken from the same vessel for drinking and all other domestic uses, includ- ing washing after defecation, it is likely to be exposed to pollution. Water is also frequently removed from the storage vessel by all the members of the extended family who live together and by visitors from outside. The unwashed hands of children and sick people can easily contaminate such water with faecal matter or infectious nasopharyngeal mucus.

Water in open jars is also affected by all kinds of wind-borne pollution and may be defiled by thirsty goats and dogs. Material found in water from such badly maintained jars has been shown to comprise soil and air-born genera and bacteria from the mouth and intestinal tracts of humans and warm-blooded animals.[41,42]

Yet it is wrong to dismiss traditional clay jars on principle as old-fash- ioned and unhygienic. Keeping water in old petrol barrels or plastic jerrycans is no satisfactory alternative, because the water is not cooled and they are very difficult to clean properly.

Low-cost project for improvement

Within the framework of a project on domestic water treatment with tradi- tional natural coagulants, which was sponsored by the GTZ (Deutsche Gesellschaft fur Technische Zusammenarbeit, the German agency for tech- nical co-operation), we developed low-cost technical improvements for hygienic water storage and cooling based on traditional clay containers.[43]

The idea of fitting clay jars with a tap to remove water came from Egypt. *Quinauwi* water jars from Upper Egypt were purchased for the Sudanese railways and private schools. This ware is strong but expensive and has poor cooling properties. However, *E. coli* counts performed on water stored in such jars from Camboni and the Sister's School in Khartoum carried out for us in 1977 by Mrs Fatima Abdel Qadir from the Mogren Water Works Laboratory showed that there was no contamination.[41] Some attempts were made to fit Sudanese cooling jars with a tap. Frequent breakages while

*Design for a jar
holder using a
tripod made from a
tree-trunk, with
detail of tap
mounting plate*

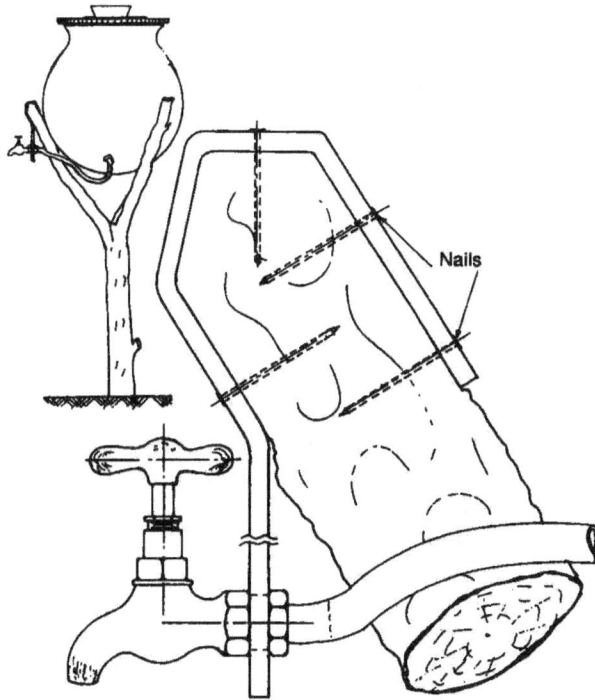

mounting the tap and the necessity of replacing both the clay vessel and the tap if only one of them functioned, made such solutions uneconomic, and even wealthy customers gave up after a single trial.

The benefits of a protected storage system can be obtained for a reasonable price if the tap is fitted to the jar holder. The jar is then no longer exposed to rough treatment during use and repair. Replacement of the clay vessel or the tap can be carried out independently. Jars shaped on a potter's wheel or made by hand are equally suitable for the models we designed. A loose tubing connection was made between the jar and the tap by drilling a hole in a ready-made clay vessel. Alternatively, the potter has to make a hole by pushing the iron connecting piece through the sun-dried clay wall before firing. We found it useful to cover the opening with a thin layer of clay to avoid breakage during firing. This seal can later be easily knocked out.

Water is removed from the jar via a plastic hose attached to a connecting piece fitted to the jar. This connecting piece consists of a 50mm-long iron tube pushed onto a second tube of galvanized iron (90mm long) leaving 10mm overlap on one end. Both the overlapping edge and the other edge of the covering tube are pierced by between seven and nine slits, each about

10mm long. A circular rubber washer is then pushed onto the outer iron tube and the overlapping ends of the outer iron tube bent backwards over the washer in the shape of a star. The connecting piece is now complete and can be inserted into the hole of the jar from the inside, so that the washer is pressed onto the inner wall of the jar. After that, a second rubber washer is fitted onto the connecting piece from the outside of the jar and the ends of the covering tube bent back to fix this second washer to the outer wall. Finally, both fixed washers are covered over with cement mortar.

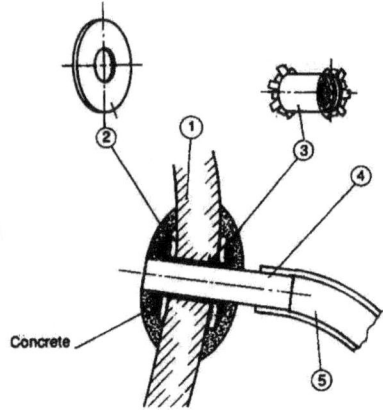

Assembly for outlet: 1 - Wall of clay jar; 2 - Rubber washer; 3 - Outer tube; 4 - Inner tube of galvanized iron; 5 - Plastic or rubber hose.

A similar outlet at the bottom of the jar can be used to drain it for cleaning. The tap for removal of the stored water can thus be mounted on any type of traditional jar holder built of wood, iron or bricks and concrete, or even screwed onto a simple holder made from a tree trunk.

A further precondition for keeping water bacteriologically safe is that the clay jar is cleaned regularly inside and out and that it is closed immediately after filling. The importance of a proper lid for complete protection from bacteriological contamination was also confirmed experimentally.[42]

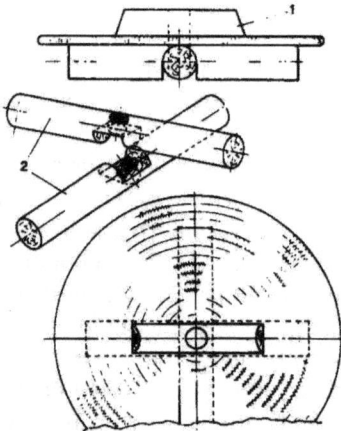

How to assemble a fitted cover for a traditional water jar. 1 — Handle; 2 — Bamboo or wooden sticks.

The cover can be made from different materials. Aluminium covers, which have been suggested for amphora-shaped jars,[42] need careful workmanship and may not fit if the jar is changed. It is much cheaper to attach two crossed-over sticks of bamboo or wood, corresponding in length exactly to the diameter of the mouth of the jar, to a plate made of wood or coiled basket-work. In addition, this provides the lid with a handle. Rural women from an adult education class were very enthusiastic about learning how to make lids from palm leaves. They decorated them according to taste.

The jars can best be filled with tap water through an opening in the handle, which also pierces the lid. The opening in the handle can be sealed with a cork once the hose is removed.

Water and usage

In our experiments, we used chlorinated water from the Khartoum waterworks, but any source of treated water can be improved by cooling storage. This includes water that has been treated with coagulants by women in rural areas, even if it is not 100 per cent bacteriologically pure.

Ideally, people should try to carry their own bottle of purified water, but where this is not possible, each person could have a cup of their own from which to drink, so that they do not touch the tap of the water storage vessel with their lips.

Interestingly, experiments with an even simpler arrangement than the tap described here, which would have cost even less, were not successful.

Chemical laboratories often use a system of removing liquids from large storage bottles via a rubber hose, which is simply clamped at the free end rather than being fitted with a tap. Using this idea, we obtained plastic connecting pieces to attach one end of a hose to a jar (one inside and one outside). The pieces are removable so that they can be transferred to another jar if the first has to be replaced. Fitting the plastic pieces was not easy to do without leaks, and although the holes could be filled by rubber washers or rubber cement, this would prevent the connecting pieces being re-used. Unskilled artisans would not be able to do this unaided in villages.

Furthermore, when we tested the arrangement with illiterate women in a village north of Omdurman, they were unwilling to try to remove water because they were unfamiliar with handling a clamp and were afraid they would spill a lot. Some of them also pulled the hose very roughly when they had problems opening or closing the clamp.

On the other hand, all the village women liked a jar with a tap. Inexperienced users in Sudan have been known to turn a tap in the wrong direction by force, but in areas recently provided with piped water, even older men and women and small children have quickly learnt how to use one. Therefore, taps have become a status symbol for rural development.

(*Watelines* Vol. 4 No. 1, July 1985)

Building the Thai jumbo water jar using a brick form

BRIAN LATHAM

The Thai water jar — or *ong* as it is called in Thai — is graceful, functional and affordable. What more could you ask for in water storage?

Used in Thailand, Kenya and other countries to store collected rainwater for drinking, the basic cement mortar model has grown in size from the traditional but relatively small 250-litre model that Watt described[44,45] to wire-reinforced 7-10m³ jumbo jars that I inspected with Professor Thamrong Prempridi of Bangkok's Chulalongkorn University. Although jars this large are a rarity, the 1.8m³ tank is very popular throughout Thailand's north-eastern region. Professor Thamrong has seen a rapid increase in their numbers in the three years they have been in use in areas such as Chaiyapum.

The jumbo jar's popularity is due to many factors. First, the price is low. Commercial varieties are available for 500 Baht (US$23) delivered. The price per cubic metre is below that of other types of water tanks as shown in Table 1. Secondly, storage can be bought when the villagers can afford it. Houses may have as many as five jumbo jars, each one bought when cash was available, such as after a harvest. Third, the jar is of transportable size and weight so that small local factories can build it. Alternatively, it can be built on the spot, in which case it can be larger than 1.8m³.

All in all, a beautiful piece of technology — but the next question is how to build it.

Construction techniques

Watt reported on a technique involving a hessian sack that was filled with sand as a mould. He illustrated the method for the 250 litre size and it was left to the reader to expand the hessian sack to 4m³. In practice, however, it

Table 1. Costs of individual small water-storage tanks (in Baht)

Type	Volume m³	Materials Total	Materials per m³	Full price Total	Full price per m³
Jumbo jar	1.8	300	165	500	280
Bamboo-reinforced concrete	11.3	4,200	370	7,000	620
Plastic (commercial)	1.1			3,500	3,200
Glass-fibre reinforced concrete (commercial)	1.8			3,600	2,000

is difficult to find and handle 2 to 4m³ of material and give the sack sufficient rigidity and strength to construct a jumbo jar.

Now, a method has been devised to build jars from 1.5m³ upwards and is being widely used in Thailand.

With the support of groups such as the Siam Cement Co, the government departments for Non-formal Education & Community Development, and non-government agencies such as the Appropriate Technology Association (ATA) and the Iodine, Iron & Clean Water Project (IICWP), people are being taught how to build the tanks. Local jar factories such as the one I visited with Jean-René Rinfret of Canadian Universities in Service Overseas (CUSO) south of Khon Kaen, have spring up as a cottage industry. Trained local technicians are building tanks on a private contract basis in some villages and many have been built under government seasonal employment programmes.

The method used involves a number of specially produced cement bricks as temporary forms. Dr Canchai Limpiyakorn, director of ATA, suggested using 11 different layers of 8 bricks each, each layer having a brick with a different curvature! Dr Romsai of the IICWP and the commercial factory used a single design of brick, bevelled at the edges and curved on the outside face. About 90 bricks are needed for each jar.

The construction sequence is as follows:
1. A base 1m in diameter and 50-60mm thick is poured. This may be flat but is often raised in the middle by 30-50mm. Number 8 wire (0.5-0.7mm) was used in a star pattern for reinforcing the base in the agency tanks but not in the factory jar.
2. After the base has hardened (24 hours), the bricks are assembled to give the desired shape. Part bricks may be needed.
3. The top of the form is made of small pieces of available lumber (300-450mm by 60mm) stacked to taper to the opening whose 650mm diameter is shaped by a galvanized metal ring.
4. A mud of non-organic soil is mixed up and used as a temporary mortar between the bricks, which are not closely butted together. Bands of light wire can be used to hold the bricks in place.
5. The skeleton is covered with the mud and smoothed to shape. The mud will be thicker in some places because the standard brick's curvature will not match the jar's curvature at all heights.
6. Construction then proceeds in the same way as Watt described. Concrete is applied to the mud form in two layers of 20mm each. Wire reinforcement is applied between layers. ATA advise using a vertical/horizontal grid at 150mm intervals but the factory used a spiral with loops 150mm apart. Some jars have bamboo reinforcement.
7. In 24 hours, when the concrete has hardened, the form is easily removed from the inside because the mud starts to give way. Bricks and mud are removed for re-use.

8. The interior and exterior are finished with a cement slurry, the opening is finished with a thick lip, and a decorative moulding is applied to the top edge. The slurry is usually coloured red or black, again for decoration.

9. The tank is allowed to cure in the shade for a week and is delivered by truck. With little or no reinforcement, the jars would not be expected to stand the rigours of delivery, but the tanks were rolled about the factory and skidded onto trucks without apparent damage.

Additional features of the jars are galvanized metal covers and an optional tap for removing the water. This can be set into the base and contents gauges can also be included.

The quality of jar construction varies greatly. The factory jar that I saw was made to minimum standards of concrete strength and reinforcement. Similar complaints about variation were also mentioned about the jars built by local or travelling artisans. The purchaser has obvious difficulty in determining how the jar was made.

The form bricks are an ideal means of constructing the jars as they involve a minimum of handling of form materials compared to the filled gunny sack. If there are delays in construction for any reason, the form will not adhere to the concrete. The bricks are relatively inexpensive and can be made of any light cement mixture because they do not have to be built to high tolerances. They are also re-usable so their initial cost is spread over a number of jars. The speed of construction is increased as well. The factory could produce about 1 jar per worker per day.

Further information

Professor Thamrong Prempridi. (Civil Engineering Department, Chulalongkorn University, Bangkok, Thailand) has done research on many types of village technology. He is very familiar with the north-eastern region and sits on the board of the Appropriate Technology Association.

Dr Romsai Suwanik, (Iodine, Iron & Clean Water Project, Faculty of Medicine, Mahidol University, Bangkok 10700, Thailand.) The IICWP is particularly interested in correcting iodine and construction project as well.

Dr Chanchai Limpiyakorn, (Appropriate Technology Association for Development, 125/3 Soi Santhipap 1, Suph Road, Sripharya, Bangkok, Thailand.) Dr Chanchai is a professor at Chulalongkorn University. The association is a training group in the appropriate technology field. It trains people in bamboocrete construction methods as well as jumbo struction methods for water tank construction as well as jumbo jar construction.

Jean-René Rinfret (Small Scale Water Resources project, c/o Civil Engineering Department, Khon Kaen University, Khon Kaen, Thailand.)

This project deals mostly with small-scale irrigation, but has built a number of ferrocement tanks.

Population & Community Development Association (PDA) (8 Sukumvit Road 12, Bangkok 10110, Thailand.) This group is known for its bamboo-reinforced poured-concrete tank. But some jumbo jars are built in Mahasarakham province, where some villagers cannot afford the tank and where roofs are below the tank's 3m height. However, it has built some jumbo jars in Mahasarakham province where some villages cannot afford PDA's usual type. The roof height of their houses is also traditionally less than the 3m height of the PDA tank, so that rainwater could not be collected.

(Waterlines Vol.3 No.1, October 1984)

Water purification with *Moringa* seeds

FROM DIAN DESA*

In developing countries, many villagers, since they have no alternative, have to consume surface water either from rivers or rain-fed ponds. The purity of these sources cannot be guaranteed.

Dian Desa adapts or refines known technologies and processes to fit local conditions, working in co-operation with self-motivated villagers. A part of the organization's success is that it maintains a close and direct contact with the community where it has a village development programme.

One of Dian Desa's activities is improving drinking-water supply for rural people. Since 1979, the NGO has been working in a hilly lime-stone area of Southern Central Java, developing and disseminating rainwater catchment tanks (ferro-cement and bamboo-cement) in the area.

In spite of this, however, many of the people still have to take their drinking-water from rain-fed ponds and underground caves. As these ponds seem to be the only water sources, many activities such as washing, bathing and bathing cattle are carried out there, while the villagers take water from the same pond home in tin cans for domestic uses such as drinking and cooking. The water is therefore polluted and Dian Desa water purification staff tried to find ways to provide potable water for the villagers.

Methods such as slow sand filtration and disinfection with iodine dispensers were tried out, but they were not workable at the village level. Colloidal solids soon clogged up the filters of the iodine dispenser.

Several aspects need to be considered when working at the village level.

---

*Dian Desa is an Indonesian non-governmental organization (NGO), which was established in 1972 to work for rural development.

In relation to water treatment technology, the following should be considered:

O The method of treatment should be simple.

O The cost of the material and equipment needed for the treatment should be within the economic capabilities of the villagers.

O Materials should be easily available locally.

Seeds as a coagulant

Dian Desa had heard about the power of *Moringa oleifera* seeds as a coagulant to temporarily precipitate solids, including bacteria, from dirty water. And it was found that, in Indonesia, *Moringa oleifera* is a well-known species called kelor. To further prove and test the usefulness of the seeds, a laboratory test was carried out with the following results:

	Percentage of total weight
Skin	35.08
Seed	64.92
Calcium	0.18
Phosphorous	0.69
Protein	36.00
Fat	32.09

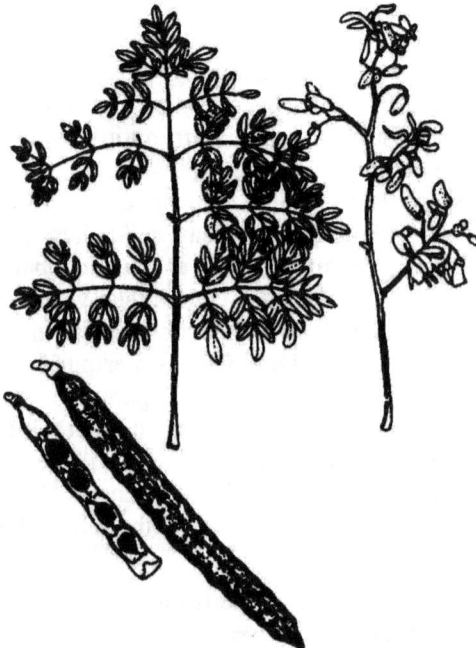

Sketch of leaves (left), fruit (right) and pods of Moringa oleifera, or kelor. Each seed is composed of three paper-thin beige wings and a dark brown rounded shell. (Diagram from Common trees of Puerto Rico and the Virgin Islands, *Little & Wadswort, Washington DC, USA, 1964)*

After mixing one powdered seed in 1 litre of turbid water, almost all the solids had coagulated and fallen to the bottom of the container after two hours. By then, 98 per cent of the coliform bacteria had been removed from the water. Coliform bacteria indicate pollution from faeces.

No side effects were identified: kelor was not poisonous to laboratory mice even at a dosage of 50g per 100ml of distilled water. Now that Dian Desa was sure that the seeds had no side effects, Djoko Srihono, who was responsible for the project, began to look at the possibilities of disseminating this water treatment technology to rural people. This was not so simple even though the technology seemed to be appropriate.

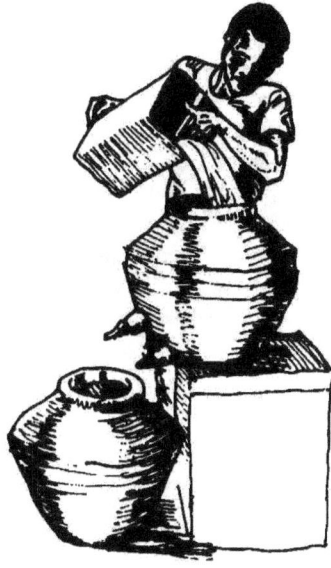

Pouring turbid water into the first pot for treatment.

Perceptions and dissemination

In most villages in Indonesia and also in many other developing countries, villagers do not seem to care about the condition of the water they consume. Accordingly, they do not treat the water either. In such a situation, it would be useless to try to disseminate water treatment technology because the people do not see the need for it. So, the priority for Dian Desa was to find out some of the villagers' perceptions about water.

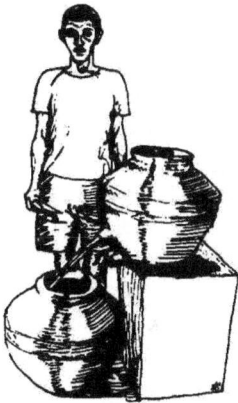

The bung is removed from the outlet of the first pot and clarified water is stored in the second. The lower outlet is used to drain the jar.

Pouring turbid water into the first pot for treatment.

O Do the villagers think that the water they consume is dirty?

O Do they want cleaner water?

O Do they know the danger of drinking polluted water?

O Have they ever tried to treat the water they consume and how?

O What do they think of kelor trees? Are there any constraints on the

Extract from a comic book illustrating the use of seeds in water purification.

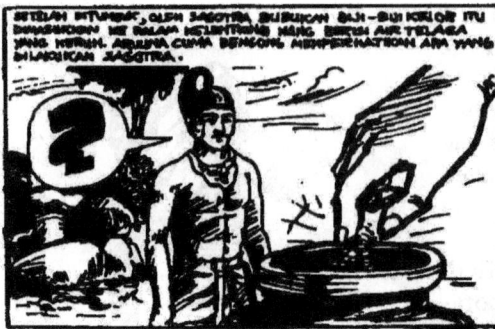

use of kelor trees, such as a taboo on consuming the species?

O How do they react to an explanation of how kelor can be used?

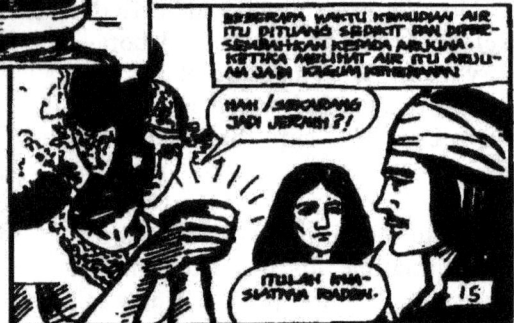

In the test village, Sumber-wungu in the Gunung Kidul area, very few villagers realized the danger of consuming polluted water in spite of their eagerness to have clean water available. So, the first thing to be done was to develop some educational materials and conduct some health education in the villages to change people's perceptions of dirty water, and to make them realize the danger of consuming it by discussing the kinds of diseases which might be caused by dirty water.

Villagers were also told about the advantages of consuming clean or treated water. They were then briefed on water treatment using kelor seeds. A cartoon booklet using the traditional stories of the Ramayana to illustrate the theme of using a seed to cleanse water was produced and distributed.

It was only after the villagers really understood about all the aspects mentioned above and showed interest in the water treatment technology that Dian Desa began to introduce kelor seeds.

Introduction and dissemination was done either through group demonstrations or by going from house to house. First, the technique was demonstrated using two glass jars. The two jars were filled with dirty pond water, then the water in one of the jars was mixed with powdered kelor seeds and stirred. The villagers could then see the process at work and the difference between the appearance of the treated and untreated water. Villagers' main concern was that water should be clear rather than turbid. When the villagers accepted the technology as demonstrated, they were introduced to the equipment needed for day-to-day use.

Two clay jars are used. The settling occurs in one and the clarified water is stored in the second. Jars are modified slightly by the addition of an outlet to siphon the treated water. This is because the protein in dissolved kelor seeds will start to ferment and smell after about 12 hours.

When the jars are ready, the villagers are taught how to grind the seeds. The equipment needed and the method of grinding is exactly the same as that by which they grind their spices, so there is nothing really new about it. What is important for villagers to know is that they should grind the seeds before using them. They are also taught how to dispose of the sediment in the first pot.

In the meantime, kelor cuttings are distributed to the villagers to be planted in their yards or even to be used as fences. This is so that the villagers have easy access to the kelor seeds at no cost. It is a very important aspect of supporting the development of the technology, and involves transplanting kelor shoots from an existing source 50km away.

So far, the villagers seem to accept the kelor techinque and are quite enthusiastic in practising it. So Dian Desa hopes to further disseminate this water treatment technology using *Moringa* seeds, so that it can be utilized by rural people all over Indonesia and in other countries.

(Waterlines Vol.3 No.4, April 1985)

Boiling drinking-water: a critical look

DEWOLFE MILLER

Reasonable access to a safe water supply is still a problem for the vast majority of the rural populations of Africa and Asia. This shortfall in water quality improvement often leads programme planners, aid agency officials, local health authorities and other government personnel — especially during periods when enteric disease out-breaks are reported — to try to encourage the affected villagers to boil their water before drinking it.

This is not a new phenomenon. Boiling water for drinking is an ancient practice. Villagers and other rural peoples had been periodically advised to boil their drinking-water long before the IDWSSD was announced. In the face of the shortfall in supply and in immediate solutions to the control of water-related disease, administrators have argued that villagers have little or no alternative to boiling their drinking-water. Besides chemical disinfection, boiling drinking-water was and continues to be a common choice of action by administrators, not only for the villagers, but also for ensuring the safety of their own drinking-water.

Efforts to make villagers boil drinking-water have met with some, rather limited, success. Recent surveys of the knowledge, attitude and practices (KAP) of rural peoples have shown that in a measurable percentage of the homes surveyed, boiling water for drinking is practised. Data from a 1982 KAP survey in Swaziland reported that 12 per cent of the rural families boiled their drinking-water.[46]

Swaziland had had a recent cholera outbreak, just prior to the KAP survey, yet 5 per cent reportedly boiled their drinking-water on some regular basis. In the Micronesian islands of Kosrae, Ponape, Yap and Palau, which are located near Guam in the western Pacific, 38 per cent reported boiling their drinking-water, but 80 per cent thought the water supply was safe to drink.[47]

Data from KAP surveys are based on interviews in which the villager may misunderstand the interviewer or may want to provide the 'right answers' and, therefore, may not be entirely accurate. It would be impractical, however, to determine by simple observation whether people boil their drinking-water. Nevertheless, it appears that boiling drinking-water is not an unknown practice and that people boil their water because they have been advised to do so by the government, rural health clinics or other villagers.

There are no epidemiologic data that qualitatively show a decrease (or any change) in relative risk to any water-related disease due to a programme of drinking-water boiling. To the author's knowledge no such studies have been reported, and, although they should be pursued if these programmes are to be continued, some of the questions may be somewhat academic. This article proposes that there are a number of negative aspects to drinking-water boiling programmes, the extent of which may override the above considerations and may result in a reconsideration of this approach to water quality improvement.

Water temperature and pathogen survival

The typical recommendation for disinfecting water by boiling is to bring the water to a rolling boil for 10 minutes. At higher altitudes, 15 to 20 minutes may be recommended. Although the female head of household, who is most likely to carry out this chore, will have no way to tell the time in a typical village, a rolling boil of 100°C of even a few moments will kill most pathogens.

The thermal death point for Giardia lambia cysts has been reported to be between 50 and 64°C. Other enteric cyst-forming protozoans appear to be equally sensitive to these temperatures in clear water. Enteric bacterial pathogens are most often represented by the faecal coliforms or *Escherichia coli* specifically, and have a thermal death point equal to or less than the protozoan cysts. Enteric viruses tend to be more resistant to high temperatures but also have thermal death points of less than 100°C, with the exception of the *Hepatitis A* virus.

There is some evidence (mostly epidemiologic) that this virus can remain infectious to humans after the water containing it is raised to a boil; such water would have been heavily polluted and very cloudy. It is well known that suspended particles provide heat sinks that absorb heat and shield the micro-organisms from the destructive effects of high temperature. Nevertheless, in excess of 99 per cent of the virus would probably be inactivated in a few moments at 100°C, which would be sufficient in less-polluted water to reduce the dose to a non-infectious level. Hepatitis A, although a disabling disease in adults, is less severe in children and is not considered a 'killer disease' among the water-related diseases.

The other organisms that would most likely survive high temperatures are helminth ova. *Ascaris* ova appear to be more sensitive to high temperatures than the enteric viruses. The conditions depicted are for survival in night soil and sludge, and may be somewhat different for water. For schistosome larvae, these fragile organisms perish at temperatures well below those for most of the other organisms and are inactivated at temperatures greater than 38°C.

Unfortunately, little is known about the survival characteristics of the rotaviruses in water, which potentially are a major cause of dehydrating diarrhoea. There is no epidemiologic evidence that these viruses are markedly different from the other enteric viruses in their ability to persist in the environment. Most likely, rotaviruses are more fragile than Hepatitis A virus.

Data on survival of pathogens in cloudy or muddy water are not readily available. It is conceivable that some pathogens may survive significantly longer at significantly higher temperatures in muddy water. Although there may be villagers who, perhaps, because of a drinking-water boiling campaign, would go to the trouble of boiling muddy water, this would surely be a rare group of people. KAP surveys have demonstrated that villagers do have indigenous attitudes regarding water quality, and muddy water was never indicated as one. The author has been unable to find any evidence that villagers like muddy water, nor seen this practice in the field.

The evidence available suggests that most pathogens would be destroyed very quickly at temperatures below boiling, especially in clean water. The recommendations of boiling water for 10 minutes, therefore, provides a significant safety factor for the destruction of water-borne pathogens. However, bringing water to a boil and holding it for 10 minutes may be unaffordable.

Cost of boiling water

Boiling drinking or other domestic water has an associated cost. In relation to other items that would be heated over the village home fire or stove, water has a high specific heat. That is, more calories of heat are required to raise one gram of water by 1°C than most foods.

There is a separate issue of deforestation and desertification in many developing countries. Domestic cooking and heating fuel demands have exacerbated this crisis. There is also the problem of indoor air pollution generated by the stove. Data from India and Nepal indicate that the village stoves, used solely to cook food, generate in the home very high levels of harmful air pollutants such as carbon monoxide, suspended particulates, sulphur oxides, nitrogen oxides and hydrocarbons.[48] Boiling drinking-water programmes would aggravate these problems.

Reconsideration of the boiling water recommendations may be required simply to address the problem of cost and ecological impact.

Recontamination

Given that the family's drinking-water is boiled, how is it stored before consumption and how is it consumed? The opportunity for the boiled water to become re-contaminated before consumption or during consumption is great. A limited amount of information on storing water in the village home is available and confirms that either the stored water was already contaminated, became contaminated in the storage vessel in the home, or is hygienically unsound.

A storage vessel may not be covered or may be cleaned only rarely. The pottery water storage vessels of the Middle East, known in Egypt as 'Zirs', are difficult to maintain hygienically. In one study, 81.3 per cent of the Zirs sampled had *Entamoeba* cysts and 15 per cent had *Ascaris* ova.[49] All domestic water supplies in Egyptian villages were found to be stored in the Zir before the water was used or consumed.[50]

Therapy with Oral Rehydration Salts (ORS)

One rationale for boiling drinking-water in the home is to have un-contaminated water for the preparation of oral rehydration salts solution. Treatment with ORS solutions has had a major impact on reducing mortality due to dehydrating diarrhoea, especially in infants and children, and can be prepared in the home using locally available ingredients.

Several studies have addressed the issue of using untreated locally available drinking-water for the preparation of ORS.[53] The first problem is to avoid the risk of using a solution that is not free of pathogens, and, secondly, there is the possibility of enteric bacterial growth in the nutrient-rich solution. Certain enteric bacterial pathogens are known to grow in the ORS solutions and others grow in ORS solutions that have been prepared with local water which contains organic matter and nitrogen.[46] Significant growth usually does not occur until 12 hours after preparation.

A remarkable observation was reported from The Gambia. In a study of children with diarrhoeal disease, no difference in recovery from diarrhoea was observed between children who were treated with ORS solution prepared with either clean water or contaminated well-water.[51] This observation suggests that the ORS therapy, namely rehydration, is the single most important aspect in controlling the child's diarrhoea, and the control of exposure to additional enteric pathogens is a secondary consideration. The implication of these findings is that boiling water for preparing ORS may not be as critical as one might assume. It is not known how widely accepted the results from this study have become, but repeated observations would be needed before those who teach the preparation and use of ORS would abandon the recommendation of using safe — usually boiled — water.

Other disadvantages

In addition to some of the problems mentioned above, recommendations for drinking-water boiling programmes may undermine the push for good water-supplies and water-supply improvement projects. In effect, the officials who recommend or initiate drinking-water boiling programmes may be misled into believing that action has been taken and that the crisis of unsafe water supply has been met by such a solution. As mentioned, there is no evidence that drinking-water boiling programmes are effective in controlling water-related disease outbreaks or in reducing the transmission of endemic water-related diseases. Therefore, such quick solutions have the potential for delaying or, perhaps worse, obscuring the need to press forward with good water-supply projects. Certainly a drinking-water boiling programme should never be considered a solution in the absence of reasonable access to a safe water supply. This disadvantage, the quick-solution attitude, can be a much greater problem than the other more technical disadvantages mentioned above.

Another major disadvantage is that this type of intervention addresses only water-borne infections and none of the other water-related diseases, especially water-washed ones. In most water-related disease outbreaks or in endemic situations, the transmission of these diseases may not be solely water-borne. Water-washed diseases, many of which can also be classified as water-borne, are reduced by an increase in water availability. This is based on the principle that domestic or personal hygiene is not possible or is severely curtailed if the family does not have enough water to wash or clean themselves and their immediate environment. A drinking-water boiling programme does not address this aspect of water-related disease transmission, but such a programme may adversely affect the practices of water use in the home.

Drinking-water boiling programmes are rarely combined with health education on water-related diseases, and are inherently contradictory to the promotion of good water-supply projects and community participation. It is obvious that drinking-water boiling programmes are directed at individuals and at best the family rather than the village community. Moreover, the available KAP surveys do not suggest that village people boil their drinking-water because they have a solid understanding of germ theory and water-related disease transmission. If such knowledge were widespread, perhaps the Decade's goals would be greatly facilitated.

A closer look at the benefits and disadvantages of boiling-drinking water is needed, but the priority of such endeavours should not preceed the development and implementation of water-supply improvement projects. The results of such investigations could well demonstrate that the disadvantages of drinking-water boiling programmes outlined here are understated.

Further reading:
Kalbermatten, J.M., Appropriate technology for water supply and sanitation technical and economic options (World Bank, 1980).
Tomkins, A.M., 'Water supply and nutritional status in rural Norhern Nigeria',Transactions of Royal Soc. of Trop. Med. and Hyg., 72 No.3, 239-43 (1978).
Watkinson, M., Lloyd-Evans N. and Watkinson, A.M., 'The use of oral glucose electrolyte solution prepared with untreated well water in acute non-specific childhood diarrhoea', Transactions of the Royal Soc. of Trop. Med. and Hyg., 74, 657-62 (1980).

(Waterlines, Vol. 5 No. 1, July 1986)

UNICEF's upward-flow water filter

LAURIE CHILDERS AND FRANS CLAASEN

The upward-flow water filter is a family-size filter suitable for removing suspended particles of soil or organic matter which discolour or pollute drinking-water. It is particularly useful in rural areas where surface water of doubtful quality is often used.

The filter is inexpensive, easy to construct, simple to use and can provide clean water for a family or a group of about 10 people. Depending on the quality of the water source, it will operate for up to one year before cleaning is required.

Raw water is poured into the storage tank on top of the filter and flows down plastic tubing into the base of the filter. The water in the storage tank pushes this water upwards through the filter media and out of the delivery tube at the top. The filter traps the suspended particles in three filter beds of fine sand and crushed charcoal. A bed of gravel is placed at the bottom of the filter to allow any water entering to spread evenly across the base. The filter will deliver the same volume of water as that poured into the storage tank. The maximum recommended capacity is approximately 40 litres per day.

Making the tanks

The method of constructing the cement tanks is explained in the UNICEF leaflet on cement jars (available free from the UNICEF Technology Support Section*). The recommended volume of the filter tank is between 175 to 200 litres, while the untreated water storage tank holds about 40 litres.

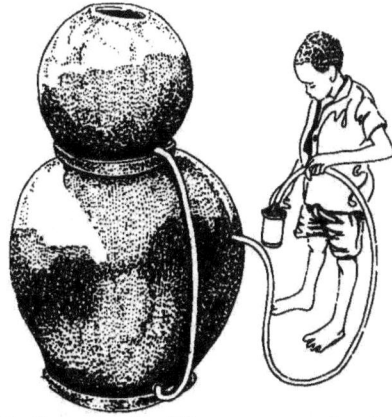

This inexpensive filter can supply clean water to ten people

The following modifications to the cement jar design are required to make it suitable for use as a filter tank:

O The base of the jar requires strengthening because of the additional weight of the filter media. This is done by building a concrete foundation 5cm deep which extends 10cm from the side of the jar's 60cm base. The jar can then be built on top of the foundation in the usual way.
O While the cement mortar of the jar is still wet, two short pieces of 1.25cm-diameter galvanized-iron water-pipe are inserted to form the inlet and outlet. The pipes are wrapped loosely with wire to strengthen the joint formed with the mortar of the wall. The outlet pipe is curved downward slightly to maintain a constant water-seal on the outlet, which will guard against the entry of unwanted insects and dirt from outside.
O The opening at the top of the filter should be of a size suitable to allow the base of the untreated water storage tank to fit tightly and securely within it.

Selecting the filter media

A few stones, 5cm in diameter, are required to prevent the inlet pipe from becoming blocked. Sufficient gravel to form a layer 5cm deep is needed. The stones and gravel should be washed in water to remove loose surface dirt and allowed to dry in the sun on a clean surface.

The lower sand-bed is made from clean, unsifted river-sand. The sand should contain a range of particle sizes (0.3 to 1.3mm), and little or no plant material. Sufficient sand is required for a layer 20 to 25cm deep across the

*UNICEF Technology Support Section, Eastern Africa Regional Office, PO Box 44145, Nairobi, Kenya.

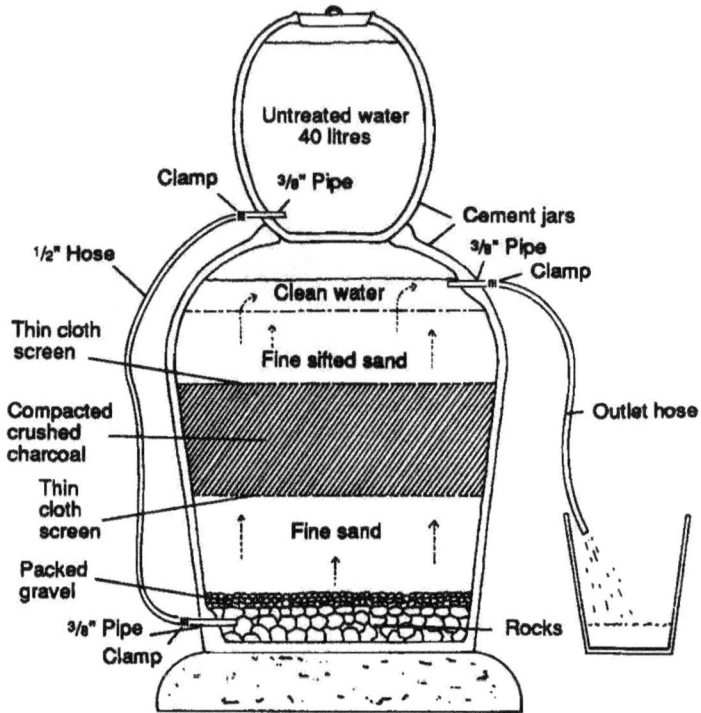

All of the media needed for the filter are readily available and most are free.

jar. The sand should be washed and spread on to a clean surface to dry in the sun. The upper sand-bed consists of clean, sifted river-sand. The screen used to sift the sand should be as fine as mosquito mesh. The sifted sand is also washed and dried in the sun.

Charcoal is pulverized into very small chips or grains about 5mm in diameter. This can be done using a double-walled hessian sack half-filled with charcoal, which is hit with a stick. Sufficient charcoal is required to form a 25 to 30cm layer, when tightly compacted. The charcoal must be washed and the dust removed by immersing the grains in a bowl of water, and then tipping off all floating matter.

Making the filter beds

When the dirty-water storage tank and the filter have been made and allowed to cure, the next step is to make the filter bed. For the lower bed, stones are placed around the inlet to prevent blockage, and gravel is packed across the base to form a 5cm layer.

It is important to check that this and subsequent filter beds have been properly packed. This is achieved by placing the untreated water storage tank on the ground (or on a low table) and connecting it, by hose, with the inlet of the filter. A small quantity of water is allowed to flow from the storage tank to the filter tank until it reaches the top of the filter bed being checked. It should rise evely across the bed. This procedure should be repeated after each bed has been inserted and compacted. If this is not done, the air trapped around the filter media will bubble out when water is added and the filter beds will be disturbed.

Above the gravel layer, sand is laid and compacted to form a bed 20 to 25cm deep. Following testing, the sand-bed is covered with a thin cloth or sheet of fine gauze to separate it from the next layer.

The compacted charcoal bed is laid to a depth of 25 to 30cm and is also covered with a thin cloth or gauze sheet. The cloth is weighed down with a small amount of fine sand to prevent the charcoal from shifting during the flow testing.

The uppermost bed, above the charcoal layer, consists of a 20 to 25cm layer of finely sifted sand, which should then be tested as before.

Operation of the filter

If the filter beds have been correctly inserted in the tank, they should already be completely immersed in water. In use, the filter beds should remain immersed, as this ensures the survival of a layer of bacteria which develops on the charcoal chips. These bacteria help to remove certain types of disease-carrying micro-organisms from the water.

To establish the filtering action of the filter beds, the same water is allowed to flow through the tank some 10 to 20 times until the outlet water begins to clear. The untreated-water inlet hose is then disconnected from the filter tank for a short time to allow the worst of the sediment to flow back out at the bottom. When this water no longer looks dirty, the pipe is reconnected. The top 5 to 10cm of the upper sand-bed must be removed and replaced with clean sifted sand. Water is passed through the filter several more times to re-establish the filtration action and the filter is then ready for use.

To maintain the proper action of the filter, the pipe between the untreated water tank and the filter should not be removed. Frequent back-washing of the filter will damage the filter beds. It is best to seal the untreated water-storage tank to the top of the filter tank with a mud or cement collar. The top surface of the layer of fine sand must be checked regularly to see whether the filter beds need cleaning. When sediment shows, the top 5 to 10cm must be removed and replaced with clear sifted sand. When changing the top layer of sand no longer has the effect of re-establishing good filtration, all the filter beds must be removed and replaced.

(*Waterlines* Vol. 5 No. 4, April 1987)

CHAPTER 4

Safer Water for the Community

In his article, Barry Lloyd recognizes the problems of effective surveillance programmes for drinking-water supplies in developing countries. The latest developments on water-quality control, including his work at the University of Surrey; are the theme of Chapter 5; here he concentrates on basics. He discusses the simple sanitary survey as a powerful tool for the observation of water quality to establish possible health risks to the consumer. The ancillary check-lists taken from various references are invaluable. For surface-water sources, he sets out recommendations for household disinfection and storage. His comments on boiling should be read in conjunction with the more recent thoughts of Dr Miller in the previous chapter. Although groundwater is generally of superior quality to surface water, he lists important queries to be considered for wells and springs.

Springs are an especially advantageous underground source as no effort is required to raise the water to the surface. It is vital, though, to protect the spring from possible contamination. Tim Rous describes how the people of Boga in Zaire protected their spring source.

For surface sources, protective measures are necessary upstream to prevent bathing or animal access. Inevitably, the water will be contaminated to a degree depending on the extent of the land area and its use upstream. In certain localities, some natural purification can be achieved through infiltration galleries constructed adjacent to the banks of the surface source. Wellpoints may be used alongside sandy banks. Alternatively the Cansdale sandfilter with pump may be considered, buried in the sand bed of a stream. All of these systems require careful installation, operation and maintenance.

Slow sand filtration is effective with raw water of relatively low turbidity, less than about 15 NTU. The International Reference Centre for Community Water Supply & Sanitation in the Netherlands has investigated slow sand filtration as a simple, cheap and reliable method of treating surface water for domestic use. Their Research and Development Project clearly demonstrates the feasibility of this technology for rural watersupply. The performance of slow sand filters in refugee water supplies in Somalia is discussed by Nigel Graham and Hans Hartung using a treatment package developed by Oxfam and Imperial College (London). Results indicate that the final treated water quality comes close to WHO standards. Where turbidity exceeds about 15 NTU, some form of pre-settlement and/or roughing filter is necessary. Martin Wegelin and Roland Schertenleib of the International Reference Centre for Waste Disposal (IRCWD) in Switzerland present a simple filter combination of horizontal roughing filters preceding slow sand filters.

Water quality surveillance

BARRY LLOYD

Few developing countries have effective surveillance programmes for drinking-water supplies.

Surveillance is the continuous public health assessment of the safety of water supplies. It involves the routine physical, chemical and biological quality-control of water from source to consumer together with sanitary inspection to ascertain the proper functioning of all components of the water treatment and supply system. These practices, and guidelines for them, are laid down by the World Health Organization, but their application is not always followed even in the capital cities of some developing countries. In a majority of provincial towns and throughout the rural areas in the Third World, surveillance of drinking-water quality is rarely if ever undertaken.

Safe water

In the absence of adequate funding, trained personnel and the organization to undertake routine technical tasks, are there any practical steps which can be taken to try to ensure that small community water-supplies are safe to drink? To answer this requires a definition of 'safe drinking-water'. Safe drinking-water is that which is 'wholesome and not prejudicial to health'. Implicit in this definition is the requirement that the water is without risk of causing chemical irritation or intoxication and microbial infection.

To establish whether water sources and supplies are safe requires the facilities of a quality control laboratory. Such facilities are almost non-existent throughout the rural areas of the developing world. The nearest approach would be a regional hospital laboratory which might have the

Table 1 Classification of water supplies.

Class of supply	Coliforms per 100 ml	Faecal coliforms (E. coli) per 100 ml	Permitted annual deviation (per cent)
1: Excellent	0	0	0
2: Satisfactory	1-3	0	5*
3: Doubtful	4-10	0	5*
4: Unsatisfactory	10	0	-

* Limits can only be applied when routine annual data are available (50 samples/annum). Water entering the distribution should always be Class 1. Ref: Bacteriological Examinations of Water Supplies. Report No. 71. HMSO (1982)

equipment to do some chemical and biological testing. The most sensitive surrogate test for the detection of disease-causing micro-organisms (pathogens) in water is a count of bacteria which indicate contamination with excreta. It is universally agreed that the most reliable technique currently used is to quantify the number of intestinal bacteria from a group called the faecal coliforms of which *Escherichia coli (E. coli)* is usually the most common member in the human intestine. Rapid and relatively simple procedures have been developed to recover faecal coliforms, but to be of any value the test must be carried out regularly (Table 1, page 83). Furthermore, the test is costly; depending on the methods, number of tests and equipment used, it may cost hundreds to thousands of dollars each year.

Untreated supplies

In most rural areas of developing countries the water supply is neither piped nor treated. In Bangladesh, for example, most villagers use river or pond water for gargling, ablution, washing clothes and cooking. Tubewell water, if available, may be used for drinking purposes and stored in pots in the home. The following data (Table 2), collected at the start of a sanitary survey in a Bengali village, are typical.

In the examples used for Table 2, the rural poor have a choice of grossly contaminated pond water and generally good quality tubewell water. In Bangladesh, there is an abundance of surface water and groundwater, but ironically there is still an extremely high incidence of water-related disease, even in those areas with tubewell supplies. The reasons for this have been hotly debated, but it is probable that a combination of factors, including high population density, poor nutrition and primary health care, together

Table 2 — Faecal coliform counts (100ml at 44°C) for water used in a Bengali village (1980)

Weekly Sample	Ponds		Tubewells				Water in pots in homes*	
	1	2	1	2	3	4	1	2
1	2,800	3,000	0	0	0	2	8	4
2	3,000	3,000	0	0	0	6	9	10
3	8,000	5,000	0	0	0	4	8	2
4	4,000	2,000	0	0	0	0	7	10
5	5,000	4,000	0	0	0	0	5	17
6	6,000	5,000	-	0	-	8	13	5
7	-	-	-	-	-	2	-	-
8	-	-	-	-	-	-	-	-
Mean	4,800	3,600	0	0	0	3	8.3	8

*Water drawn from tubewells.

with bad hygienic practices and living conditions, all conspire to defeat the hard-won improvements in water supply.

These examples pose a number of difficult questions:

O Are the hoped-for improvements in the quality of water supplies likely to be sufficient to warrant routine surveillance?

O Are the international guidelines for drinking-water realistic?

O What quality standards or guidelines, if any, are appropriate for small, untreated rural supplies?

O What type of training is appropriate for the operation and maintenance of small rural supplies?

In an attempt to answer these questions we can argue as follows:

O If improvements have been made, then some effort must be made to evaluate them in terms of assessing maintained quality improvements. Unfortunately there is no alternative to bacteriological testing and to *E. coli* counts in particular. Therefore the manufacturers of *E. coli* test-kits bear a real moral obligation to lower the cost of their equipment and to design kits for use at the village level at realistic prices. The market for this equipment is obviously immense, and there must surely be businessmen with sufficient imagination and designers with the skills to meet this need. The technology is no more complicated than the transistor radio.

O Current WHO recommended standards are regrettably not realistic. Guidelines such as those indicated in Table 1 are rarely met in developing countries even where supplies are filtered and chlorinated.

O More realistic quality standards are tentatively suggested for unchlorinated rural supplies in Table 3. As with Table 1, judgement on the quality of the supply should never rest upon a single sample but on regular tests

Table 3
Suggested bacteriological quality criteria for drinking-water from unchlorinated rural hand-pumps and other sources

Mean count* 44°C 100ml E. coli count	Category	Comments
0	A	Excellent
1-10	B	Acceptable: but make regular sanitary checks on status of equipment
10-50	C	Unacceptable: look for structural faults and poor maintenance of pump and plinth
<50	D	Grossly polluted: look for alternative source, or carry out necessary repairs and disinfect well.

*Limits can only be applied when routine survey data are available, eg. 5-10 consecutive weekly samples.

and regular sanitary inspection of water sources and the devices used to treat and supply water.

For the foreseeable future many millions of rural inhabitants will be dependent on untreated supplies in regions where the logistics of routine quality control, even if the funds were available, would make the task of routine water testing impossible. It is therefore far more important to concentrate limited resources on basic improvements, maintenance and sanitary inspection.

For rural populations, improvement in water supply is unlikely to mean the provision of a conventional, treated, chlorinated supply. If a village is lucky and large enough, say with a population of 1,000 plus, it might qualify for a slow sand filtration plant. But in India, 23 per cent of villages have populations of 500-1,000, and 56 per cent less than 500; what quantity and quality of improvements can be hoped for? At best, if the geology is right, tubewells may be a possibility. Open wells and springs will hopefully be curbed and protected from outside contamination.

Appropriate training

When these modest improvements are achieved then routine maintenance of rural water supplies is essential.

Training centres should be established for environmental/sanitary inspectors, maintenance mechanics and plumbers. The prime requirement is for the training of a dedicated 'Jack-of-all-trades' who clearly understands his responsibilities for all aspects of simple water supplies for a number of villages. He will need transport for the tools of his trade and eventually perhaps for the transfer of water samples to the district hospital laboratory where basic, routine bacteriology and chemistry can be executed.

But in the interim, without the back-up of a laboratory service, we return to a fundamental question: how can one attempt to ensure that water supplies are safe? Regular sanitary surveys will make a major contribution to this.

Sanitary surveys

The sanitary survey is an on-site inspection and evaluation of the water-supply system. With routine bacteriological testing, it can become a powerful tool for the observation of water quality.

The aim of the survey is to establish whether any part of the system, or any practice relating to the operation of the water supply, could present a health risk to the consumer. Sanitarians (public health inspectors) would reasonably claim that this task requires their professional personnel. However, successful surveys have been undertaken in small communities by personnel with a limited education and who have undertaken intensive practical courses.

It is clear that one of the greatest needs for the Water Decade and beyond is for the setting up of provincial training centres and the design of comprehensive practical instruction manuals for such people.

It is beyond the scope of a short article such as this to lay down detailed guidelines for the inspection and control of water-supply systems. However, it is pertinent to summarize the more obvious investigations and actions which a health worker can carry out in order to improve and protect the quality of water used by those rural communities which have no treatment plant and distribution system. Water resources can be divided into surface and ground water.

Surface water sources

Surface water is invariably contaminated by large numbers of micro-organisms (see pond samples in Table 2) washed in from the soil and including those from human and animal excreta. Such water must always be regarded as unsafe and alternative sources sought whenever feasible. Lowland rivers, streams, canals, ponds and lakes are usually visibly dirty (turbid). Where there is no alternative to such polluted sources, the certain ways of rendering these waters safe, on a small scale, are by boiling, disinfection and household filters.

In poor communities, routine boiling may be considered too troublesome or costly on fuel; but where feasible, and particularly for infants before, during and following weaning, the health worker should strongly advise mothers to boil drinking-water and water intended for incorporation into foods vigorously for 3-5 minutes minimum. Further advice should be given that the water should be stored, out of reach of animals, in clean, covered pots. Boiling is, in some respects, preferable to disinfection, since it is easy to control and very effective.

Disinfectants such as sodium hypochlorite, an ingredient in bleach, tend to lose their potency rapidly in tropical climates. Furthermore, water which is turbid will 'mop up' much of the disinfecting action, leaving some potentially infectious micro-organisms alive. On the other hand, water which is clear is readily disinfected by a dose of 1 to 2mg/litre of chlorine, or 2.5mg/litre of bleaching powder. Providing that the disinfectant is thoroughly mixed and dissolved, almost all micro-organisms will have been destroyed in several minutes, but, to be certain, the water should be left for 20 to 30 minutes.

After the disinfection of a container of water has been carried out, a small residue of disinfectant will usually persist in the sample for at least a day, when stored in clean, cool, dark, covered pots. This has the advantage of continued modest protection against recontamination arising from poor domestic hygiene. As little as 0.2mg/litre of residual chlorine (in solution as hypochlorous acid) can be tasted by the majority of people. This is a useful rule-of-thumb in as much as being able to taste this residual trace of chlorine almost certainly signifies that it is microbiologically safe. However, there is the chance that consumers will find chlorinated water unpalatable.

Many household filters are inappropriate for rural use as they are expensive and require a mains or pressure supply to the unit. However, several companies sell filters for the purification of small quantities of water, to which water must be transferred manually or by hand pump.

Surface water from upland streams and lakes may appear clearer and cleaner than lowland sources, but it must be remembered that clear water is not necessarily safe water. Water which is transparent may contain ten million bacteria per litre or more! Therefore, if such water is used untreated, the collection site should:
O Preferably be near the watershed, where contamination is likely to be light.
O Be sparsely inhabited and protected by fencing to prevent animals and people from entering the source.
O Consistently yield clear water.

To ensure these points, the catchment area should be frequently inspected and the community instructed to avoid polluting upstream of the communal collection site.

It is obvious that untreated surface waters carry an inherent high risk of infection by waterborne pathogens. The foregoing suggestions are thus the minimum action which can be taken where there is little opportunity for major improvement. Where communities depend on this type of untreated surface-water source, every encouragement should be given to the formation of action groups to apply for government and aid agency funds and to develop a community water-treatment, storage and supply project.

Groundwater sources

Groundwater is generally of superior quality to surface water in terms of clarity and microbial quality. Factors which affect water quality include:
O Geology
O Distance from sources of pollution.
O The method of construction and maintenance of wells and springs, to avoid surface contamination.
O Abstraction rates which may lower the ground water table and convert springs into water table pollution points.

Therefore in surveying wells and springs, in order to evaluate their sanitary quality, important general questions to ask are as follows:

O Are the aquifers (water-bearing strata) shallow or deep?
O If shallow, is the water source near to a source of pollution? It is suggested, for example, that pit latrines should be sited at least 30m away from a well, [52] and further away in highly permeable soils. Whether it is shallow or deep (more than 20m), is the aquifer likely to be fissured, as in limestone or chalk, and hence hazardous?
O Is the aquifer overlaid by alluvial deposits (fine silt and sand)? These provide effective percolation and hence probably good quality water, as demonstrated by the tubewell samples in Table 2.

Checklist for water sources

The common rural constructions which allow groundwater to be drawn for domestic use include open dug wells with steps or windlass and bucket, tubewells and protected springs. A survey of their potential and real sanitary defects should indicate the simplest and most cost-effective improvements that could be made. A minimum investigation should include the following specific questions:

Step wells

1. Is there an impervious platform or hardstanding (apron) of concrete to exclude surface water?

2. Is there a parapet to prevent users and animals from entering the water?

3. Could a parapet or cover be constructed and the well converted into a drawn or pumped well?

4. Are ropes and buckets permanently installed and hygienically stored?

5. Could well water be pot-chlorinated?

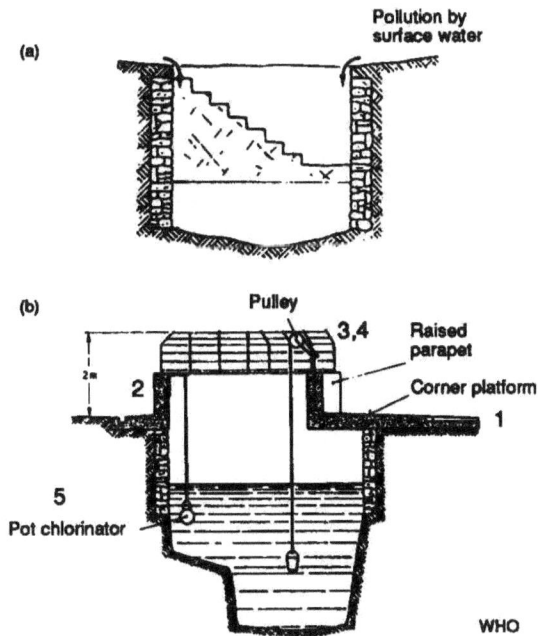

Figure 1. Step well (a) and (b) improved step well. (From Rajagopalan and Shiffman.[53])

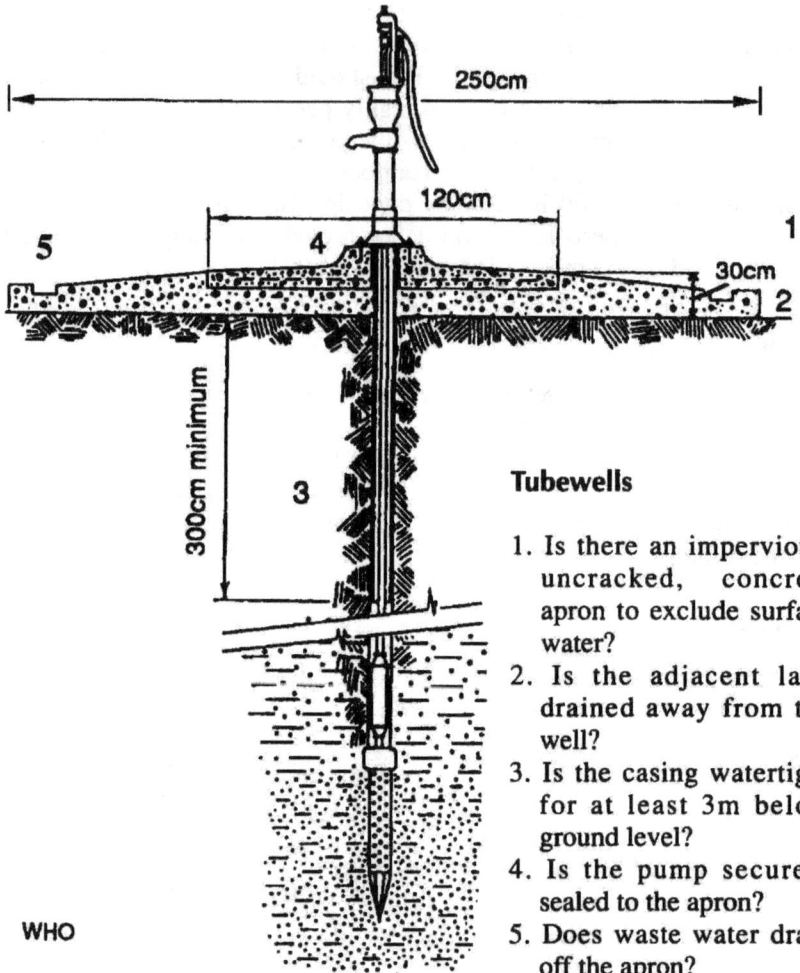

Tubewells

1. Is there an impervious, uncracked, concrete apron to exclude surface water?
2. Is the adjacent land drained away from the well?
3. Is the casing watertight for at least 3m below ground level?
4. Is the pump securely sealed to the apron?
5. Does waste water drain off the apron?

Figure 2. Section through tubewell.

Dug wells with windlass

1. Is there an impervious, uncracked headwall and concrete apron to exclude surface water, and is it adequately drained?
2. Are the sides of the well-shaft sealed and not cracked for at least 3m below ground level?
3. Is there a lining at the base of the well which allows clear water to enter through the sides at the same time as protecting the well from collapse?
4. Is the surrounding land drained so that waste water does not run into the well?

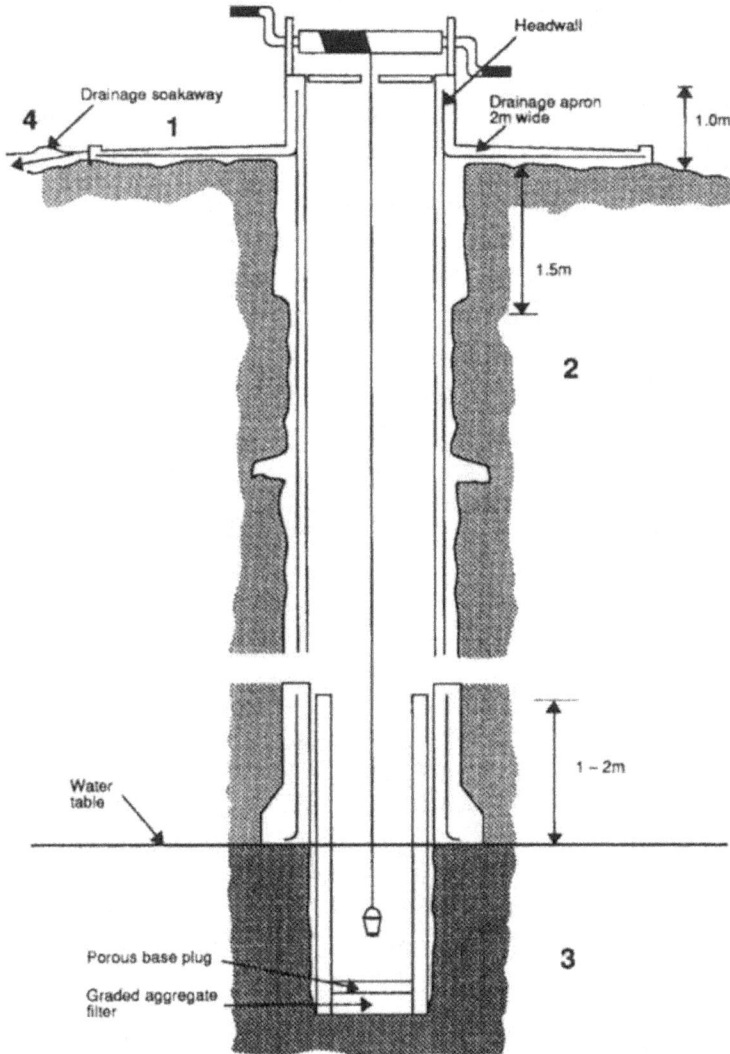

Figure 3. Dug well with windlass. (Adapted from Watt and Wood.[54])

5. If provision is made for clothes washing and livestock watering, is it at a distance from the well to prevent contamination?
6. Can the well and its immediate surroundings be fenced for additional protection?
7. Are the bucket and rope mounted so that contamination by users is minimized?
8. Is the well mouth covered when not in use?
9. Could the water be pot-chlorinated regularly?

Protected spring source

There are many different designs, but the principles for protecting the
   spring are the same. Figure 4 shows a protected spring feeding a piped
   gravity supply.
1. Is there a diversion ditch around the spring to divert surface water?
2. Is the collection structure inaccessible to users and animals?
3. Is adequate drainage provided below the outlet and overflow pipes?
4. Are animals effectively excluded by fencing the spring area?

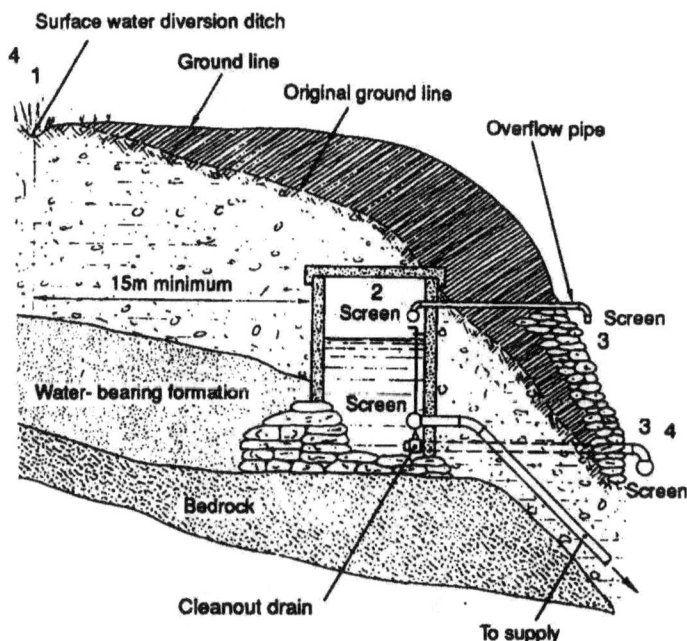

Figure 4. Protected spring source (after Rajagopalan and Shiffman.[53])

Further reading
Surveillance of drinking water, WHO, Geneva, 1976
Wagner and Lanoix, *Water Supply for rural areas and small communities*,
WHO, Geneva, 1959
R E Brush, *Wells construction*, Action Peace Corps.
Manual for rural water supply, SKAT (Swiss centre for Appropriate
Technology)/Helvetas (Swiss Association for Technical Assistance, SATA),
St Gall University, Switzerland, 1980
Jordan, Thomas, *Handbook of gravity-flow water systems for small commu-
nities*, United Nations Children's Fund (UNICEF), Nepal, 1980

Protecting a shallow seepage spring

TIM ROUS

In Boga, Haut Zaire, there are a large number of seepage springs in soft ground which should provide clean water. But the water is dirty because animals walk in it, children play in it and insects lay their eggs in it. The water looks clean, but people using it may suffer from diarrhoea or worms, as well as other illnesses.

To stop this happening, the people at Boga have started to protect their springs. That is, they put a pipe in each spring, protecting the end from silting up with a small screen. The screen is then covered with gravel, sand and stones. They put earth over the stones and the pipe so that nothing that is likely to cause disease can get into the water.

Anyone can do this, as is explained below:

Method of construction

O Choose a good shallow spring. It must be one that does not dry up, even at the end of the dry season. Make sure that there are no latrines within 50m of the spring. Make sure that the land slopes downhill, so that the water can flow away from the spring.

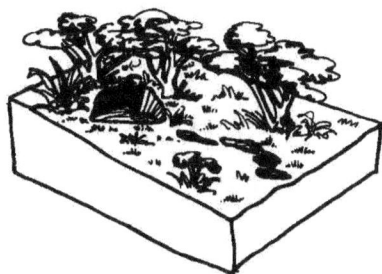

O Talk with all the people who use the spring. Make sure first of all that they want work to be done on the spring so that their health will improve. Also make sure that they are willing to help dig and collect materials. Clean out the spring, removing vegetation from its path. Dig a long deep trench level with the bottom of the eye of the spring and at least 3m long and about a metre wide so that all the water which comes into the spring can flow freely out again.

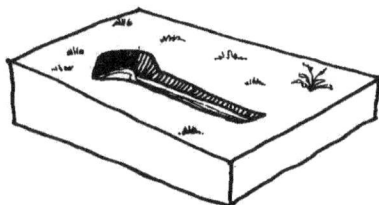

O If the spring is on a shallow slope, the trench will have to be much longer than it it is on a steep slope. Start digging the trench at the end furthest from the spring, and

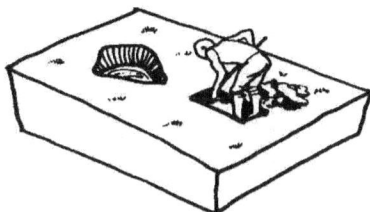

digging towards it, so that you will be working in very little water.

O If you start to dig the trench downhill from the spring, you will be standing in deep water, as the water from the spring will be filling up your trench.

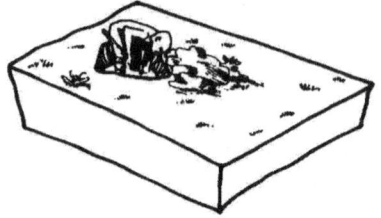

O Dig a second trench, 1m deeper than the first one, extending from the downhill end of it.

If you did not have the second, deeper, trench, there would be no space for people to put their containers below the pipe from the spring, which will be at the bottom of the first trench. Sometimes people make the second trench much wider than the first at the point where the pipe finishes, with steps going down into it. Making a water-collecting area like this makes it much easier for people to get to the end of the pipe, collect their water and leave the trench again by the steps.

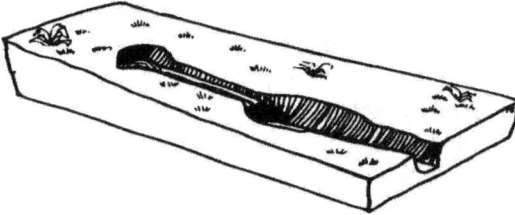

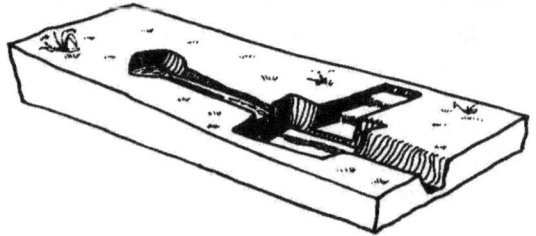

If it is not possible to do all the excavation below the spring, it is sometimes feasible to excavate from the spring into the hill above the spring. Uncovering the source in this way may improve the yield.

O The next stage is to install a screen. This can be bought or made locally (as described in the next section).

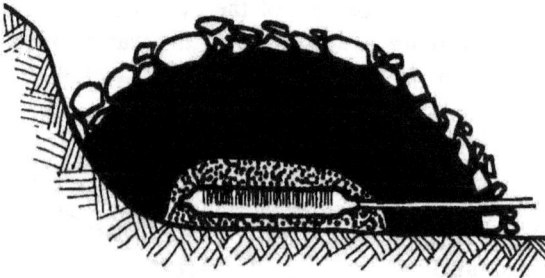

First, put some clean, washed gravel where the filter will lie in the eye of the spring. The individual pieces of gravel should be between 5 and 10mm across. Lay the screen in and join it to the outlet pipe (also described later). The pipe should be long enough to overhang into the deeper trench by about 20cm. Check that the water flows through it freely. Cover the screen with about a bucketful of gravel. This material must have particles too large to get inside the slots of the screen. Cover the screen and the gravel with a layer of sand at least 30cm deep. Grain size should be between 2 and 5mm. If sand or gravel is not available, you can use crushed charcoal if you crush it to the same grain sizes.

Place large stones over the sand, being careful not to break the filter. Fill up the eye of the spring to within 50cm of the top with more stones. If there are no stones nearby, this stage can be left out.

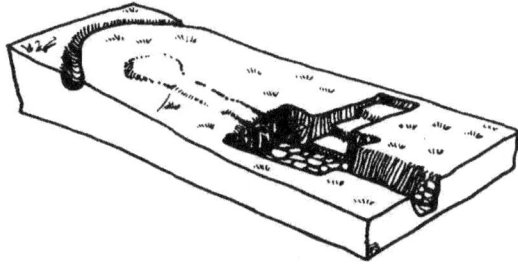

O Dig a third trench around the uphill side of the source. This is to stop rainwater flowing down into the spring, and taking dirt in with it.

O The next stage, another measure to prevent the spring becoming contaminated, is to cover the stones with soil. Put enough soil on the stones so that the soil is slightly higher than the ground around it when it has been thoroughly pushed down.

O Cover up the pipe in the shallow trench with soil. Plant grass over the spring right up to the water collection area to stop rain-water washing away the soil. If the pipe through which the water flows is not high enough above the bottom of the water–collection area, dig the floor of this area deeper, and excavate the rest of the deeper section of the trench further.

O Strengthen the sides of the water collecting point with stones or wood, if necessary. Pave the floor of the water collecting area with big flat stones so that people using it can keep their feet dry.

The screen and pipe

Whether you buy the screen or make it yourself, remember that it is just there to stop sand getting into the long pipe. It does not clean the water: this happens as it passes through the sand and gravel.

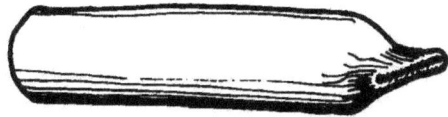

To make a screen, take a length of wide plastic pipe. It may be as wide as 10cm across. Heat the end of it gently by a fire, and squash the last few

centimetres flat. Cool the
pipe in water.

Cut off about 50cm of
the pipe. This will be the
screen. Heat up the other
end of the screen. When it becomes soft, mould it round the end of the pipe
which will take water from the spring to the collection point. Cool the
screen in this shape. It does not matter if the fit is not perfect.

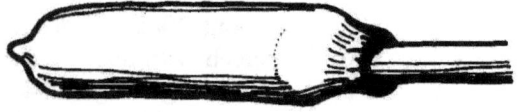

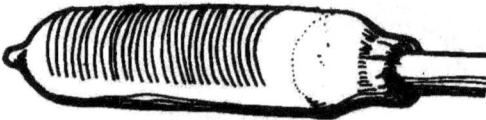

The pipe mentioned
above may be of metal or
plastic. It should be
between 12.5mm and
50mm in diameter. The
wider it is, the better.

With a fine-toothed wood saw, make many slots across the pipe. Each
slot should be about 2mm wide, and they should be 5mm apart. Each one
should only cut through three-quarters of the thickness of the pipe: leave the
rest to hold the screen together. The slots should not go right to the ends of
the screen.

If you can buy plastic glue, use it to stick the screen to the end of the long
pipe.

Other materials can also be used to make the screen. You can use a tin
can with holes punched in it or you can bore a piece of bamboo down the
centre and slot it, as described in *Waterlines* in Technical Brief No 5, July
1985.

But some materials last for longer than others. If you use a bamboo
screen, you may have to replace it once a year. A plastic screen will last a
lot longer. The screens we used in Boga, Zaire, were obtained from SWS
Filtration Ltd, based in Morpeth, Northumberland, UK.

When the work on the spring is finished, you may find that the water
tastes slightly different, because it is flowing through new sand and stones.
In Boga, for instance,newly-protected springs taste of iron, a mineral
contained in the local rocks. If the spring has been properly protected, the
water should taste good after about two weeks.

If the filter blocks after a while, first try cleaning it by back-washing it:
that is, by pumping or pouring water backwards through the pipe into the
spring. If this washes away the sand that is blocking the screen and the
spring starts flowing again, you must wait 10 days before you can drink the
water without boiling it. If you cannot clear the screen by back-washing, it
will probably be necessary to dig the screen out and replace it.

(*Waterlines* Vol. 4 No. 2, October 1985)

IRC's slow sand filtration project

JAN TEUN VISSCHER,
R. PARAMASIVAM
AND M. SANTACRUZ

The need for a simple and reliable method for treating surface water for domestic use was the stimulus for the International Reference Centre for Community Water Supply and Sanitation (IRC) in the Netherlands to initiate, in close collaboration with institutes in six developing countries, the Integrated Research and Demonstration Project on Slow Sand Filtration (SSF).

This project embraces applied research, demonstration programmes and the transfer of information on SSF. The applied research on the engineering aspects of SSF has been done by institutes in India, Thailand, Kenya, Sudan, Ghana and Colombia. Useful starting points for the research were experiences in Europe, where slow sand filters are an essential element of water treatment, on works in European cities like London and Amsterdam.

After proving the reliability of the process for tropical conditions, the second phase demonstrated the effectiveness of SSF as a simple purification technique in villages and developed guidelines for design. The importance of the non-technical elements and the important role of the users were also recognized at this point. The communities in the villages were involved in the planning, construction, operation and maintenance of the schemes, and a health education programme was run at the same time.

In the third phase of the project, national and international seminars were organized to transfer the information generated and to encourage the wider application of this technology. Recent developments in Colombia, for

Figure 1. Major components of a slow sand filter.

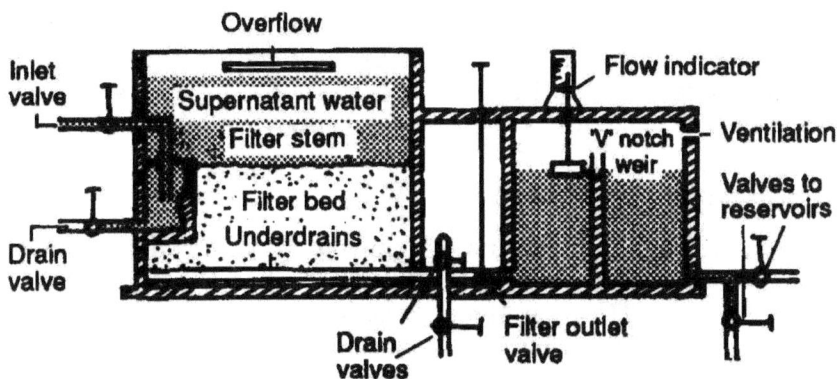

example, clearly show that such an intensive transfer of information pays off. As a result of a seminar, two participants, both staff members of the University of Valle, started developing SSF in Valle and Cauca in consultation with the National Health Institute and IRC. So far, two new plants have been built and nine more are in the offing.

One of the proposed plants in Colombia will be sited in Condote and is most interesting as it will replace an existing rapid sand filter plant which did not function because of problems with the procurement of chemicals. This particular design makes full use of the structural components of the abandoned rapid sand filter plant and is therefore relatively low in cost.

Treatment process

In a slow sand filter, the water percolates slowly through a porous sand bed. During its passage, the physical, chemical and biological quality of the raw water improves considerably.

Impurities are removed by a combination of filtration, sedimentation, (bio-)chemical and biological processes. Shortly after the start of filtering, a thin layer of slime forms on the surface of the sand of the filter bed. This thin layer, known as the filter skin or *schmutzdecke*, is the most important element of the filter. It consists of a great variety of biologically active micro-organisms which feed on organic matter and bacteria. This layer also reduces the size of the pores between the sand particles at the top of the filter bed, which improves its efficiency in straining out suspended inorganic substances.

Because of the straining process, the load of suspended solids in the filter skin will grow and its resistance will increase. After several weeks or months, the resistance will reduce substantially the amount of water which can pass through the filter skin. The filtration capacity can then be restored by scraping off the top layer of the filter, including the filter skin. The reformation of the filter skin takes some time. At the start, it will only contain a few micro-organisms and many of the bacteria present in the raw water will be able to pass through it. However, the number of micro-organisms will gradually increase and after some days (one or two for filters which have been cleaned, some 10-20 for a completely new filter), virtually all bacteria will be removed from the water as it passes through.

Controlling the rate of filtration

The rate of filtration is extremely important. When treating reasonable quality surface water with a turbidity level of 10-20 Nephelomatric Turbidity Units (NTU, a way of measuring suspended solids in the water), a rate of filtration of 0.1-0.2m/hour is appropriate. Higher rates would make the filter clog rapidly. A constant rate of filtration is preferable because strong and rapid fluctuations lead to a deterioration in the quality of the water flowing out.

The National Environment Engineering Research Institute (NEERI) in Nagpur, India, compared the efficiency of purification of surface water with a turbidity of 10NTU at three rates of filtration: 0.1,0.2 and 0.3m/hour. Although up to standard for all, it was somewhat better at higher rates. But the average filter run (the time between cleanings) was 45 days at 0.1m/hour, 26 days at 0.2m/hour and only 13 days at 0.3m/hour. Thus, a low filtration rate does not increase efficiency of filtration, but reduces the need for maintenance.

The rate of filtration can be controlled either at the inlet or at the outlet of the filter. Both methods have advantages.

In an inlet-controlled filter, the rate of filtration is set by the inlet valve (see Figure 1). Once the desired rate is reached, no further manipulation of the valve is required. At first, the water level over the filter will be low, but gradually it will rise to compensate for the increasing resistance of the filter skin. Once the level has reached the scum outlet, the filter has to be taken out for cleaning.

Inlet control reduces the amount of work which has to be done on the

Figure 2. Outlet structure.

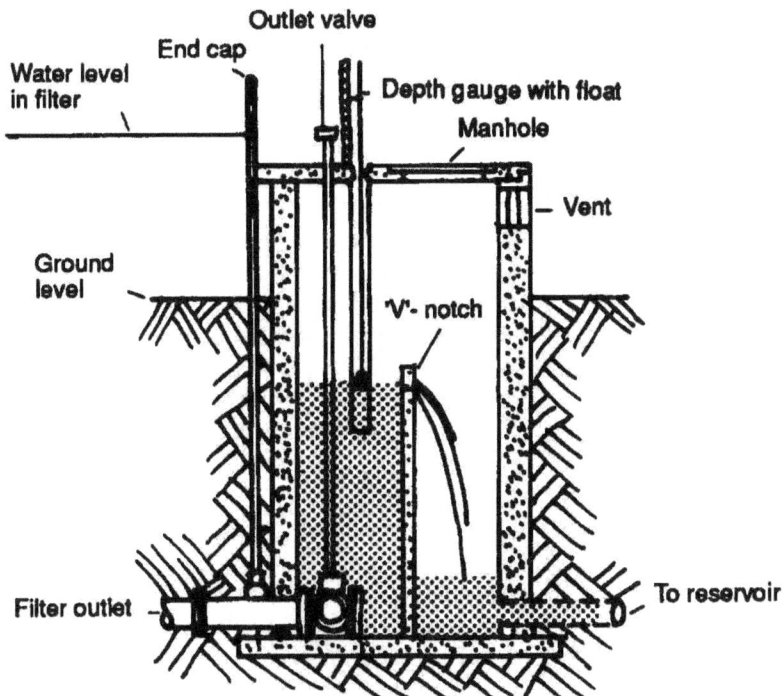

filter to just cleaning it. The rate of filtration will always be constant with this method, and the build-up of resistance in the filter skin is directly visible. On the other hand, the water is not retained for very long at the beginning of the filter run, which may reduce the efficiency of treatment.

In an outlet-controlled filter, which is more common, the rate of filtration is set with the outlet valve. Daily or every two days, this valve has to be opened a bit further to compensate for the increase in resistance in the filter skin. The disadvantage of this method is that the outlet valve has to be manipulated on a regular basis, causing a slight variation in the rate of filtration. Thus, the operator is forced to visit the plant at least every day, otherwise the output will fall. The water is retained for five to 10 times longer than in the inlet-controlled filter at the beginning of the filter-run, which may make purification more efficient. Removal of scum will also be much simpler than with inlet-controlled filtration.

In many countries electricity and diesel fuel are not available all the time, so existing SSF plants sometimes only function for part of the day. Research has shown that this leads to a serious deterioration in the quality of the out-flowing water and must be avoided. If electricity for working pumps is likely to be intermittent, either a raw-water storage reservoir, which can feed water to the filters under gravity supply, can be built, or 'declining rate filtration' should be used. That is, when the raw water is stopped, all valves remain in the same position and filtration continues at a declining rate as the water level in the plant falls. When the raw water supply is restored, the water standing over the sand bed will rise to its earlier level. Where declining rate filtration is used, a larger filter is needed.

Pre-treatment systems

Periods of high turbidity are common in many surface waters in developing countries. Unfortunately, SSF cannot cope very well with water high in turbidity, and pre-treatment may be required (Figure 3). Simple pre-treatment systems which have been applied in the IRC's SSF project are:

O River bed filtration. This is a very suitable method for rivers which have fluctuations in turbidity between 10 and 200 NTU and peak values over 400 NTU. An interesting test of a river bed filter using corrugated PVC pipes is in progress in Chorro del Plata in Colombia under the supervision of the University of Cali.

O Allowing the solids to settle out.

O Storing the water for a long time. This is suitable for turbidities over 1,000 NTU.

O Horizontal roughing filtration. The water is passed through gravel of different grades. This method is suitable for turbidity levels up to 150 NTU. (See the last article in this chapter.)

RAW WATER QUALITY   TREATMENT REQUIRED

Turbidity < 1 NTU *E.Coli* MPN < 10/100 Guineaworm or Schistosomiasis *not* endemic	**YES** → No treatment: if possible safety chlorination

NO ↓

Turbidity < 1 NTU *E.Coli* MPN < 10/100 Guineaworm or Schistosomiasis endemic	**YES** → Slow sand filtration: if possible safety chlorination

NO ↓

Turbidity < 10 NTU *E. Coli* MPN 10-1000/100 ml	**YES** → Slow sand filtration: if possible safety chlorination

NO ↓

Turbidity < 50 NTU or > 50 NTU for only a few weeks a year *E. Coli* MPN 10-1000/100 ml	**YES** → Pretreatment advisable Slow sand filtration: if possible safety chlorination

NO ↓

Turbidity < 150 NTU *E. Coli* MPN 10-10,000/100 ml	**YES** → Pretreatment Slow sand filtration: if possible safety chlorination

NO ↓

Turbidity < 150 NTU *E. Coli* MPN >10,000/100 ml	**YES** → Pretreatment Slow sand filtration: chlorination

↓

Detailed investigation required

MPN — Most probable number
NTU — Nephelometric Turbidity units

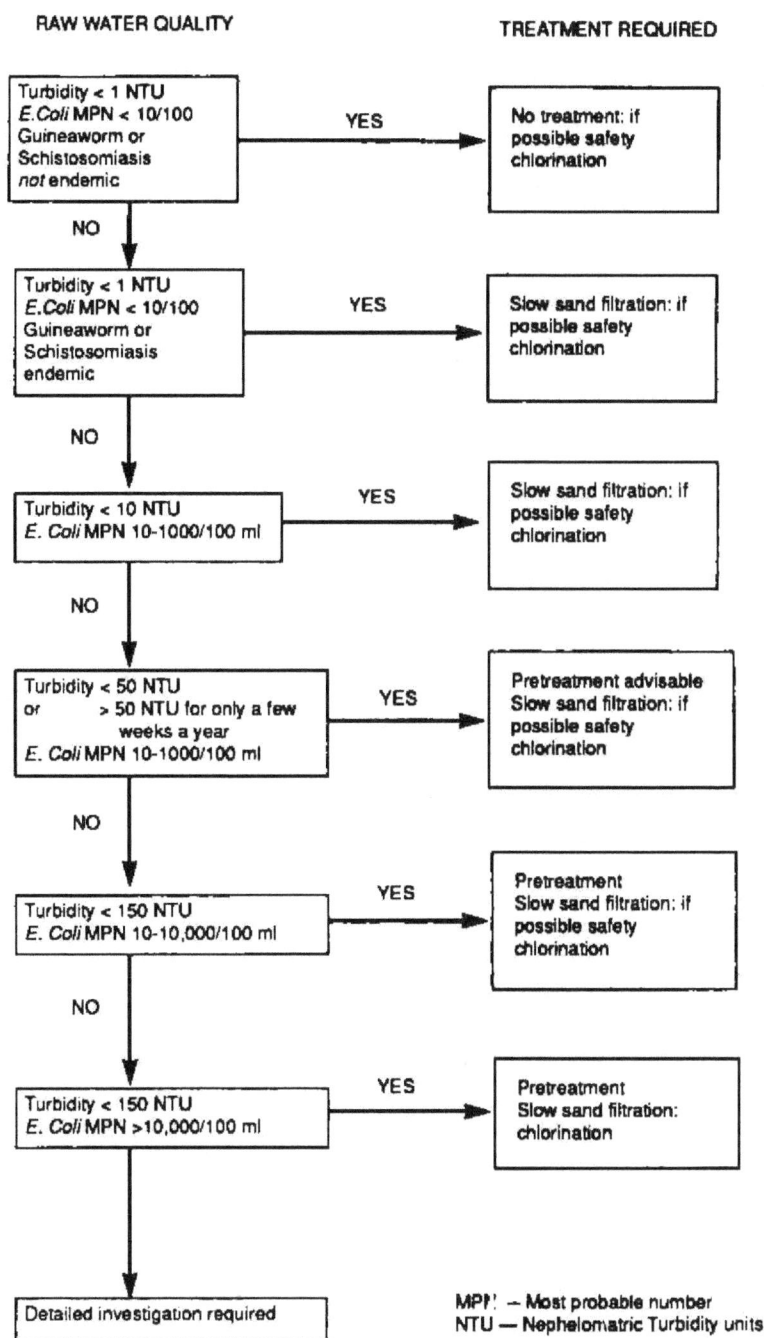

Figure 3. Guidelines for selecting a treatment system for surface water.

Cost of construction

The cost of construction is primarily determined by the cost of materials (cement, sand, gravel and steel). Labour is the second most important component. The construction cost of small and medium-sized slow sand filters often will be less than that of other types of treatment. Table 1 gives an example of a comparison of the construction cost of slow sand filters and rapid sand filters in India (1983 prices).

Table 1. Construction cost of slow sand filters and rapid sand filters in India (NEERI, 1983)

Capacity in m³/day	cost in US$1,000	
	SSF	RSF
1,000	50	60
1,500	60	80
2,000	80	90
3,000	120	120
4,000	150	140
5,000	190	160
7,000	250	190

Construction of a slow sand filter in India is less expensive than a rapid sand filter up to a capacity of 3,000m³. However, if recurrent costs for operation and maintenance are taken into account, the balance shifts to 8,000 m³. When cheaper materials are used, for instance ferrocement and cheaper drainage systems, the cost of SSF will fall. Often the cost of land only represents a small part of the total; less than 1 per cent in rural India. However, the somewhat larger areas required for slow sand filter plants are a problem in densely populated areas.

The cost of sand can form an important part of the total cost because large quantities are involved. In practice, sand for SSF plants does not have to meet high specifications. Often locally available sand will be suitable, which can save money. A minimum depth of 0.5m is required.

General design criteria

Based on research results, IRC has formulated general design criteria for slow sand filter plants (Table 2). Special attention to the design of some parts is essential to ensure that the plant works properly. The inlet must be constructed as indicated in Figure 1 to prevent the incoming water damaging the filter skin. The outlet has to be designed in such a way that the water level in the filter cannot fall below the sand surface under normal condi-

Table 2. Design parameters for slow sand filters in developing countries

Parameter	Time
Design period	10-15 years
Period of operation	24 hours per day
Rate of filtration	0.1m/h (0.1-0.3m/h)
Number of filter beds	Minimum of 2
Height of supernatent water	1m (1-1.5m)
Initial depth of filter bed	0.8m (0.8-1.2m)
Minimum depth before re-sanding	0.5m
Depth of underdrains	0.2-0.4m
Specification of filter sand	Effective diameter 0.15-0.35mm, uniformity coefficient 2-5

tions. It is also important to install a proper flow-measuring device (Figure 2).

When properly operated and maintained, slow sand filters can produce water that is safe to drink. Therefore caretakers have a very important, but not too complicated, task. An example of a maintenance schedule is set out in Table 3. For each plant the schedule will be different, as it depends on site-specific variables, such as how much suspended solids there are in the

Table 3. Typical operation and maintenance schedule for slow sand filters

Daily
Check the raw water intake (some intakes can be visited less frequently)
Visit the slow sand filter
— verify and adjust the rate of filtration
— check water level in the filter
— check water level in the clear well
— sample and check water quality
Check all pumps
Keep the logbook of the plant up to date

Weekly
Check and grease all pumps and moving parts
Check the stock of fuel and order if needed

Check the distribution network, check taps, repair if needed
Consult with community members
Clean the plant site

Monthly or less
Clean the filter bed(s)
Wash the sand removed from the tap

Yearly
Clean the clear water well
Check that the filter and the clear well are water-tight

Every two years or less
Replace the sand in the filters

raw water, the size of the plant, and the type of supply. It is very important to draw up the maintenance schedule in co-operation with the caretaker(s) at the end of their training.

Caretakers can be selected from the village or be employees from the water agency. Formal education is an advantage, but not really necessary to operate most village water-supply systems. Other factors such as their being likely to stay in the job for a decent length of time, having the respect of the community, receiving sufficient reward in cash, kind or in a rise in status, and being trained, are far more important. Also, the caretaker must have back-up and supervision when he needs it.

Community participation

Water-supply systems not only have to be well-designed, constructed and operated, but they must be used as well! Even the best quality water will not give a health benefit if some households continue to use other water sources. Continuous and correct use will be more likely when all the villagers, or at least members of all sections of the community, have been able to express their needs and their points of view during local planning and have been actively involved in decision-making and in putting the scheme into practice.

Although the degree of community participation will vary greatly in

Table 4. Subjects for community involvement

Project phase	Subjects for community decisions and involvement
Planning	Selection of type of systems e.g. standposts or house connections, including siting of taps Contributions of cash and kind Site selection and preparation Selection of reliable and motivated caretaker(s) Establishment of local committee for management
Construction	Contribution in cash or kind and services Timing of the construction period
Operation	Prevention of water wastage and pollution Payment of water tariff
Maintenance	Provision of labour support to caretaker Contributions in cash or kind for major repairs
Evaluation	Occasional checks on users' satisfaction through informal discussions

different countries and cultures, an attempt has been made to define major decisions on water supply in which the community should be actively involved (see Table 4).

Villagers, in particular the women, have expert knowledge on the local situation, which can help to prevent mistakes being made. For example a beautiful purification plant was constructed on an island in the Caribbean, but it cannot be used for 3 months of the year because the source runs dry. Consultation with the population and better preparation could have prevented this.

The people in some of the SSF project's demonstration villages actively participated in the construction of the water-supply system. This proved particularly feasible where the community benefited directly from their participation.

Hygiene education

Both motivation for community participation and the health of the new water supply can be increased considerably by a hygiene programme in which the relationship between hygiene and disease prevention is demonstrated.

A water-supply system has to deliver water that is safe to drink to the consumers. In the case of yard connections or public taps, this safety is not easy to guarantee. Often the safe purified water is stored before it is used. The water can be recontaminated before drinking, wasting the time and effort spent in treating it.

The local community not only has to understand and appreciate the need for safe water but also must have the means to prevent it from being recontaminated. Proper hygiene education is a prerequisite, as well as close collaboration between the agencies involved in the project in the fields of water, health and community development.

The result of IRC's health education effort and the impact of the new supply were evaluated by comparing the knowledge, attitudes and practice of the community, and examining stools before and after the scheme was put into practice. In general, experimenters found an increased knowledge of water-related diseases and better acceptance and use of the water from the slow sand filters: 80 per cent of the villagers indicated that they used the water for drinking and cooking.

In Alto de los Idolos in Colombia, a 60 per cent reduction in diarrhoea and a 30 per cent reduction in skin diseases was reported, however the study did not include control villages. Therefore we cannot rule out the possibility that the positive findings are not entirely due to the installation of a new water supply and to the health education that was given.

The education programme also included general information on sanitation, but did not adopt a participatory approach. It did not take local habits and constraints on improving the existing facilities for water transport, water storage and waste disposal, into account. Thus, many ways of transmitting disease were not eliminated. It is expected therefore that the health impact of the water-supply system could be further increased by placing greater emphasis on the local situation in the health education programme. Such a programme should focus on developing solutions for common hygiene problems, in co-operation with the community.

Conclusion

The Research and Demonstration Project on Slow Sand Filtration clearly demonstrates the feasibility of this technology for rural water supply.

However, close consultation with the community is required and the introduction of a new water-supply system should be combined with a hygiene education programme to increase the health impact and make the investment really worthwhile.

Further reading

H. van Dijk and J. Oomen, *Slow sand filtration for community water supply in developing countries, a design and construction* manual, Technical Paper No. 11, IRC, The Hague, 1978 (being revised).
L. Huisman and W.E. Wood, *Slow sand filtration*, World Health Organization, Geneva, 1974.
Guidelines for operation and maintenance of slow sand filtration plants in rural areas of developing countries IRC, The Hague, 1983.
Evaluacion del impacto de un servicio de agua tratada en una zona rural, Alto de los Idolos, Huila, Colombia, IRC, The Hague, 1984.
B.B. Sundaresan and R. Paramasivam, *Slow sand filtration research and demonstration project - India*, NEERI, Nagpur, India, 1982

Performance of slow sand filters in refugee water supplies in Somalia

NIGEL GRAHAM AND HANS HARTUNG

In April 1986, there were 39 refugee camps in Somalia supporting a total refugee population of approximately 700,000 people. These refugees are concentrated in four regions: Gedo, Hiran, the Lower Shabelle and North West (see map). The responsibility for providing water supplies for the camps lies with the Refugee Water Supply Division of the National Water Development Agency; this operates through a Northern Refugee Water Unit (North West Region) and a Southern Refugee Water Unit (SRWU) for the Gedo, Hiran, and Lower Shabelle regions.

Since 1983, the Ecumenical Relief & Development Group for Somalia (ERDGS), an ad hoc church aid organization, has been working in close co-operation with the United Nations High Commission for Refugees (UNHCR) and the Somali National Refugee Commission on medium-term relief and development programmes, including the provision of water-supply facilities in the southern regions. The main activities of the ERDGS/SRWU have been the installation of appropriate water facilities at the 26 camps in southern Somalia and the setting-up of the manpower and organization to operate and service these facilities.

The overall situation regarding the provision of water supplies in the southern Somalia refugee communites is shown in Table 1. Generally, the refugee camps in the Hiran and Lower Shabelle regions obtain their water supplies from the River Shabelle, while camps in the Gedo region collect their supplies from the River Juba. In both the Hiran and Gedo regions, a number of camps obtain water from drilled wells, and the water is abstracted by electrical pumps (diesel- or solar-powered) or wind-pumps. Groundwater supplies receive neither treatment nor chlorine addition.

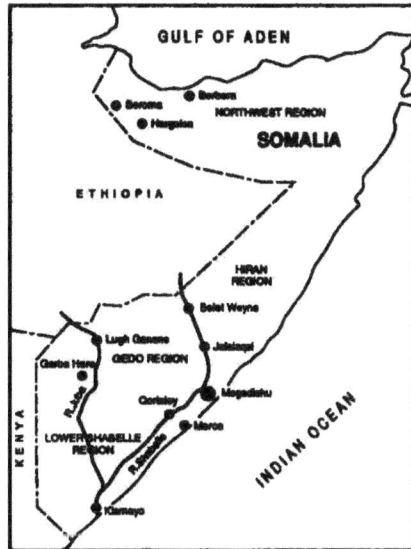

Treatment systems and performance

Treatment systems for river-water supplies include either river-bed filtration, chemical flocculation and settling, or package slow sand filter units. The systems using chemical flocculation and settling were originally installed between 1980 and 1981 during the emergency phase of the relief programme, and continued to be used by ERDGS/SRWU in 1983 using polyaluminium chloride (PAC) as the chemical coagulant. It was clear to ERDGS/SRWU that the continued foreign-exchange requirement for the purchase and importation of PAC (approximately US$1 per 10m³ of water) together with the logistical support needed for its ordering and distribution did not make it a desirable long-term solution. Consequently, alternative treatment methods were considered and an extensive programme of installing river-bed filters at 12 camps was carried out.

After a promising start, many of these units were abandoned either because of contamination by the highly saline local ground-water or because of unstable river-bed conditions. In 1981, as another alternative to the chemical treatment system, it was decided to install the Oxfam package slow sand filter units at the Maganey, Horseed and Qorioley II refugee camps on a trial basis. Following the general success of these units it was decided to begin a programme of replacing all the chemical treatment systems with package slow sand filter units.

The treatment package, developed by Oxfam and Imperial College (London), consists of two raw-water storage tanks which feed two slow sand filter tanks. A complete description of the equipment can be found in the Oxfam field manual. Treated water from the treatment package is designed to discharge into some form of storage vessel prior to distribution: at the camps in southern Somalia, 22m³ steel-sheet tanks were used for this purpose.

The source-water quality of the Rivers Juba and Shabelle is highly variable in two principal parameters: dissolved solids and suspended solids. The dissolved solids' concentration is sensitive to local surface run-off, and, consequently, the concentration can be unacceptable on occasions (electrical conductivity > 5,000μmhos/cm) during the rainy season (particularly March, April and May), when the river rises after an extended low period. The suspended solids' concentration can also be excessive during the rainy season, and concentrations greater than 5,000mg/litre have been recorded in the River Juba. The suspended solids are mineral in nature, and water samples show no discernible colour, but a considerable degree of faecal contamination is present.

In conventional water treatment, it is clear that no single unit process can reliably produce a water treatment that comes within WHO guidelines from a source of widely varying quality. In developing countries, the importance of slow sand filtration as the basic component of the water-treatment process is becoming increasingly realized, particularly so for small-scale rural water supplies. The difficulties in ensuring adequate chemical disinfection of water supplies places emphasis on the inclusion and proper operation of slow sand filtration because of its capacity to remove micro-organisms.

In general terms, when slow sand filters are operated at conventional flow rates — that is between 0.1 and 0.2m/h — they can achieve a one-log reduction in turbidity and between a one- and two-log reduction in faecal coliform concentrations. Thus, to achieve water quality that approaches WHO standards, the influent turbidity and faecal coliform concentrations should not generally exceed 10 NTU and 100 organisms per 100ml. Since turbidity and faecal coliform concentrations in raw waters are typically greater than these values, some type of pretreatment process is usually necessary, or, alternatively, disinfection of the treated water is required to destroy residual faecal coliform concentrations.

With the exception of the units at the Qorioley refugee camps, which take their raw water from lagoons, all the camps with package slow sand filters pump the raw water directly from the river via a floating intake into the raw-water storage tanks of the package system. The raw-water storage tanks are therefore the only form of pretreatment prior to slow sand filtration, and, although the storage tanks were not intended to serve in any treatment role, some lessening of the pollution load on the slow sand filters was evident. The possible problems of high solids and microbiological loadings on the slow sand filters were mitigated, to some extent, by the presence of a synthetic fabric layer on the sand and by the low filtration rates being used, for example, 0.04 to 0.06m/h.

Nevertheless, the absence of water disinfection following filtration meant that the complete absence of faecal coliforms in the water supplied to the refugees could not be guaranteed.

The Southern Refugee Water Unit (SRWU) does not have water-quality testing facilities at the refugee camps. This means that routine and frequent monitoring of the performance of the individual water-supply systems has not been possible. However, the SRWU water chemist carries out periodic tests on samples at the camps using portable testing equipment, which includes the determination of turbidity, electrical conductivity, total and faecal coliforms. For those camps where hypochlorite dosing is practised, free residual chlorine is also measured. The performance data collected are consequently limited in extent and this prevents a full and detailed evaluation of each of the treatment units. Nevertheless, if the individual data are considered collectively, it is possible to make a relative assessment of the performance of the package units.

Effect of raw-water storage

River water is typically delivered to the raw-water tanks of the package plant via a floating intake and diesel-engine pump; pumping is carried out for a few hours either in the early morning or evening. The tanks are not ideally suited as sedimentation tanks since, for hydraulic reasons, the raw water enters at high level and exits at low level. Nevertheless, the limited data from three camps, Maganey, Horseed and Bur Dhubo, suggest that a significant reduction in particulate concentration does occur. The data show that influent turbidities to the raw-water tanks varied between 10.5 and 250NTU.

From these values, and the corresponding effluent turbidities, an overall mean reduction in turbidity of 37 per cent was calculated for the tanks at the three camps. Sizeable reduction in faecal coliform concentrations were also found in the raw-water tanks, due partly to sedimentation and partly to natural die-off; average water temperatures at the time of sampling were 30°C±2. For example, influent faecal coliform concentrations were in the range 1,080 to 2,400 per 100ml, and reductions across the tanks were between 43 and 84 per cent.

Caution was exercised in the interpretation of individual results of turbidity and faecal coliform removal determined from influent and effluent samples taken at the same time, since, theoretically, the tanks have flow residence times of approximately 1.5 to 4 days.

Experience showed that the accumulation of settled solids in the raw-water tanks could be quite rapid; at the Maganey camp, 33cm of sediment was found after one year of operation. Periodic opening of the tank drain-valve was found to be insufficient to remove the deposited sediment, and it was recommended that the tanks should be emptied and the sediment flushed out yearly.

Run times and filtration rates

It is clear from the water quality data collected that the turbidity and faecal coliform concentrations in the influent water to the slow sand filters are very variable and can be well above the guideline maximum values of 10NTU and 100 organisms per 100ml necessary for satisfactory treatment. It is not surprising, therefore, that the filter run times for each unit also show great variability. At the time that the package units were originally designed, it was anticipated that the sand filters would operate for periods in excess of two weeks at the design filtration rate of 0.084m/h, given that the influent water quality was reasonably consistent and low in turbidity and coliforms.

At all six refugee camps where filter run times were recorded, the actual filtration rates were significantly lower than 0.084m/h, and this, in general, should have given rise to an improved filtration performance. Mean filter run times for individual slow sand filters ranged between 35 and 79 days for the camps in North Gedo and between 17 and 24 days in South Gedo. Since there are no available long-term data on the quality of the River Juba in these areas, it is not possible to speculate whether differences in filter run times between the two regions are due to differences in raw-water quality. However, it is worth noting that the filtration rates of the slow sand filters in South Gedo are generally higher than in North Gedo; this may be contributing to the difference in mean filtration runs. The variation in the filter run time for a given filter was generally large, and this is the direct result of the variable river quality as well as differences in the efficiency of filter cleaning. For example, for the Maganey and Horseed camps, where the filter run times were recorded continuously over 18 to 20 months, minimum filter runs were between one to two weeks and maximum filter runs between 12 and 20 weeks.

The treatment performance of the slow sand filters has generally exceeded the performance expected, given the nature of the influent water quality. This may in part be due to the low filtration rates. Again, it should be noted that the data gathered for individual filters represent influent and effluent water quality measured within hours on the same day. Since the flow residence time within the filters may be of the order of one day, the direct comparison of influent and effluent data was considered to give a close approximation of filter performance.

Meeting the needs

Actual effluent turbidity values were, with two exceptions, within WHO guideline values for drinking-water despite influent turbidities in North Gedo being far in excess of 10NTU. Effluent faecal coliform concentrations were less than 10 per 100ml (cf. 200 to 900 per 100ml in influent) which, in the absence of final disinfection, do not quite meet the WHO guideline criterion of 0 per 100ml. However, two of the eight effluent samples indicated that no faecal coliforms were present, and, taken together, the faecal coliform data demonstrate that a high treatment efficiency was being achieved by the slow sand filters.

With the change of approach in 1983 from short-term emergency support to longer-term self-help development projects, the adoption of the Oxfam package treatment system on a trial basis was an interesting decision since its design philosophy is that of a temporary facility using non-indigenous components and materials. However, the appropriateness of the treatment process in terms of simplicity, reliability and avoidance of chemicals has so far been borne out. Furthermore, the equipment costs have proved to be well within the US$5 per capita guideline value originally specified as an appropriate target value. The durability of the equipment, particularly the tank membrane linings, remains uncertain and will obviously depend on the degree of wear and tear experienced, but a lifetime in excess of 10 years is expected.

One aspect of the general water-supply provision observed in the refugee camps in southern Somalia is significantly different to the assumptions made originally in developing the Oxfam package system. This is the actual per capita water demand, which was estimated in 1985 to be between 5 and 10 litres for the Maganey, Horseed, Bur Dhubo and Qorioley II camps; this is considerably lower than the design value of 23 litres for the Oxfam package system. This difference is not important since the original design value was arbitrary and based on individual experience. However, lower water demand, if typical, will benefit the treatment system since it gives rise to a longer storage time in the raw-water tanks — and therefore a higher degree of particle settlement and bacterial die-off — and a lower hydraulic loading on the sand filter beds. A lower hydraulic loading should increase filter-bed performance in terms of both water quality and filter run time; the performance of the Maganey and Horseed filters is consistent with this.

Overall, the treatment performance of the package units in the North Gedo and South Gedo (Bur Dhubo) refugee camps has considerably exceeded expectations based on the studies of a prototype unit in 1982. Despite the lack of any authentic pretreatment process, the package units in general have been producing a water quality very close to WHO drinking-water standards (turbidity< 5NTU, faecal coliforms < 10 counts per 100ml) which in the context of short-term facilities/communities is very acceptable. In addition, filter run times have been satisfactorily long and even minimum run times have generally been around two weeks. Current work at Imperial College is evaluating more appropriate fabric materials that might replace the type currently being used on the slow sand filters and this may reduce some of the variability in the filter run length and further extend the run time.

The high quality of the water produced from the package units has meant that the practice of hypochlorite dosing is no longer necessary at camps using the units. This has brought cost- and labour-saving benefits, but post-filtration recontamination has been detected in the open treated-water tanks and in refugee water bottles. This aspect needs further study.

(Waterlines Vol. 6 No. 3, January 1988)

Horizontal-flow roughing filtration for turbidity reduction

MARTIN WEGELIN AND ROLAND SCHERTENLEIB

Slow Sand Filtration (SSF) is a simple but efficient process for the treatment of surface water [55,56]. In reality, however, SSF still faces many operational difficulties. Apart from the inappropriate design of such filters and the lack of trained caretakers, the raw water turbidity affects the filter operation very seriously.

Reasonable filter operation is only possible at turbidity levels of less than 10 to 20 NTU. Since periods of higher turbidities are very common in surface water in many developing countries, pretreatment of the raw water is often necessary. Plain sedimentation commonly fails to separate the fine solid matter, chemical treatment (flocculation) can be difficult or unreliable, and prolonged storage may not be feasible due to local (topography, geology, climate) and financial circumstances.

The solids can, however, be separated by filtration. River bed filtration is usually combined with the raw water intake. Unfortunately, such installations are difficult to clean and maintain. Horizontal-flow roughing filtration (HRF) represents another, more promising, pretreatment method. The following article is an abstract of the HRF manual[57] recently published by the International Reference Centre for Waste Disposal (IRCWD) in Switzerland and is meant to introduce the technology to a wider audience.

Historical background

Even during the last century, coarse media filters were used for raw water pretreatment prior to the development of slow sand filters in England and France. For the past 25 years, gravel pre-filters have been used in combination with sand beds for artificial groundwater recharge in Germany, Switzerland and Austria. [58] More recently, investigations on coarse-media pre-filters were carried out at the Asian Institute of Technology in Bangkok, Thailand, [59] and the University of Dar es Salaam, [60] Tanzania, to examine the treatment efficiency of these filters with highly turbid water. In 1982, IRCWD, attached to the Swiss Federal Institute for Water Resources & Water Pollution Control (EAWAG), in Duebendorf, Switzerland, started extensive laboratory investigations on HRF. [61] The investigations were followed up by a demonstration project involving construction and monitoring of village schemes and sponsored by the Swiss Development Co-operation. Its objective is to introduce the HRF technology in different developing countries and to gain more practical experience in how to use this process.

Figure 1. Main features of a horizontal-flow roughing filter

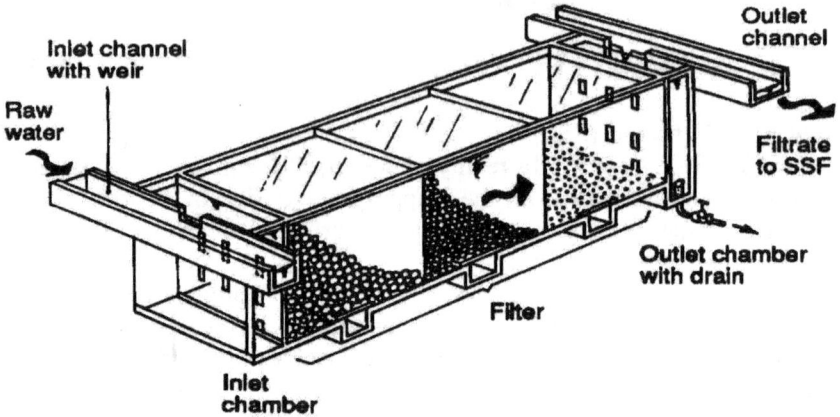

Filter composition

HRF basically comprises three main parts (as illustrated in Figure 1): the inlet structure, the filter bed and the outlet structure. The inlet structure is composed of a weir which leads the raw water into the inlet chamber. The outlet structure consists of a chamber located upstream of the outlet weir. The inlet and outlet structures are flow-control installations required to maintain a certain water level and flow along the filter, as well as to establish an even flow-distribution across the filter. The filter bed is composed of three or four sections filled with filter media of different sizes arranged from coarse to fine in the direction of the water flow. The coarsest material should be around 15 to 25mm and the finest gravel not smaller than 4mm. Each fraction is usually separated by perforated vertical elements, or an open-jointed masonry wall to avoid mixing during cleaning. The filter bed is usually also provided with an under-drainage system to enable hydraulic sludge extraction to be carried out after a certain running period without too much difficulty.

The raw water falls over a weir into an inlet chamber, where coarse solids settle and floating material is retained by a separation wall. The water passes through the perforated separation wall and flows in a horizontal direction through a sequence of coarse, medium and fine filter material. The pretreated water is collected at the filter end by an outlet chamber and then discharged over a weir.

The bulk of solid matter in the raw water will be retained by the first coarse filter pack. The last filter compartment should act as a polisher and remove the last traces of solid matter in the raw water. Each gravel pack becomes gradually loaded with retained solid matter until its respective filter efficiency is exhausted.

Longitudinal section HRF

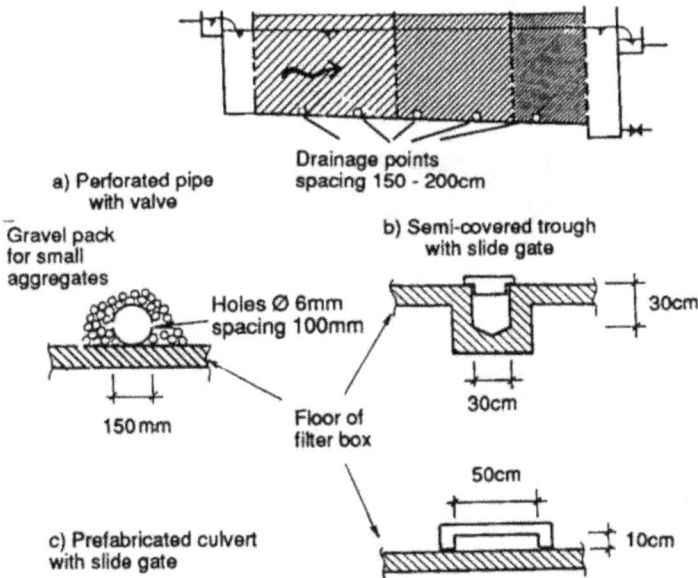

a) Perforated pipe
with valve

Drainage points
spacing 150 - 200cm

Gravel pack
for small
aggregates

b) Semi-covered trough
with slide gate

Holes Ø 6mm
spacing 100mm

30cm

30cm

150 mm

Floor of
filter box

50cm

c) Prefabricated culvert
with slide gate

10cm

Figure 2. Three different drainage systems.

In HRF, sedimentation is the main process responsible for the separation of the solid matter from the water. The filter acts as a multi-store sedimentation basin, thus providing a large surface area for the accumulation of solids that will settle. The solids accumulate on top of the collectors, and later on they drift as small heaps to the filter bottom. This drift regenerates the filter efficiency of the upper gravel layers and enables the accumulation of a considerable amount of retained material. Depending on the organic characteristics of the raw water, other processes such as biological oxidation or adsorption of solid matter at the slimy filter surface might also occur. Drainage facilities, as illustrated in Figure 2, are required for filter efficiency regeneration and filter cleaning. Hydraulic cleaning consists of a fast filter drainage and a slow refilling of the filter with water. Perforated pipes, troughs or culverts are placed perpendicularly to the direction of flow at the filter bottom. Each drain should discharge into an open channel to allow people to see the results of any cleaning operation.

Filter operation and cleaning

Unlike SSF, HRF acts as a physical filter and does not depend on a continuous supply of nutrients. Hence, intermittent operation is possible without a marked deterioration of the filter, provided smooth restarting of the filter

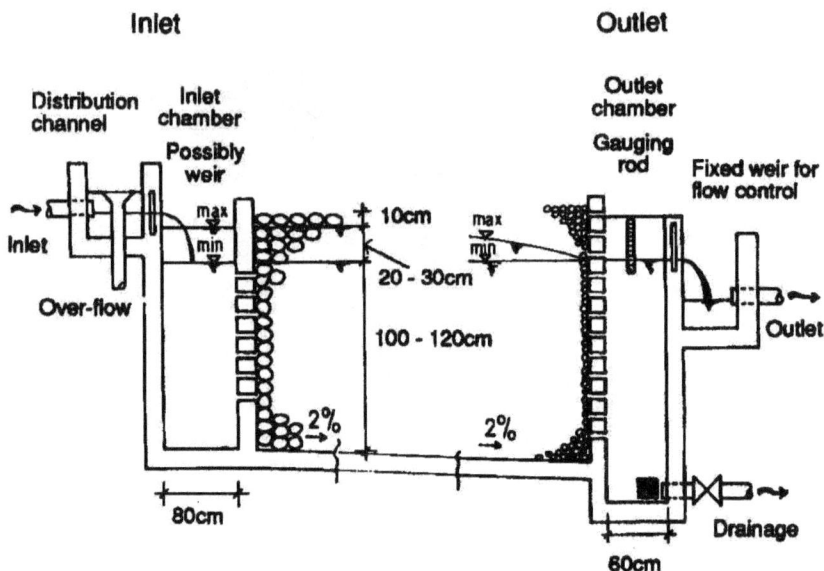

Figure 3. Inlet and outlet structures of horizontal roughing fileters.

operation is observed. Due to the relatively small water volume stored in the HRF, it is not reasonable to operate the HRF at a declining filtration rate to enable SSF operation at a constant filtration rate.

A continuous filter operation makes the best use of the installations, provides maximum production and a constant flow pattern. However, full gravity flow will be required for such an ideal situation. In case of a pumped scheme, a raw-water balancing tank is required. Removal of the coarse solids is a positive side-effect of such a tank.

Filter efficiency decreases with progressive accumulation of solid matter in the filter. Hence, periodic removal of this accumulated matter restores filter efficiency and keeps the filter in good running condition. An HRF can be cleaned in two ways, either hydraulically or manually.

Hydraulic cleaning assists the mechanisms of self-regeneration already discussed. The natural drift of accumulated matter towards the filter bottom can be enhanced by filter drainage. The retained solids are washed down when the water level in the filter is lowered. The upper part of the filter bed is thereby cleaned and regenerated while accumulation of solid matter takes place at the filter bottom. These solids can be flushed out of the filter by an adequate drainage system at initial vertical drainage velocities ranging preferably between 60 and 90m/h.

The annual hydraulic cleaning schedule has to be adapted to the annual fluctuation of the water quality. High turbidity loads are preferably treated by relatively clean filters to prevent the solid matter breaking through, which would badly affect SSF operation. The HRF should therefore be thoroughly cleaned before peak loads (for example, before the start of the rainy season). Hydraulic cleaning can be handled by the caretaker and should not require help from anyone else.

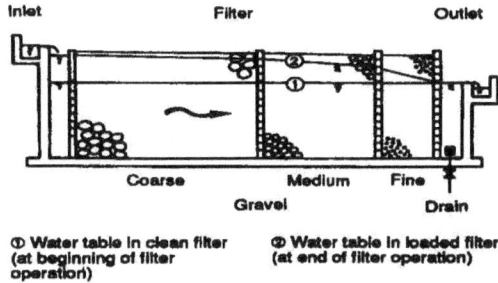

① Water table in clean filter (at beginning of filter operation) ② Water table in loaded filter (at end of filter operation)

Manual cleaning must be done when the

Figure 4. Flow control and head-loss development

solids accumulated at the filter bottom or at worst, all over the filter, can no longer be removed by hydraulic cleaning. This occurs if a drainage system is absent under the filter bed, if proper hydraulic cleaning has been neglected, or if solid matter has cohered to the filter material or at the bottom. A slimy layer might cover the filter material if there is biological activity in the filter caused by high loads of dissolved organic matter in the water. This biological layer will most probably increase the filter's efficiency at the beginning, but will subsequently hinder the drift of deposited material towards the filter bottom, and impair self-regeneration of the filter. Finally, retained material in silted, but drained, filter beds will also dry up and form a crust around the filter material. Thus, HRF should never be allowed to dry out unless the filters are properly cleaned in advance.

Manual cleaning consists of excavation, washing and reinstalling the filter material. The filter material can be excavated from a drained filter. The coarsest filter material is usually cleaned first. The filter box compartment must be washed and the cleaned filter material can be refilled afterwards.

The washing of the filter material is best achieved by mechanical stirring of the aggregates in the wash-water basin as mechanical friction rubs the impurities off the surface of the aggregates. Wash-water can be saved and a good efficiency achieved if small filter material loads are stirred with a

Figure 5. Water treatment plant layout.

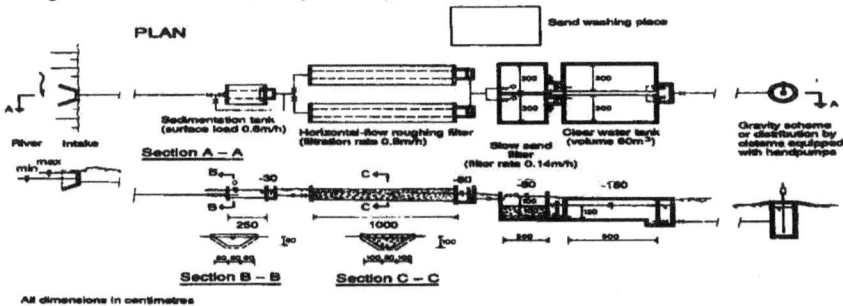

All dimensions in centimetres

shovel in a first tank to remove the biggest impurities before they are transferred to a second tank for a final wash. Centralized cleaning, however, involves transportation of the filter material. Use of the open draining channel located along the HRF is an alternative to the washing place which requires less efforts to move the gravel.

Manual filter cleaning involves a great deal of hard work, which is often beyond the caretaker's capacity. Additional manpower must be mobilized either by contracting local casual labourers or by involving the community. Careful planning is necessary when manual filter cleaning is carried out with village participation. The cleaning should be scheduled for a convenient time.

Adequate material and tools must be provided to the caretaker for efficient filter operation and maintenance. Simple and sturdy test equipment is necessary to monitor the flow and performance of a treatment plant. Such equipment is presented in more detail in the HRF manual.[57]

Examples of HRF in action

With the financial support of the Swiss Development Co-operation, the practical phase of the HRF project was begun by IRCWD in 1984. The HRF technology is expected to be introduced by constructing and monitoring demonstration schemes in different developing countries, and then compiling the results.

Cocharas in Peru rehabilitated its water treatment plant with the assistance of Del Agua and CARE. The work was carried out with extensive community participation, and therefore the specific construction costs for the HRF could be kept small. The respective costs amounted to approximately US$40 per cubic metre of daily capacity.

The HRF in Kasote, Tanzania, was set up by the local authorities with the assistance of NORAD. The high specific construction costs for the HRF of approximately US$130/m³ were partly caused by the transport costs required for carrying the construction materials to the remote village located near Lake Tanganika. The first trials have been promising. The filter resistance in the SSF was recorded at 60cm after the first rainy period, and a filter running time of four months. None of the filters had to be cleaned until then.

Fau 5 is a refugee camp in the Sudan set up by the Swiss Disaster Relief Unit. The water treatment plant for this camp includes two sedimentation tanks and four HRF units. The treated water is disinfected before distribution. Earth basins with inclined walls and earth dams constructed with bags filled with soil were installed. The filter boxes were therefore coated with a plastic lining and filled with gravel. The first practical experience with the

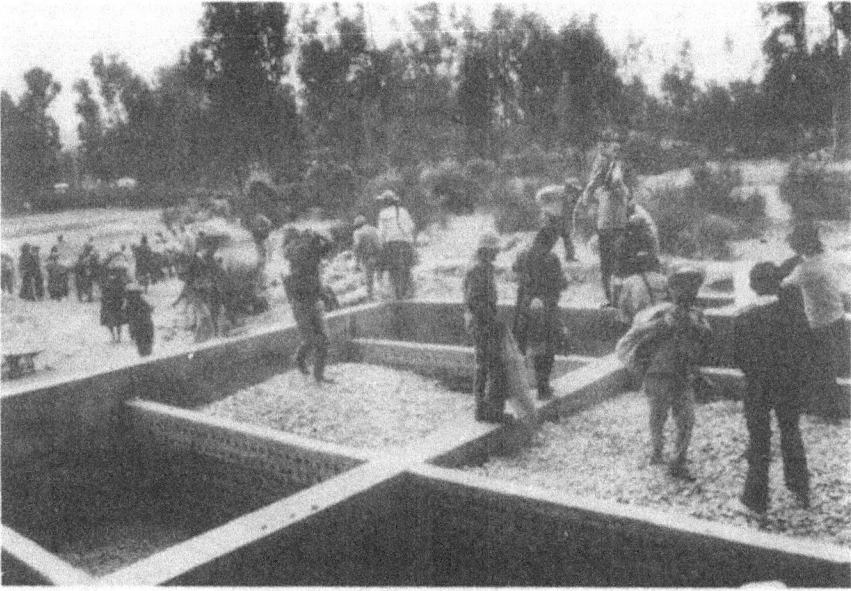

A Peruvian community participates in preparing pre-filters in Cocharcas. (Robens Institute/J. Bartram)

An Environmental Health Technician checking water quality in Jauja, Peru, using a portable testing kit. (Robens Institute/J. Bartram)

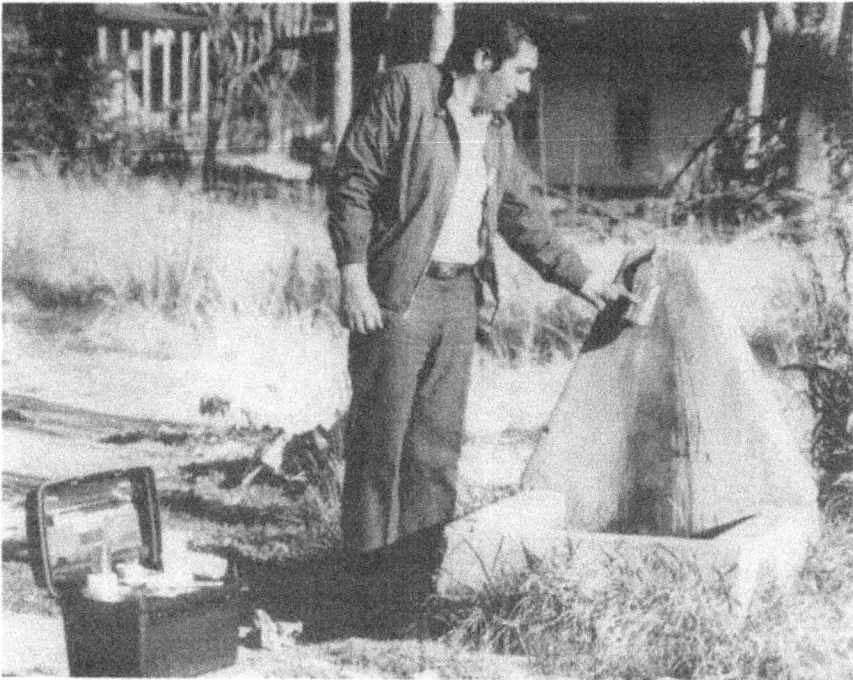

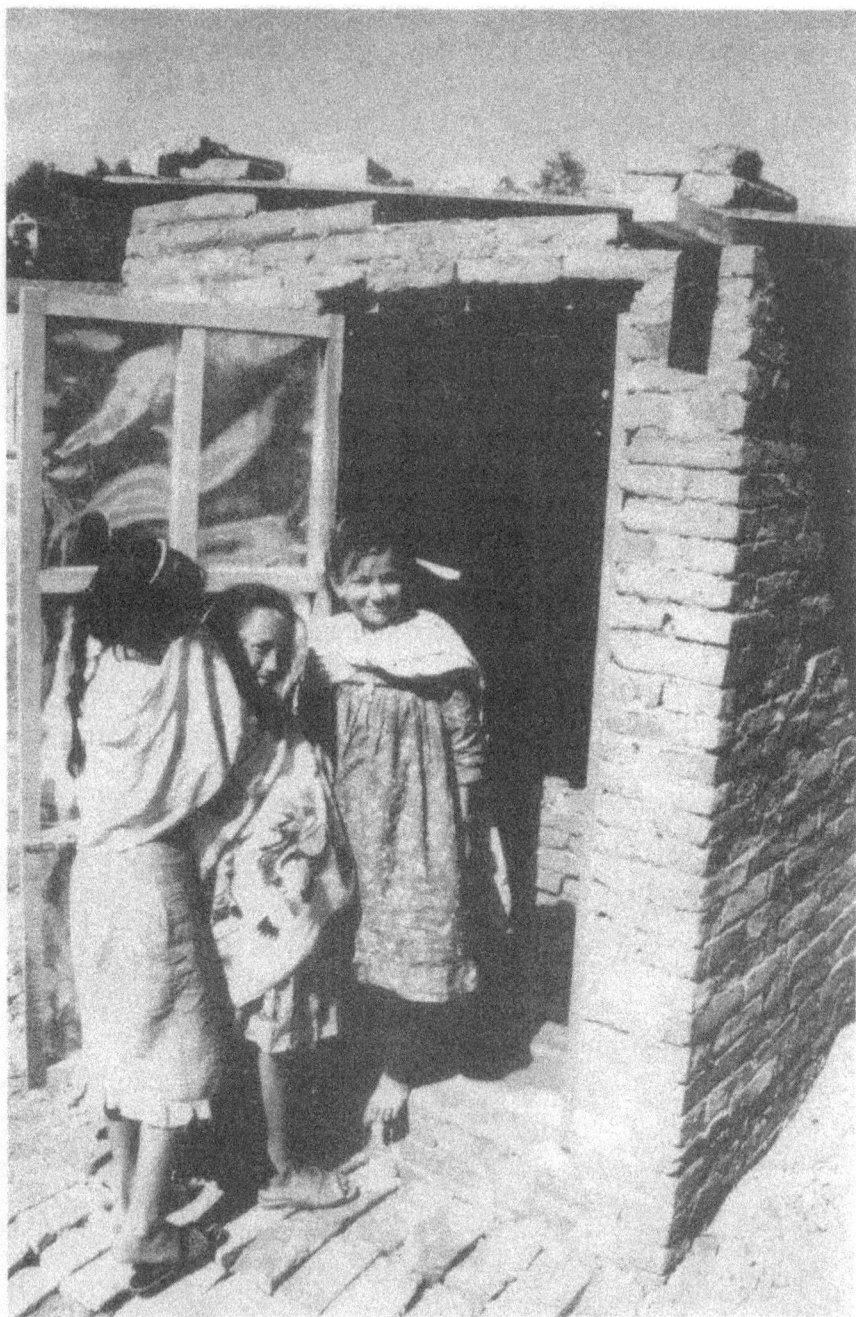

A pour-flush latrine structure in Nepal. (WaterAid)

treatment plant revealed that the raw water turbidity of 2,000NTU could be reduced to 1,000NTU by the sedimentation tanks, and then down to 5 to 20NTU by the HRF.

Conclusion

The simplicity of construction, operation and maintenance, as well as the nature of the filter combination of HRF with SSF make this treatment technology suitable for application in the water supplies for rural areas and small towns in developing countries.

Pretreatment of turbid water with HRF can solve operational problems experienced with so many SSF plants. Hence, this filter type will play a major role in the rehabilitation of water treatment plants using SSF, and will commonly enhance a broader implementation of SSF. Once tested under local conditions and introduced through demonstration schemes, the HRF/SSF technology can be reproduced with the use of local resources with very little difficulty. IRCWD in Switzerland offers any technical advice required for HRF implementation.

(Waterlines Vol. 5 No. 4, April 1987)

CHAPTER 5

Water quality control

This chapter looks at the provision of safer water for the community through water quality control. All these articles were in the January 1989 theme issue of Waterlines co-ordinated by Barry Lloyd and David Wheeler, respectively Head and Deputy Head at the Environmental Health Unit of the Robens Institute, Surrey University.

Richard Helmer of the WHO Division of Environmental Health provides the background to the WHO Guidelines for Drinking-water Quality[62] and the WHO dual strategy for country-wide improvements to drinking-water quality. The country projects described in the remaining articles in the chapter are introduced in this context.

Rural water-supply in Indonesia is characterized by many hundreds of thousands of public and private unpiped facilities. Barry Lloyd and Sri Suyati describe cost-effective methods developed for the sanitary inspection of these facilities. The methodology of the pilot surveillance project in Java is proposed as a working hypothesis for field evaluation in other project areas in Indonesia. This article is very relevant to Chapter 11 — Strategies for improvement, as are those that follow in this chapter.

Poverty, coupled with war, has left 86% of Nicaragua's population without a safe water supply. CIIR, with funds from Oxfam and Christian Aid, has been helping the national water authority to set up a National Programme for safe water-supply.

In 1985, the Western Province of Zambia was selected by WHO for the development of a rural project on the control of drinking-water quality, concentrating on bacteriological tests. Hans Utkilen and Sally Sutton set out the experience and results from this project.

The Ministry of Health in Peru began a programme of water surveillance for rural communities with support from WHO and ODA to reduce the risk of water-borne disease. One of the conclusions from the diagnostic surveys was that slow sand filtration plants had failed to reduce critical contamination to safe levels. Rehabilitation including gravel prefiltration is now in progress.

Drinking-water quality control: WHO cares about rural areas

RICHARD HELMER

The importance of water as a vehicle for the spread of diseases has long been recognized. Most of the illnesses which prevail in developing countries, where water supply and sanitation are deficient, are infectious diseases caused by bacteria, protozoa, viruses or intestinal parasites. The prevention of any communicable disease requires that the cycle of disease transmission be broken.

Depending on the principal transmission route, different interventions in water supply and sanitation may be required. Bacterial and viral diarrhoeas and epidemics of cholera and typhoid for example, are frequently transmitted primarily via drinking-water, thus making the quality of drinking-water a crucial health factor. Any improvement in personal and domestic hygiene, can of course often be even more important in halting the spread of pathogens and disease.

In all instances, basic requirements have to be met to ensure the bacterial and chemical quality of water, the quantities available, the convenience of the source, and the reliability of the supply. It was established at the United Nations Water Conference at Mar del Plata, 1977, that 'all peoples, whatever their stage of development and their social and economic condition, have the right to have access to drinking-water in quantities and of a quality equal to their basic needs'.

Much has been said about the relative importance of water quantity and quality in safeguarding human health and reducing the incidence of communicable diseases. Both are important and complementary. There is no question, however, that the first priority is to provide water. Water is essential to sustain life and must be made available to consumers even if the quality is not high. Larger quantities, sufficient for adequate personal hygiene and household uses, reduce disease transmission by person-to-person spread and through food contamination.

Which intervention first?

There is no question that breaking the cycle of water-borne disease transmission requires the availability of drinking-water that is safe and free of contamination. It should always be kept in mind that an essential priority is to maintain, and where necessary to improve, the microbiological and biological quality of the water consumed. Drinking-water should be free of pathogenic bacteria and viruses as well as of protozoa and helminths.

There are three main types of intervention employed to safeguard drinking-water quality:

O The protection of water sources from direct faecal contamination and from secondary pollution caused by leaching from pit latrines, septic tanks, cesspools etc. Because water from small-community installations is often not chlorinated, source protection is the first and most important means of providing hygienic drinking-water.

O The treatment of source water prior to supply is an obvious fall-back position where protection measures have failed. It may also be an essential technical intervention to make the water potable at all, in for example the treatment of surface waters from rivers, canals or reservoirs, where the removal of suspended material and pathogenic organisms is vital.

O Health education is a mandatory companion to any technology-based intervention, if only to guarantee proper use and maintenance of the facilities. Consumers must be made aware of the links between water and health. The use of safe water supplies has to be explained to prevent people reverting to water of questionable microbiological or biological quality. The contamination of drinking-water may also occur during handling and storage. This factor must be included in educational programmes.

The control of microbial and biological contamination inevitably takes the dominant role in any rural water-supply programme. Chemical contaminants are not normally associated with acute effects and are thus of lower priority than microbial contaminants, the effects of which can be immediate and drastic. There are instances where excessive levels of certain chemicals such as fluoride, arsenic and nitrate in drinking-water constitute a threat to human health, and must be controlled. In the Rift Valley, for example, not only dental but also crippling skeletal fluorosis is prevalent, so the chemical quality of water there assumes particular importance. In most cases, however, microbiological quality will be of greatest concern.

The WHO Drinking-Water Guidelines

The threats to human health associated with poor drinking-water quality were critically assessed by WHO in Guidelines for Drinking Water Quality.[62]

Securing safe drinking-water for small populations scattered over large geographical areas poses tremendous logistical problems for which standards or guideline values can at best provide a reference point. What is the use of a comprehensive list of international standards when there are just a few district hospital laboratories available, often with limited capacity for analysing water samples? There, concern for water quality has to be brought back to its essentials, namely the safeguarding of the microbiological quality of the water supply. Although the recommended guideline values for bacterial quality of drinking-water provide a target, the approaches and means to attain them should be tailored to the situation in each country.

As part of the development of the current WHO Guidelines, a meeting was convened in late 1982 in Bangkok (sponsored by DANIDA) to deal specifically with drinking-water quality surveillance for small communities in rural areas. Unlike water quality surveillance schemes which have been applied successfully to large urban water supplies, little had been achieved in rural areas and small communities. As a first step, methods were identified that allowed for a cost-effective application of the Guidelines in sparsely populated areas. This required that not only simple monitoring and control methods be made available, but also that the responsible health authorities at national, state and district level should be ready to adopt and implement them.

Current Decade strategy

WHO's strategy for the last years of the Decade leading into the post-Decade period, is based on a dual strategy for drinking-water quality.

First, where the existing infrastructure and resources permit, national drinking-water quality standards should be formulated to support country-wide improvement of drinking-water quality. The implementation of such standards must be accompanied by practical and feasible surveillance, and with the provisions and means to take remedial action when required.

Secondly, in rural areas and small communities where standards have little meaning, action plans need to be developed and implemented to improve the protection of water supplies from bacteriological contamination. This requires regionally- or locally-based systems linked to primary health care for raising public awareness of the problem and possible solutions, including the implementation of minimal water quality surveillance and remedial measures relying on appropriate technology and community participation.

In translating the strategy into practical action programmes, field experience was sought from country initiatives in places as far apart as Peru, Papua New Guinea, Indonesia and Botswana. (Some of these are described in detail later in this chapter.) When comparing the design, implementation and results of these and other projects, common elements emerged which were clearly necessary for any such action programme. They included the following:

O Careful planning is necessary for surveillance and control, including the design of a workable organizational structure, the assessment of local conditions, and the proper handling and use of information.

O Sanitary inspection is a crucial part of any surveillance programme and needs to be carried out by trained people at the community or regional level. In many very poor areas, this may constitute the only feasible form of routine surveillance.

O In the case of chlorinated water-supplies, the routine checking of residual chlorine is essential and field methods are provided. This can be applied at the community level with a minimum of training.

O Immediate remedial measures as well as long- and short-term preventive action are absolutely essential for achieving control of drinking-water quality. Only if sanitary deficiencies identified during surveillance are remedied will the effort put into the programme render its full benefits.

O Community education and involvement are mandatory components of an effective surveillance programme. The active participation of members of the community is a vital prerequisite for safeguarding drinking-water, particularly in remote areas with small and scattered communities. Much of the local health education should be implemented within the framework of primary health care.

Water quality control responsibilities should be shared between water-supply agencies and health authorities. The latter, in particular, have overall responsibility for ensuring that all drinking-water in their area is safe. All too often, however, health authorities have neither the necessary resources nor the qualified staff to carry out such surveillance activities.

Proper surveillance involves both sanitary inspection and the sampling and analysis of public water supplies. Ideally, this should be based upon legislation and regulatory standards, and be supported by codes of practice, trained staff, laboratory facilities and community health initiatives. However, a programme may be started with only basic support.

WHO's programme areas

WHO's programme for drinking-water quality control is based on three specific areas. These three key areas are technology, the running of pilot projects and training.

Technology needs

Since the early years of the Decade, techniques and equipment for water quality surveillance have undergone in-depth re-evaluation with the purpose of making them simpler, cheaper, and more appropriate to the needs of small communities and the level of technology and skills available to health and water authorities in rural areas. Two avenues were explored: the basic district laboratory; and, as an alternative, the field kit for on-site water testing.

The design of conventional water laboratories at basic, intermediate and central agency levels was outlined in a WHO guidance document entitled "Establishing and Equipping Water Laboratories in Developing Countries". This document is of great help in selecting the necessary tools and equipment and planning the targets in terms of samples processed and analytical results obtained. Costs of installation and operation, as well as staff and skill requirements, are indicated on the basis of experience with country projects.

With regard to field kits for bacteriological and chemical analysis, several independent research groups — in countries such as China, India and the UK — scrutinized the specifications and needs for simple field tests. The results of these efforts today include a choice of field kits on the market which are not only affordable but which require different combinations of instruments, equipment and power-supply alternatives, depending on local conditions. Workers with a suitable vehicle, such as a motorbike, will ensure that even the most remote rural communities receive a minimum of surveillance services. One fundamental aim of the WHO strategy has thus become feasible: to undertake sanitary inspection combined with sampling and basic bacteriological and physico-chemical testing of all supplies at reasonable time intervals.

The development of appropriate technology does not stop, however, with surveillance, but has to include processes and interventions for correcting faults and eliminating the contamination of water supplies. Simple treatments for sediment removal have been designed and constructed, including horizontal-flow filters and other types of roughing filters to protect slow sand filters and perfect their performance. Experience in the Blue Nile Health Project area in Sudan and from the Andes in Peru confirms the suitability and validity of their conceptual design. In other situations, however, disinfection by chlorination is the ultimate means of guarantee of the hygienic safety of the water supply. Simple dosing mechanisms have been developed and much progress has been achieved in developing electrolytic chlorinators and similar processes for the in-situ generation of disinfectant. Trials have been supported by WHO in order to test the various disinfection technologies under field conditions.

Pilot projects

In implementing new approaches, experience is vital to test the principles on which they are based. The World Health Organization and the United Nations Environment Programme therefore joined forces in 1984 to launch a project in support of the application of WHO's *Guidelines*. The project's long-term objective was 'to support the aims of the International Drinking Water Supply and Sanitation Decade through the promotion of effective control mechanisms for safeguarding drinking-water quality'. The immediate aims were:

O To apply and field-test methods for the surveillance of drinking-water quality under the conditions of rural areas.
O To establish demonstration areas for the effective control of drinking-water quality in small community supplies.
O To train technical staff of national and local authorities responsible for drinking-water quality.
O To field test and, as necessary, improve upon WHO's Guidelines for the Surveillance and Control of Drinking Water Quality in Small Community Supplies.

The success or failure of the pilot activities, would largely be determined by human factors, most importantly the competence and dedication of all participants. Therefore, the responsible health authorities and water agencies were to be brought together in working sessions during which approaches and methods were introduced, and technical as well as manpower requirements for the establishment of the pilot surveillance schemes discussed. Thus, a common basis was generated for active participation of staff at all levels. The incorporation of village health workers, sanitary inspectors, public health officers and district hospitals in varying geographic, demographic and administrative settings was one of the prime challenges in developing each pilot area programme.

Preparatory discussions with several interested countries and external support agencies led in 1985 to the designation of pilot areas in three countries, each located on a different continent. The three programmes — in Peru, Indonesia and Zambia — each received consultancy experts supported by WHO and other agencies. The Peruvian project started as a pilot enterprise in one health region, but has grown to the extent that it now covers almost one-third of the country, as described in the article by Lloyd, Pardón and Bartram. It was the substantive financial support by the UK's ODA as well as the professionalism of those at Del Agua which were responsible for this success. In Indonesia, a pilot area was designated in the Gunungkidul regency on Java. The article by Sri and Lloyd describes the difficult hydrogeological conditions of this area. The Mongu district in western Zambia was chosen as a pilot area typical of many rural settings in the Zambesi river basin. Close co-operation of the health and water sector, as well as NORAD's support, were main ingredients in today's operational surveillance scheme, as described by Utkilen and Sutton in their paper.

The other country project described by Katherine Wedgwood was not part of the WHO-UNEP project, but followed very similar lines and worked toward the very same basic objectives. In Nicaragua, the conceptual approach originated from the same 'source' as did the Peruvian pilot project.

Training

Following the dual philosophy of drinking-water quality surveillance and control, both the water-supply agency and the health authority responsible for the area should train their staff for the tasks involved. The importance of the human resources was recognized early in the Decade and has since evolved into a multitude of training activities at every level.

An example was set by the WHO Eastern Mediterranean Region, where a series of national seminars was held to bring together all working people from health and water sectors to discuss the WHO Guidelines. Thus, the way was paved for the drafting of national drinking-water quality standards. This initiative was followed up by national training courses for laboratory technicians responsible for analytical work. A training manual supports these courses and is available for similar courses in other countries.

Together with DANIDA, WHO regularly holds regional training courses, which are attended by participants from the host and neighbouring countries. The participants are district health inspectors and water authority personnel together with relevant central agency staff. All elements of drinking-water quality are covered from planning to the application of preventive and remedial measures for the maintenance of safe water supplies. A training manual prepared jointly with the Technical University of Denmark is used in these courses and provides for practical demonstration and interpretation of WHO Guidelines in rural areas.

The international and regional seminars, training courses and workshops are important fora at which to present new techniques, to verify the applicability of methods under varying hydrological and socio-economic conditions, and to stimulate innovative approaches to resolving water quality problems. Thus the train-the-trainers concept is enhanced, and the researchers and technicians receive their share of training in the application of new solutions to the old problems of safeguarding water quality in rural areas.

Achievements in surveillance

The many activities described above have brought together professionals from all sectors of environmental health and have mobilized human resources as well as co-operation and understanding between the health and water sectors. The University of Surrey in the UK has played an important role in the conceptual and technological development (see *Waterlines*, Vol. 1, No. 2, 1982) and its Robens Institute has now been designated as the WHO Collaborating Centre for Protection of Drinking-Water Quality and Human Health. This centre will certainly enhance international co-operation in the subject area, provide guidance, and promote the exchange of relevant experience.

Development workers must consider the sheer magnitude of the task ahead, bearing in mind the fact that today only a few developing countries actually do serve their rural areas with an effective infrastructure for drinking-water quality surveillance and control. This task is certainly one which goes beyond the Decade. Many more projects, such as the examples described in this chapter, are needed to make a measurable impact on drinking-water quality, and to make improvements in the health status of rural peoples on a global scale. This ambitious target can only be reached through the common efforts of water suppliers and health service providers in the rural areas, national administrations and external support agencies.

(*Waterlines* Vol. 7 No. 3 January 1989)

A pilot rural water surveillance project in Indonesia

BARRY LLOYD AND SRI SUYATI

In 1985, the Directorate General for Communicable Disease Control & Environmental Health of the Ministry of Health in Indonesia was made responsible for ensuring that drinking-water supplies do not present a health risk. Water surveillance for rural supplies was initiated as a pilot with support from UNEP and the World Health Organization in the province of Yogyakarta, central-southern Java, in 1985. It is intended that surveillance should be phased in elsewhere on an incremental basis over the next five to 10 years using the lessons learned and the strategies developed in Yogyakarta. Consequently, the principal objectives of the project were the following:

O To develop, test and evaluate the methods described in WHO's *Guidelines for Drinking Water Quality, Vol.3, Water Quality Control for Small Communities.* [62]

O To develop a surveillance infrastructure at sub-provincial level to ensure that drinking-water supplies are kept under continuous public health assessment.

O To provide a scientific basis for strategies of remedial action that will protect the consumer from the risk of water-borne disease.

Phase 1

One of the most important preparatory planning activites in surveillance is the development of comprehensive inventories of all water-supply facilities in the area under consideration. This is necessary to define the water-supply coverage and existing levels of service. The district selected for the project,

Gunung Kidul, has a population of 702,000 of which 560,000 (about 80 per cent) live in the rural areas. The magnitude of the problem of providing any form of surveillance service became clear at the outset of the project, when 21 sanitary technicians began to prepare inventories of the supplies for all the villages in the district. For the 144 villages and 1,421 hamlets, over 21,000 public installations were recorded. It was clear that the total number of facilities, principally private unprotected wells, could easily amount to four times this number.

This brings us to the next planning step and raises the question of how to select installations for inspection and testing. It has therefore been recommended that the first priority must be given to public facilities serving the larger populations. The inventory of the different types of public water sources was as follows:

Piped supplies	13
Artesian wells	2
Rainwater tanks	11,027
Protected springs	45
Shallow wells with handpumps	459
Deep wells with handpumps	808
Dug wells	9,204
Surface water sources	91
Total number	**21,649**

After completing the inventory, 21 sanitary technicians and laboratory staff were trained, equipped and sent out to begin water testing and inspecting a selection of these facilities.

At the end of the first year of the project, 2,546 samples had been collected and analysed for faecal coliform contamination, but complementary sanitary inspection had not been done. The analytical results for the first year demonstrated that 86 per cent of facilities were faecally contaminated and classified as bad.

Phases 2 and 3

The results of bacteriological analysis were classified as good or bad, and sanitary inspection also classified the facilities as being in a good or bad state in a somewhat subjective manner. A bad bacteriological result was considered to be any sample from which at least one faecal coliform was recovered from 100ml of sample and/or the total number of coliforms exceeded 10/100ml.

In the second year of the project, 500 facilities were sampled and tested, and 77 per cent were classified as bad. In addition, the sanitary inspection suggested that 72 per cent of these same facilities were bad.

In the third year, 1,012 facilities were surveyed of which 66 per cent had a bad bacteriological result and 67 per cent had a bad sanitary inspection result. Unfortunately, faecal contamination did not correlate statistically with the bad result suggested by sanitary inspection.

The lack of association between observed sanitary risk and measured bacteriological risk was particularly worrying since so many of the facilities were grossly contaminated. It appeared that the majority of facilities were in need of improvement or rehabilitation, but there was no rational basis on which to build an improvement strategy.

Retrospectively, it is clear that there were three principal errors. First, it was wrong to expect sanitary workers to come to an objective decision about the sanitary status of a facility without clear guidelines on what was good or bad. Second, the sanitary inspection form was not designed to permit quantitative assessment of the status of the facilities, and it was not possible for the supervisors to evaluate the most important points of risk of contamination. Third, there was no distinction between high, intermediate, low or no faecal pollution, and so the majority of sources were simply graded as bacteriologically bad.

New procedures for Phase 4

It is extremely discouraging for sanitary workers to find that the great majority of systems, which they may have helped to construct, are functioning as badly as suggested by the surveys in Phases 1 to 3. It was proposed, therefore, that a more elaborate grading of the level of faecal contamination be developed, as well as a quantitative evaluation of the number of points of risk of pollution of the supply as judged by sanitary inspection. However, it should be emphasized that the purpose of these revised classifications is not primarily to give comfort to depressed sanitary workers, but rather to assess more accurately the health risk attributable to each drinking-water installation in order to plan remedial action.

None of the rural supplies in the pilot project area is chlorinated, and it is inevitable that the majority will contain large numbers of total coliform bacteria which may have limited faecal significance. It was decided to base the classification scheme primarily on 44°C thermo-tolerant faecal coliform bacteria.

Sanitary inspection report forms

A sanitary survey form was designed for each of the main types of facility listed in the inventory. The objective was to establish a reporting system which could be rapidly but accurately completed at the site at the same time that the bacteriological sampling was carried out. The report form was intended to serve several purposes:

O To identify all the potential sources of contamination to the supply.

O To quantify the level of risk attributable to each facility.

O To provide a graphical means of explaining the risks of each facility to the users (hygiene education).

O To provide clear guidance to the user, and a record for the health centre supervisor, as to the remedial action required.

To meet these needs, double-page report forms (Figure 1) were designed to improve upon the models provided in the 1976 WHO publication.[63]

The sanitary workers should first inspect the facility and complete the check-list on the report form with the assistance of the owner or community representatives; this can take half an hour. The number of risk points can be immediately totalled to give a sanitary inspection risk score in the range 0 (no risk) to 10 (very high risk).

The sanitary worker should then circle each of the points of risk on the diagram, preferably in red ink. The diagram should be separated from the report form and given to the owner or community representative together with instructions and an explanation of what needs to be done to improve the facility. The recipient should sign the report form, which the sanitary worker retains for the health centre records.

The sanitary worker should take a water sample in a sterile sample bottle for bacteriological analysis. This may be analysed there or sent to the district hospital laboratory in a cold box for analysis the same day. It is most cost-effective for the sanitary worker to make at least a half-day per week available for the surveillance activity so that at least four inspections and samples can be done in that time.

Figure 1.

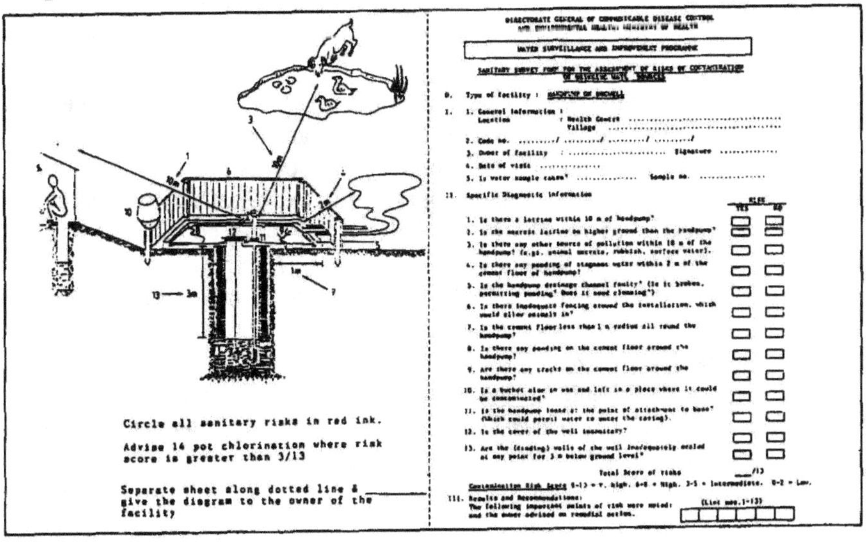

Phase 4

The procedures described were applied in the pilot project area for the first time from June to September 1988. At the time of writing, 328 facilities have been bacteriologically analysed and, of these, 244 inspected. Using faecal coliform counts, systems may be classified as A=0/100ml, B=1-10/100ml, C=11-100/100ml, D=101-1,000/100ml and E=>1,000/100ml. Tubewell water is least contaminated, with 86 per cent of shallow wells and 84 per cent of deep wells falling into categories A and B. At the other end of the scale, 9 per cent of these deep wells and 7 per cent of shallow wells fall in the very high risk grades (D and E). This contrasts with 22 per cent of open dug wells and 20 per cent of converted dug wells in the very high risk grades, while only 4 per cent of rainwater tanks were found to be contaminated at these levels.

It was considered essential to combine the faecal grading with the sanitary inspection risk score in monthly reports to the district office. Figures 2 to 4 show how the faecal coliform grades A to E and the sanitary inspection risk scores are associated for each type of facility in reports for this final phase of the pilot project. These figures provide a strategy for remedial action by order of priority by classifying each facility into one of four levels of action:

O Very high risk and hence urgent remedial action.
O Intermediate to high risk requiring action as soon as resources permit.
O Low risk.
O No risk; no action.

These figures can be used, at a glance, by the district surveillance co-ordinator not only to decide priorities for remedial action, but also for supervision purposes and for urgent re-sampling where gross faecal contamination does not correlate with a high-risk sanitary inspection score as indicated in the urgent re-sample category (see circled area in Figure 4, over page).

Figures 2 to 4 also demonstrate at a glance how the different facilities cluster characteristically. The deep tubewells are typically well protected from sanitary risks and thus low sanitary risk scores correlate well with a high proportion of A or B category bacteriological results. This is characterized by clustering of results in the bottom left-hand corner of the graph (Figure 4). By contrast, the converted dug wells (Figure 3) produce a dense cluster in the intermediate- to high-risk zone and a broad band correlation from top right to centre, but almost no facilities with no risk in the bottom left of the graph.

All the matched bacteriological and sanitary inspection data have been summarized in Table 1 (page 135). The most obvious conclusion from this is that the facilities presenting the highest risks are the 88 per cent of unimproved, open dug wells made up of the 43 per cent intermediate- to high-

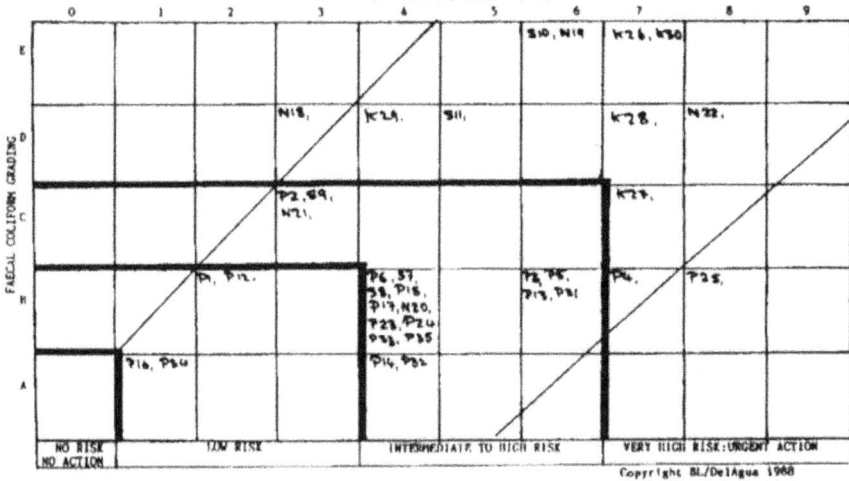

Figure 2. Combined risk analysis of sanitary inspection and faecal coliform contamination of a single point drinking-water facility.

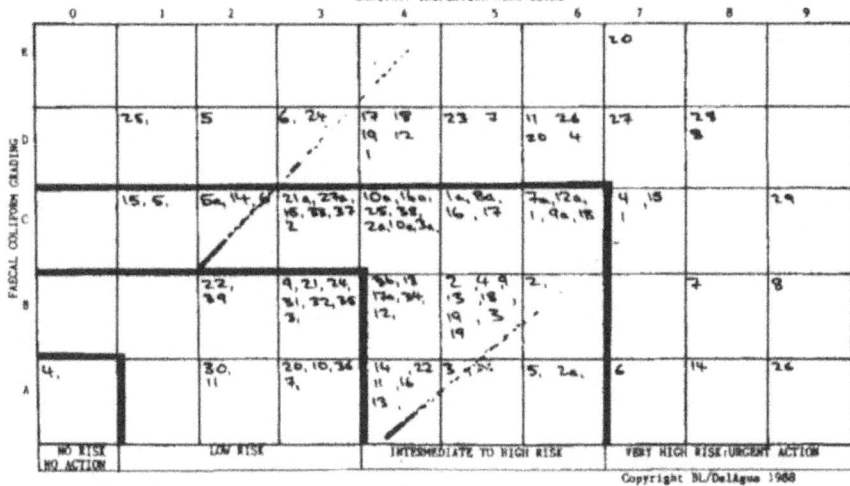

Figure 3. Combined risk analysis of sanitary inspection and faecal coliform contamination of a single point drinking-water facility.

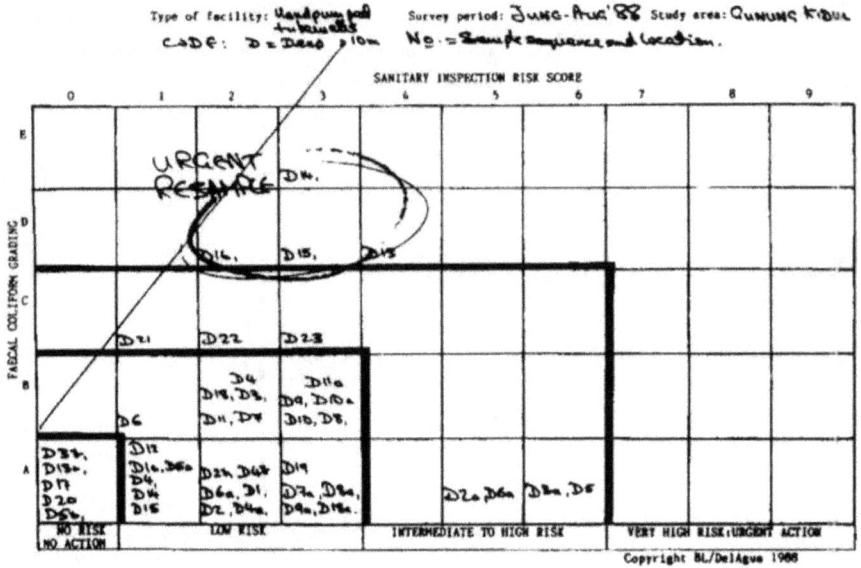

Figure 4. Combined risk analysis of sanitary inspection and faecal coliform contamination of a single point drinking-water facility.

risk and 45 per cent very high-risk categories. What is worrying is that the expense of conversion of dug wells by fitting a handpump and a 'sanitary' cover does not make a more substantial reduction in risk; 83 per cent are still in the two high-risk categories.

A significant improvement in risk reduction is achieved by shallow tube-wells, only 15 per cent of which are in the very high-risk category; however the highest proportion (80 per cent) are classed in the intermediate- to high-risk category. When we examined bacteriological quality alone it was seen that 72 per cent were in grade A (WHO guideline value) and a further 14 per cent were in grade B, making a total of 86 per cent low risk with respect to faecal contamination. The clustering of points, however, that can be observed in the cases of the shallow tubewells indicates a poor correlation between level of faecal contamination and sanitary risks. Thus the largest cluster of grade A facilties would be found in association with a high sanitary risk score of 6 (square A6). This may be due to one or more of the following reasons:

O The facilities are deteriorating structurally with age, but have not yet reached the point where they allow contamination to enter the tubewell.
O Several risk points in the sanitary inspection report form are being unnecessarily emphasized by the sanitary worker.
O The sanitary reporting procedure is perhaps over-rigorous.

Whichever reasons explain these apparent anomalies, they should be

Table 1. Phase 4 summary of combined risks for sanitary inspection and bacteriological analysis of drinking-water facilities in the pilot project area in Java

Type of facility	No risk Number(%)		Low risk Number(%)		Intermediate to high risk Number(%)		Very high risk Number(%)	
Unimproved open dug well	2	(6)	2	(6)	15	(43)	16	(45)
Converted dug well + handpump	1	(1)	15	(16)	50	(53)	28	(30)
Shallow tubewell + handpump	0	(0)	2	(5)	30	(80)	6	(15)
Deep tubewell + handpump	5	(11)	28	(62)	8	(18)	4	(9)
Rainwater tanks	0	(0)	4	(12)	16	(50)	12	(38)

Most urgent action

Total facilities under study = 244

verified by the district co-ordinator re-checking the facilities in question. Whatever the outcome, the results emphasize the considerable bacteriological source protection afforded by the drilled tubewell.

In contrast to the shallow tubewells, the combined risk analysis in Table 1 and clustering shown in Figure 4, for deep tubewells, are much closer to the situation which would be predicted from first principles. Only 9 per cent are very high-risk, and 18 per cent in the intermediate- to high-risk group, thus leaving 73 per cent in the low-risk group. This correlates well with the 16 per cent (in grades C, D and E) high-risk and 84 per cent no-risk and low-risk bacteriological grades (59 per cent A, 25 per cent B), and lends further strong support to the case for installing tubewells. The four points which are grossly contaminated but have relatively low sanitary risk scores (D13, D14, D15, D16) may represent remote contamination of the aquifer rather than defects at the tubewell; hence the need for re-sampling.

Inspection and analysis

It is important to emphasize the complementary nature of sanitary inspection and analysis. There are many occasions when the source of contamination is not visible to sanitary inspectors. In the case of groundwater contamination, for example, a tubewell with handpump may be in good repair, but the aquifer itself may be contaminated.

Contamination of the aquifer can only be detected by bacteriological or chemical analysis. On the other hand, a single water sample may be unrepresentative, and changing environmental conditions, particularly heavy rainfall or drought, may quickly alter the level of contamination of a poorly protected source. Thus the sanitary inspection should at the very least reveal the most obvious points of risk of contamination. It would be most unsatisfactory if sanitary inspection routinely underestimated bacteriological contamination.

Happily the data show that this is rarely the case, and that generally the sanitary inspection reveals more of the chronic risks of contamination that can be revealed by a single and costly bacteriological examination. We would hasten to add that this is not an argument for dispensing with bacteriological testing but rather for an economical and intelligent approach to bacteriological testing where money is limited.

The sanitary inspection procedures and bacteriological grading proposed in this article are not considered by the authors to be the definitive listings of points of risk nor an ideal model for improvement strategies. They are presented to readers, and especially to rural water-supply project staff, as a working hypothesis for field evaluation in other project areas. We are aware of inadequacies in the system proposed. In particular we would welcome comment on the equal weighting of different inspection points and suggestions for additional factors to include. We have intentionally excluded problems of operation and maintenance of handpumps, for example, although we are well aware of the risk to health imposed by breakdowns. Discussion is also needed about the importance of the radius of the concrete plinth protecting dug wells and tubewells, and the safe distance of the nearest latrine from the well point.

(*Waterlines* Vol. 7 No. 3 January 1989)

Nicaragua: rural water-quality surveillance and improvement

KATHERINE WEDGWOOD

Up to 1987, only 13.5 per cent of Nicaragua's rural population had been provided with a water supply (see Table 1). However, at the present time, there are several water supply construction programmes financed by such organizations as CARE (Canada), COSUDE of Switzerland and UNICEF. The majority of these supplies are hand-dug wells fitted with a handpump. There are some boreholes with electic pumps but the national water authority, INAA, discourages their construction because they are costly and difficult to maintain. In the mountainous Regions I and VI, there are some gravity-fed water supplies which have both spring and surface sources.

Table 1. Growth and target growth of water supplies 1980-90 (Source: INAA)

Year	Number of urban people served	Percentage of urban pop.	Number of rural people served	Percentage of rural pop.
1980	913,418	35%	77,449	6%
1987	1,581,087	77%	196,397	13.5%
1990	2,100,000	100%	750,000	50%

Starting a pilot project

In February 1986, a pilot project was initiated in the Department of Boaco with the aim of introducing the concepts of routine water-quality control and improving the rural water supplies in the area. Until then only in the capital, Managua, had routine water-quality surveillance been carried out by INAA in accordance with WHO's Guidelines. In other urban centres, sporadic water-quality checks were made. Some rural water-quality analyses were carried out in Region I, but these excluded determination of faecal contamination.

The pilot project began by training a small team of INAA community promoters and a Ministry of Health (Minsa) worker to carry out sanitary inspections of the water supplies, and use the Oxfam DelAgua portable water-quality testing kit. Six kits had been donated with some essential equipment for INAA's central water-quality laboratory as part of purchases made with funds provided by several UK non-governmental agencies including Christian Aid and Oxfam. The kit enabled a number of parameters to be determined: pH, turbidity, temperature, conductivity, and number of faecal coliforms (i.e. the most important bacteria of sanitary significance).

Diagnostic survey

A diagnostic survey of all known water systems in the department was subsequently carried out by the team. Table 2, over page, gives the results of the sanitary inspection and water-quality analyses of the 63 communities with installed supplies.

The survey revealed that preventive and corrective maintenance was totally inadequate, resulting in poor water-quality. Users lacked the basic organization, training and resources necessary to undertake rudimentary repairs and preventive maintenance: many also lacked a clear understanding of the relationship between water and health and the measures necessary to prevent contamination of drinking-water.

Given the general level of development in Nicaragua and an economic crisis exacerbated by war, it was felt that the INAA could not be expected to provide comprehensive maintenance of all rural supplies. Part of the burden

Table 2. Results of the 1986 diagnostic survey

System	Physical state				Water quality**			
	Number	Abandoned	In need of major repair	In need of minor repair	A	B	C	D
Hand-dug well with handpump*	46	16	8	14	7	6	12	4
Borehole with electric pump or windmill	9		2	3	8		1	
Spring-fed supply	7		3	3	3	2		2
Surface water	1						1	
Total	**63**	**16**	**13**	**20**	**18**	**6**	**16**	**6**

*In the case of the hand-dug wells, water quality analyses were only carried out when there was sufficient water in the well. If the well was dry, analyses were carried out, where possible, in alternative sources.
** Water quality classification key
A = less than 10 faecal coliforms/100ml   C = 50-500 faecal coliforms/100ml
B = 10-50 faecal coliforms/100ml   D = more than 500 faecal coliforms/100ml

of preventive and corrective maintenance should be placed upon the users themselves.

The pilot project attempted to improve this situation. First, it sought to rehabilitate water supplies where there was sufficient commitment demonstrated by local people in a series of meetings held in the community. Secondly it began to develop a model of self-help operation and maintenance in the rural sector of INAA, combining within the model routine water-quality monitoring, sanitary inspection and corrective action.

Getting communties involved in rehabilitation

Every community visited in the initial survey was sent a report of the results of the analyses, pointing out the likely causes of contamination and recommending necessary repairs and improvements. Public meetings were held in each community to discuss the reports, to promote the rehabilitation and to encourage the re-establishment of elected drinking-water committees (CAPs). Such committees had been formed during the construction phase to organize the work carried out by the community. Sadly, most had subsequently disbanded instead of going on to assume maintenance responsibilities. Community response was mixed. Wherever the users were receptive, rehabilitative work went ahead. A CAP was formed and remedial work began.

In the pilot project, it was decided that, wherever possible, users should provide local materials and pay for spare parts, cement and reinforcing steel. This policy was adopted for three reasons: to be less paternalistic; to overcome INAA's lack of available funds; and to try to deepen a sense of community ownership and responsibility for the water supply.

The CAP organized the collection of sand, gravel and stones by the community, and the project transported the cement and steel purchased from the town council. Spare parts and handpumps were obtained from the stock left over from a previous programme. The rehabilitation was carried out by the users under the technical supervision of the community promoters, who simultaneously carried out a programme of basic, sanitary education involving both adults and children. To aid this educational work a video recorder was purchased along with appropriate educational videos. Illustrative posters were developed, which were particularly useful in communities without electricity.

Typically, the rehabilitation of a well includes the installation of a new handpump or the repair of a broken pump, repair of the well lining and platform, improvement of drainage, construction of a stock-proof fence and a sanitary inspection cover, and repair of existing bathing and clothes-washing facilities. In the spring-fed gravity water supplies, the rehabilitation typically consists of repairing inspection covers, leaky valves and taps, covering air vents and overflow pipes with fine mesh and improving the construction of the public standpipes. Upon completion of work, the supplies are disinfected using a 50 mg/l solution of nationally produced sodium hypochlorite. The final requirement is that the CAP and any other interested users attend a workshop on operation, maintenance and administration of the supply. The importance of basic sanitation and water-quality are once again emphasized in these workshops.

Operation and maintenance

During the rehabilitation stage, it became clear that keeping those systems in working order needed continuing attention from INAA. Recognizing this, INAA created a Unit of Operation & Maintenance (UNOM). In Boaco, this had comprised one community liaison officer, called a promoter, who was part of the pilot project from its inception. Subsequently, two further promoters were appointed, so each was responsible for about 20 systems.

A community promoter is responsible for 'promoting' community action with respect to water supply. INAA tries to select promoters who have completed both secondary education and military service, and who are from the area in which they will work . In theory, a promoter, having completed initial intensive training, must work for a minimum of two years as a construction promoter, (i.e. promoting when the water supply is being constructed), before being eligible to work for UNOM. INAA has recognized that ensuring ongoing maintenance is a difficult task, made even more so in communities which did not meet their responsibilities right from the start. It is easier to interest a community in constructing a new water supply than in contributing to its subsequent routine maintenance.

The pilot project has sought to achieve the inclusion of one extra responsibility within the work of UNOM: that of routine water-quality control and sanitary inspection. The other areas of responsibility are: operation and maintenance, administration, promotion and education. To enable them to carry out their work, the UNOM promoters are provided with motorbikes, which they are able to buy from INAA over a three-year period. The project also has the use of a four-wheel-drive pick-up for transporting materials and equipment.

Once the CAP in a community has participated in the training workshop, they are expected to be able to carry out basic preventive maintenance and minor repairs unaided by the promoters. Regular cleaning, greasing and repair of pipe and tap leaks figure among their responsibilities. To do this, a CAP has to collect a monthly tariff, an amount which is decided by the users themselves in public meetings. The fund is kept and controlled by the treasurer of the CAP, who is accountable to the community. The UNOM team also has some entertainment films, which are loaned to CAPs for fund-raising events on condition that the water and sanitation videos are also shown.

The Boaco team has produced a simple manual on the basic operation and maintenance of hand-dug wells and handpumps to be distributed to all CAP members. The UNOM promoter, who plans the monthly visit to each community, has access to more sophisticated tools should they be required — for example, pipe-threading and cutting equipment and large wrenches. The CAPs will contact the UNOM office if they have a problem at any other time.

The promoter supervises the treasurer of the water committee, who keeps a record of the accounts in a simple system recommended by INAA. To try to keep up community participation and interest, the promoter and CAP organize user meetings to report and discuss changes, problems, tariff increases and the like. Periodically, the promoter also carries out educational activities in house-to-house visits, in the school, or in public meetings, using the audio-visual aids.

Monitoring and inspection

Routine water-quality monitoring and sanitary inspection are carried out in accordance with WHO Guidelines. Every three months, the promoters conduct a full sanitary inspection of the systems under their control. Appropriate inspection forms have been developed for the three most common kinds of supply. At the same time, the water quality is determined using the portable testing kit. The promoter uses the results to make recommendations for corrective action. A report of results and recommendations is given to the CAP with copies being made for regional and central INAA offices. Copies are also given to local schools and health centres, so that teachers and nurses can encourage implementation of the recommendations.

INAA's water-quality control division has decided that in the short term, the target for rural water suppplies will be less than 10 faecal coliforms per 100ml. Promoters carry out a disinfection of the system should the results exceed this level, having first eliminated potential sources of contamination. Within seven days of disinfection, the promoter checks the water-quality again. Sometimes, it is necessary to carry out a series of disinfections. On other occasions, wells must be relocated because of poor siting.

The INAA, as it is interested in chlorination of small rural supplies, has encouraged the team to experiment with continuous chlorination. There are now four wells which are being continuously chlorinated in communities which did not want to move the wells, or where there was no obvious alternative site. Public meetings were first held in these communities to explain why and how chlorination would be carried out, and to gain the approval of the users, at least in principle. Implementation has proved more difficult as many people do not like the taste of chlorine. With time and constant education about its importance, however, users are gradually coming to accept chlorination. The person responsible for chlorinating is provided with a stock of 1 per cent sodium hypochlorite solution, DPD 1 tablets and a simple comparator (pool tester). S/he is taught by the promoter how to measure the chlorine concentration every evening.

Another landmark was passed in July 1988, when the water-treatment plant for the town of Boaco was inaugurated. Previously the town had used untreated river water. The incidence of diarrhoeal disease was correspondingly high: in April 1988 over 900 cases were reported to Minsa in a town with a population of 19,000. The treatment processes now being used are flocculation, sedimentation, filtration and chlorination.

Within the plant, there is a small laboratory for monitoring the treatment processes. This laboratory has the equipment necessary to prepare material needed in the portable testing kits.

National Programme

In late 1986, a course was held in INAA's central laboratory for all UNOM promoters in the country. It introduced the concept of water quality control and field testing. Four of the six portable test kits were distributed to UNOMs in Regions I,IV,VI and Special Zone III. Regular follow-up training and supervision has been given.

It became clear that a more clearly defined strategy was required, so in May 1987, INAA produced a 'National Programme for Water-Quality Control and Rural Supply Maintenance'. This five-year programme is based on the experiences of the pilot project in Boaco. In each region, similar laboratories will be constructed and equipped. UNOM offices and workshops will have tools and spares. Extra staff will be employed and trained to ensure that the Programme fulfils its objective of monitoring all INAA water supplies, urban and rural, in accordance with WHO *Guidelines.*

Twice yearly, samples will be sent to the central laboratory for extensive physical and chemical analysis. All records of analyses carried out in the regional and central laboratories will be kept in a central data bank. It is hoped that, over time, the most important parameters to be controlled in each region can be determined. Financial resources permitting, the regional laboratories would then be equipped to carry out such analyses.

The National Programme is ambitious, and, as yet, not all the necessary funding has been approved. The original pilot project funders, Oxfam and Christian Aid, have already agreed to supply part of the funds. It is to be hoped that the Programme will achieve success in a country whose government has clearly demonstrated its commitment to the prevention of disease and the promotion of public health.

(*Waterlines* Vol. 7 No. 3 January 1989)

Experience and results from a water quality project in Zambia

HANS UTKILEN AND SALLY SUTTON

Western Province, Zambia, consists of a vast elevated and sandy plain dissected by the Zambezi and its tributaries. Woodland, bush and seasonal marshland cover most of the area of the district chosen by WHO for the development of a rural project on the control of drinking-water quality. In the central, most accessible part of the province, Mongu district is the most densely populated part of the province, but, even so, the population is only 80,000. Villages seldom exceed 500 people and groups of less than 20 houses are the norm, except along the Zambezi valley edge and in the peri-urban areas of the two main townships.

Water is not scarce, with shallow groundwater and surface water available both in the main Zambezi flood plain, and in the seasonal lakes (*dambos*), which are found within the elevated woodland areas. Traditional water-holes in the sands are the dominant source of drinking-water. As many people (45 per cent), however, take their drinking-water from the 240 or so protected sources (shallow dug wells with lining and windlass, and from handpumps on well-points and boreholes) as from the traditional scoop-holes. The remaining 10 per cent use surface water. Safe sources constructed by the Department of Water Affairs become the responsibility of the community upon completion. Thus, cleaning the source and maintaining it are community activities in which local health workers may have an advisory role.

The main aims of the project were to set up a system to monitor water quality and initiate rehabilitation where necessary. This was to be done within the framework of the existing co-operation between the health and water sectors, and, except for the appointment of the laboratory technician, did not involve any new employment.

Structure and planning

The project was represented at national, provincial and local level. The project management committee — consisting of representatives of the Ministry of Health, WHO, and the Department of Water Affairs — was based in Lusaka, some 600km away from the project area. This committee was formed in 1985, and remained unchanged during the implementation of the project.

At the provincial level, water, sanitation and health education were co-ordinated by the WASHE committee, representing all government organizations with an interest in water supply, health, education, social development, agriculture and local administration. Similar committees were being established at district level, and the plan was that the Mongu WASHE committee would provide local management of the project. This body was regarded as especially appropriate for relating the water quality surveillance output of the project to the rest of the water sector in Mongu. Unfortunately, it was not in fact established until almost the end of the project implementation.

At local level, the health assistants stationed at the 14 rural health centres were the field-workers who were to collect the samples and initiate necessary rehabilitation. They were to liaise with the laboratory that was established by the project in Mongu for water quality analysis, sending samples and responding to the results passed on to them by the supervising District Health Inspector.

Early enthusiasm for the project, which was expressed within Mongu by both health and water senior representatives, was only partially carried through to the implementation of the project. This arose partly from the year's delay in the starting of the project, and partly as a result of changes in personnel. Integration into the WASHE programme was also a limited success, both because of the lack of a district-level WASHE committee, and because the management committee for the project was at the national level, based in Lusaka where the WASHE programme was not represented. Communication between the central administration and provincial bodies was poor.

Communication problems

The project was planned by the project management committee and the liaison officer, based in Lusaka. Financial resources were disbursed at the national rather than local level. Incentives for sampling were poor, and, in retrospect, it would seem that more responsibility for the day-to-day running of the project could have been delegated to local personnel.

An opportunity to provide recognition and encouragement to the field-workers was also lost during the training courses. These were arranged at the beginning and end of the project implementation, but no certificate was given to participants. This would have helped to evaluate their understanding and given them a useful record of their developing expertise. Timing of the second workshop in the middle of the project, rather than at the end, would also have given the health assistants encouragement and given them a chance to discuss and solve some of their problems (many of which arose in the early stages) while there was still time for changes to be made.

Continuity of the staff involved at both the local and the national level was good, but, at the intermediate level, the Provincial and District Health Inspectors, whose roles were vital in the liaison between the upper and lower levels, changed five times during the implementation stage of the project. This led to difficulties in communication, as new personnel were not fully informed of the plans for the project and their role within it.

As in many parts of the developing world, the major constraint to fulfilling targets was the lack of transport. Two health assistants had motorbikes donated for other aspects of their work, but many of the centres included in the project were far from Mongu, accessible only along poor tracks in thick sands, and sometimes through swamps at seasons of high water. When this constraint was realized, plans should ideally have been changed to cope with the situation. The rural health centres from which samples could not be collected should have been told to concentrate on sanitary inspections and rehabilitation activities, which in the circumstances would have had a higher value for water quality than the sporadic collection and analysis of samples. For the health assistants it was discouraging to find that the samples (whose collection from distant villages had required several hours of hard walking in loose sand) were not collected for the next leg of the journey, and their efforts wasted.

The WHO *Guidelines* recommend a clear distinction between the roles of the surveillance agency and water supplier, but this separation may be difficult to maintain in developing countries and is unrealistic where transport is a major constraint. The project was supposed to be co-ordinated and run by both the Ministry of Health and the Department of Water Affairs, as was the case with the WASHE programme, but this did not happen, showing that much better definition was needed from the planning stage of the responsibilities of the different agencies involved.

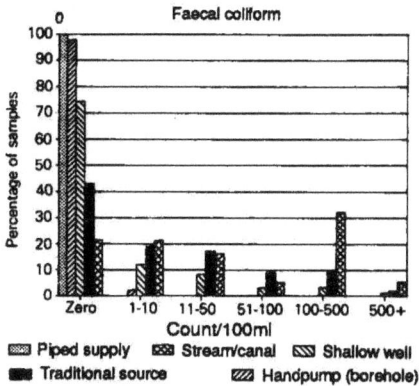

Figure 1. Drinking water from different sources.

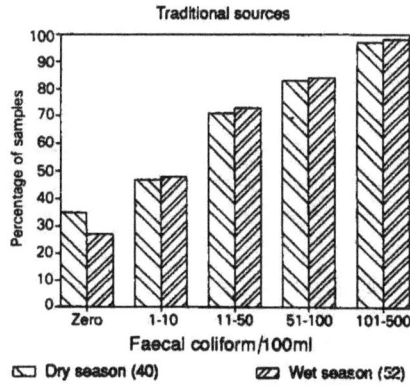

Figure 2. Seasonal quality variation.

Results of surveillance

The results from tests on bacteriological water quality show that handpumps and boreholes appear to offer safe and reliable supplies, free of faecal coliforms (see Figures 1 and 2). Shallow wells provide lower quality supplies, but are seldom prone to more than very slight pollution. More often traditional sources are significantly polluted, and one in three samples showed relatively high levels of contamination. It should be noted, however, that in general the level of contamination for both shallow wells and traditional sources is low compared with that found in many other countries. There tend to be coliforms of some sort in almost all traditional sources (83 per cent) and in 49 per cent of shallow wells. Part of the reason is probably because vegetation reaches right to the edge and often into the traditional source, and water is able to flow in. In contrast, the use of lids on most shallow wells keeps out wind-blown debris, and rings prevent the return of water.

While early sampling suggested that traditional source quality deteriorated in the wet season, comparisons with a greater number of samples did not show any real difference between wet and dry season samples (see Figure 2). This may be because the risks of returning water in the wet season are counteracted by the shallower water in the dry season and the frequent need to stand in it to fill a container. Table 1 shows that the risk of some level of contamination is higher in traditional sources than in shallow wells. The former are twice as likely to have faecal contamination and, while no shallow wells reach what might be termed 'moderate' pollution levels (>50/100ml), one in five traditional sources reached this level and one in 10 might be regarded as grossly polluted. In neither case is gross

Table 1. Percentage of water samples from different sources

Source	Number of sites	Number of samples	Percentage with no faecal coliform	Percentage with faecal coliform of <10/100ml
Handpump (borehole)	32	40	100	100
Standpipe	34	35	100	100
Handpump (well-point)	7	14	93	93
Shallow wells (SW)	98	266	78	92
Traditional sources	108	148	42	62
Springs	4	9	89	100
Streams	6	14	28	57
Unprotected SW	14	17	53	94

pollution (over 1,000 faecal coliforms per 100ml) apparent. These levels suggest that only a few sources present a permanent risk to health, but that in terms of epidemics, such as cholera or typhoid, the protected sources offer supplies with a very much lower risk of disease.

Monitoring results

Sampling by the project to measure contamination followed sanitary inspections by the WASHE programme, and it is interesting to note that these independent surveys could be closely correlated. Comparison of sanitary inspection and bacteriological results shows that of 26 protected wells with faecal coliform, all except one had previously been identified as being at risk and remedial work initiated. The combination of remedial work and community health education led to an overall improvement in water quality. Of 41 shallow protected wells regularly monitored over 18 months, 21 improved in quality, 20 had no faecal coliform at any stage, two became slightly worse, and three remained with slight levels of contamination throughout. Barring one case, handpumps were not found to be contaminated, but remedial works were carried out to ensure they did not become so.

While the WASHE programme rehabilitated all protected wells in need of repairs during 1986-7, the WHO/UNEP/NORAD project concentrated its efforts on the traditional scoop-holes. Thus health assistants initiated improvements in protection to some 30 sites, on the basis of the results they received from the laboratory. Consequent changes in quality were not, however, monitored.

By the end of 1989, some 30 per cent of the rural population will have access to supplies which offer no risk of the transmission of disease (handpumps), and a further 20 per cent will have access to sources where the risks are very low (shallow lined wells). A second phase of the WHO/UNEP/NORAD project, funded by NORAD, will now concentrate on finding low-cost technical solutions to the improvement of traditional scoop-holes, so that communities too small to qualify for new protected sources in the WASHE programme can nevertheless benefit from better water quality. This second phase will build on the experiences of the work carried out in 1986-7, working with the health assistants who were most active in the first phase, but with greater emphasis on community education and participation.

(*Waterlines* Vol. 7 No. 3 January 1989)

Improving piped water-supplies in Peru

BARRY LLOYD, MAURICIO PARDON AND JAMIE BARTRAM

The Peruvian National Plan for Rural Water Supply began in 1962, and, during the subsequent 25 years, over 1,300 piped water-supply systems were constructed for populations ranging from 500 to several thousand people. The great majority of supplies are simple gravity systems, but about a quarter are treatment plants for surface water sources. The treatment systems were built to a common design, which typically incorporated screened intake, a grit chamber, a settler/sedimenter, a pair of slow sand filters and a reservoir leading to a distribution network.

The surveillance programme was initiated with a preliminary study of 60 piped water supply-systems. The study was confined to the department of Junin, located in the high jungle and central highlands of the Peruvian Andes.

The lessons learned from the study were incorporated into a pilot regional surveillance programme, which extended its range during 1986 and 1987 to include all community water supplies in Junin. The programme has become the model for a national strategy of water surveillance, which is now being replicated and extended throughout adjacent departments.

The surveillance programme methods are based on the sanitary inspection and water analysis procedures described in the WHO *Guidelines for Drinking Water Quality, Volume 3, Drinking Water Quality Control in Small Community Supplies*.[62]

Surveillance methods

The on-site sanitary survey evolved by DelAgua in Peru uses detailed report forms to evaluate the main factors, including environmental, social, sanitation and water supply, that pose a risk to health. The largest component of the report form is that used to identify all points of risk in the water supply. After completion, the report forms are summarized to assess the critical factors which control the quality of service and its risk to health:

O Coverage: percentage of the total population served.
O Continuity: hours per day and days per year that water is supplied.
O Quantity: total water volume supplied per capita per day.
O Sanitary risk score: based on the assessment of all points of inspection from source to the tap.
O Quality: graded primarily on faecal contamination classes A-D.
O Cost: domestic tariff paid per month.

Analytical methods for quality assessment have been developed by DelAgua for application in many developing countries and include on-site analysis using the Oxfam DelAgua field test kits, which incorporate the testing of all essential parameters indicated in Volume 3 of WHO *Guidelines*. The main focus of water testing is on the detection and classification of the level of faecal contamination using standardized membrane filtration methods. Using faecal coliform counts, all systems may be classified as A=0/100ml, B=1-10/100ml, C=11-50/100ml or D=>50/100ml.

A preliminary inspection of 40 treatment plants carried out by CEPIS in Peru in 1979 indicated that they were often poorly maintained (see Table 1). The results showed that 33 per cent of slow sand filters and 37 per cent of sedimenters presented operating problems. The disinfection situation was worse: 88 per cent of systems were not being disinfected. It should be noted, however, that these results were based on sanitary inspection only. The seriousness of the situation was not, therefore, fully revealed until full diagnostics based on WHO *Guidelines*, incorporating both water quality analysis and sanitary inspection, were carried out in the Peruvian highlands and jungle.

Table 1. Preliminary evaluation of water treatment in rural communities of Peru, 1979

System component and state of unit		Number	%
Settlers	with sedimentation problems	15	37
	never been cleaned	6	15
Slow sand	bad state or not operating	13	33
filters	never been cleaned	13	33
Disinfection	not operated or maintained	35	88
Survey size		40	100

Table 2. Summary of the preliminary diagnostic survey of water treatment systems in the central highlands and high jungle of Peru, 1985

System	Sites surveyed	Systems presenting major deficiencies and problems	
		Number	%
Abstraction	18	16	89
Settlers	18	11	61
Slow sand filters	16	16	100
Disinfection	18	18	100

Note: The Ministry of Health reports a total of 28 rural treatment systems in the region.

The preliminary study of rural and urban systems showed that over 80 per cent of supplies were faecally contaminated, and none of the rural supplies was routinely chlorinated.

The survey demonstrated that the majority of treatment system components had fundamental design and operational problems which are summarized in Table 2.

The 18 filtration plants included two rapid sand filtration plants which were not working. All slow sand filters and disinfection units had major deficiencies and operating problems. The reasons for this have been examined in detail, and a clear pattern of common problems has emerged. They can be grouped in two main categories, either administrative or technical.

Administrative problems

The construction programme for the National Plan for rural water supply is the responsibility of the Rural Sanitation Division of the Ministry of Health. Systems in the National Plan are constructed with the help of the community, whose members provide the work force. The community is required to establish an Administrative Committee (JAAP) responsible for operation, maintenance and recovery of operating costs. The majority of rural schemes fall into the JAAP administrative category and herein lies a major problem in supplying safe and continuous water. The JAAP is not trained, and there are no incentives to provide a professional service. Until recently, the committees never received any professional supervision once the supplies were commissioned by the Rural Sanitation Division. Because of these problems, the national institution responsible for surveillance (DITESA) has set up a pilot project to create a training and supervisory infrastructure through the Ministry of Health.

Technical problems

Although some of the problems of treatment relate to faulty construction, the more fundamental problems are those associated with the raw-water source quality and flows for which the standard designs are inadequate. With grossly contaminated source water, it is essential to build a series of barriers to prevent contamination entering into distribution. This process of protection and treatment begins with source-water selection and abstraction. It is clear from Ministry of Health records that, although a chemical analysis is carried out on intended source waters, the more important bacteriological analysis is neglected, and no adequate design provision has been made to cope with high turbidity and high-level faecal contamination.

Thus the problems of performance of slow sand filters cannot be considered in isolation from the other components of the system. In order to provide a better understanding of the whole, the technical problems are summarized in Tables 3 and 4.

Table 3. Summary diagnostic of 18 treatment systems in the water surveillance programme, 1985

Community	Structural and maintenance problems identified						Water quality (Res + Dist)	
	Abst	Line	Sedi	Filt	Res	Dist	Turb (TU)	Bact (grade)
Huancavelica (Urban)*			+	++ (coag)	+		<5	A
Yauli			+	+ (coag)		++	15-32	D
Palian	+++		+	++++	+		15-300	D
Cocharcas	+++		++	++++			<5->250	D
San Martin de Porras	++		++	++	++ (coag)		10-20	D
Tres de Diciembre	++		+	+	+		<5	B
San Agustin de Cajas	+++	+	++	+++	+	++	15-50	D
Chaquicocha	++		++	++		+	<5	C
San José de Quero	+		++	++		+	<5	B
Huayao	+++		+++	++	+	+	<5	C
Churcampa	++		+++	++		+	<5-9	C
Hualhuas	++++		+++	++++	+	++	15-50	D
Saños Grande	++++		+++	++++	++		18-500	D
El Mantaro			+	+++	++		10-60	C
Julcan	++	+		+	+	+	<5	C
Sacsamarca	+++		++	+++	+	++	6->50	D
Tarmatambo	+++		++	+	++	+	<5	C
Pichinaki	+	+	+	+			<5	C

Key: + = Number of problems identified at each stage
Line = Conduction line. Res = Reservoir. Dist = Distribution system. Sedi = Sedimentation tank. Abst = Abstraction. Turb = Turbidity. Filt = sand filters. Bact grade: A = O, B = 1-10, C = 11-50, D = >50 Faecal coliform/100ml.
*Chlorinated with 0.3 mg/l.

Table 4. Operational problems of rural sand filters water surveillance programme, 1985

Community	Depth of sand bed (cm)	Volume of sand reserve (m³)	Distance to source of sand (km)	Actions required*
Palian	20	00	25	P
Cocharcas	00	00	5	P
San Martín de Porras	30	00	10	R
Tres de Diciembre	25	200	0.12	R,C,I
San Agustín de Cajas	55	00	3	P
Chaquicocha	10	00	10	R,C,I
San José de Quero	40	00	12	R,C,I
Huayao	50	00	1	R,C
Churcampa	00	00	?	P
Hualhuas	35	00	18	P
Saños Grande	20	00	25	P
El Mantaro	10	00	?	P
Julcan	40	00	15	C,I
Sacsamarca	20	00	50	P
Tarmatambo	35	4	55	R,C,I
Pichinaki	40	00	?	I

*NB Minimum sand depth recommended is 60cm; P = complete rehabilitation, R = complete sand bed replacement, C = cleaning, I= increase depth

Table 5. Summary of the diagnostic survey for the level of risk from faecal contamination of rural water in distribution in the central highlands and high jungle of Peru, 1986-7

System type	Number of systems surveyed	Percentage of systems presenting			
		No risk (A)	Low risk (B)	Intermediate risk (C)	High risk (D)
Gravity without treatment	273	23	43	17	18
Gravity with treatment	25	4	8	12	76
Pumped	9	11	22	22	44
Totals	307	21	39	17	23

Pilot programme results

A complete diagnostic was carried out on 307 community supplies in 1986 and 1987, and the bacteriological status of these systems is summarized by type of system in Table 5. This demonstrates paradoxically that the best quality supplies are typically those without treatment, as 63 per cent of these systems are classified as no risk and low risk, comprising 23 per cent grade A and 43 per cent grade B. The reason for this is that the great majority of untreated systems are derived from protected springs, and their quality is maintained during all flows and seasons. By contrast, 88 per cent of the treated supplies are classified as intermediate (12 per cent) or high risk (76 per cent).

Pumped systems also show a high frequency of gross faecal contamination, 44 per cent having grade D faecal contamination, despite generally superior source water. The deterioration in quality during transmission is attributed indirectly to the pumping regimes since communities can rarely afford to pump for more than two to six hours daily. As a consequence of the discontinuity in supply, the distribution networks have zero internal pressure for most of the day, and this facilitates the ingress of contaminants.

Resulting action for rehabilitation

It was concluded from the diagnostic surveys that the communities at greatest risk from water-borne disease were those with no alternatives to surface water sources. In particular, slow sand filtration plants had failed to reduce critical contaminants to safe levels. As a result, the Ministry of Health imposed a moratorium on the construction of new slow sand filter installations until pilot demonstration projects could demonstrate improved performance. It was clear that in those supplies where the raw water turbidity overloaded the filters, rehabilitation and new construction — incorporating prefiltration — was required. The systems with grade D water required immediate attention to improve both the quality and continuity of the supply.

It is hoped that the reasons for the failures have been identified, and a programme of rehabilitation of treatment plants incorporating flow control at abstraction, gravel prefiltration, enhanced slow sand filtration, and terminal disinfection is now in progress to improve the quality of these rural water supplies.

(*Waterlines* Vol. 7 No. 3 January 1989)

CHAPTER 6

Latrines for Health

There is a wide range of sanitation alternatives for low-income communities. The technical and economic options have been extensively reviewed in World Bank publications, which also present a general methodology for low-cost sanitation programme planning. Reference should be made to these publications for detailed information. The articles here have been selected for their general interest and to provide an overview of the problems and solutions in different countries.

Brian MacGarry outlines the development of the Blair VIP latrine in Zimbabwe from 1973. The essential feature is a fly-screened vent pipe, which not only reduces internal odours significantly but also minimizes fly access and breeding. Controlled experiments in Zimbabwe have shown that, over a 78-day period, some 14,000 flies were caught from an unvented latrine, but only 1% of that number from a vented (but otherwise identical) pit latrine. Simple but effective; yet 10 years were needed for this latrine to be adopted. In Chapter 10, Peter Morgan provides further information in his article on the Zimbabwe village-level sanitation programme.

Mozambique has developed an alternative to the VIP latrine for use in poor peri-urban areas. This consists of a thin non-reinforced precast concrete slab as detailed by Bjorn Brandberg. Savings were achieved by using a tight-fitting lid on the slab opening, instead of a vent-pipe, and an enclosure without a roof. In a recent report (*Waterlines*, July 1988), UNDP stated that more than 25,000 slabs have since been sold and installed benefiting over 125,000 people. UNDP and IDRC have also helped to train some 350 people, who are now employed as professional latrine constructors and community motivators, thus not only helping to improve environmental sanitation but also providing skills for employment.

Andrew Cotton and Richard Franceys discuss some of the technical, social and economic issues that need to be considered in a national latrine construction programme. In Sri Lanka, water availability is critical for latrine selection. Pour-flush latrines are preferred but, where no water is available, a VIP latrine is used. The performance of aquaprivies in Thai refugee camps is the subject of the article by Robin Biellik and Peggy Henderson. Under emergency conditions, the system performed well as a primary sewage-treatment facility, and the cultural acceptability among Khmers was excellent. However, the authors do not recommend the aquaprivy for permanent widespread use in developing countries. In the final article, Deepa Naryan Parker, a psychologist, investigated why people were not using the public toilets in the Maldives. She concludes that a mixture of three improved types are needed to satisfy diverse needs.

The development of the Blair VIP latrine

BRIAN MACGARRY

Real success stories in appropriate technology are rare; devices or techniques that not only work, but are adopted by users, so that they become responsible for the development of the technology. One such success story has been the Ventilated Improved Pit (VIP) latrine developed by the Zimbabwe Ministry of Health's Blair Laboratory. The latrine itself has been described more fully by its developers, Peter Morgan and Ephraim Chimbunde, [64,65] but its history may also interest present readers.

Before Blair's first VIP latrines were built in 1973, little systematic work had been done elsewhere on the function or operation of a ventilated pit latrine, and the value of venting was doubted by many. The Blair laboratory team showed the effectiveness of a wide (6in or so) vent-pipe with an effective flyscreen on it for both removing smells from inside the latrine and dramatically reducing the number of flies emerging from the latrine, which are a major source of disease in the vicinity of traditional unvented latrines.

The early version was a round structure with a door and a vent-pipe which was at first made of asbestos, but later more commonly of black PVC. This proved so effective that its popularity even survived its use in the 'protected villages' built by the Rhodesian regime during the later stages of the guerrilla war that led to the independence of Zimbabwe in 1980.

In 1976, the now familiar doorless VIP latrine with its snail-shell ground plan emerged and proved itself even more effective. Two features contributed to this: the vent-pipe, leading odorous vapours out through a flyscreen and thus attracting flies to that screen, through which they cannot enter the pit; and the dark interior of the curiously-shaped cubicle, which, by preventing direct sunlight from ever penetrating to the centre of operations, ensures that any flies that do get into the pit, and their offspring born inside it, can only see one light towards which to navigate when they want to escape — that coming down the vent-pipe. They therefore take that route, find their way barred by the screen and die of dehydration in the warm draught which flows up the pipe.

Need for cheapness

Complete with a plastic vent-pipe supplied by a local manufacturer, this latrine, built with walls either of brick or of concrete cast on site, could cost the average rural users about Z$60 to build for themselves. The next stage of development was directed towards making construction simpler and cheaper.

Aiming at simplicity, a commercial firm began producing a prefabricated version, which was not particularly cheap and not very efficient in use. This firm has done some serious thinking and redesigned its product, so that it now appears to be technically satisfactory.

Looking for cheapness, the Blair laboratory staff produced a cut-price version in 1980, designed to translate the proven design into locally available natural materials. The version built at the research station, which provided their test and demonstration site, and was enthusiastically adopted by the workers there, had a solid floor of thick poles instead of a concrete slab; the vent-pipe was of stout reeds, plastered outside with a cement-sand mixture; the roof was of thatch, and the walls could be of any easily available materials, for instance poles plastered with mud, or brick, or thatch. The only materials that needed to be bought were one bag of cement for Z$3-4 and a piece of plastic-coated fibreglass flyscreen material for 20¢.

Saving the local wood

The workers at this station, in a wooded area, proved effective promoters, but visitors, convinced of the fundamental soundness of the approach, did ask whether a cheap latrine could be built without cutting down so many trees. More thinking and discussion led to the conclusion that most people can afford more than one bag of cement for something as important as a latrine, even if they can't buy it all at once. Now the developers suggest that, if you can only buy one bag of cement in the first year, you use that to make a good concrete slab, saving a little to plaster the vent-pipe. The rest of the structure can be of perishable materials that will be replaced when you can afford something more durable, usually brick. Thatched roofs as a permanent feature are quite popular.

Another simplification in design emerged when the Blair team and a number of rural latrine users realized that the plastic vent-pipe, costing $16 (in 1983 it had reached $20) does not need to be black or round and can just as well be built of brick. A very smart and durable VIP latrine can thus be built with the minimum cash expenditure: most villagers can make their own bricks.

The principles on which the latrine works are now so well known in Zimbabwe (they have even been included in the primary school syllabus) that in many areas expert advice for would-be builders is locally available, often from neighbours who have built their own latrine. Even if many of the 60,000 VIP latrines built to date are now disused due to poor design or faulty materials (for example a flyscreen that does not stand up to the corrosive vapours from the vent-pipe or to strong sunlight), the design has taken off. Many new latrines are being built, and far fewer of these are defective than those built a few years ago.

Variations and developments

Developments continue: a few square VIP latrines are to be seen around the country, and as long as the interior is still as dark as in the spiral form, they are not noticeably less effective. In several districts, it has become normal to build latrines with two cubicles, where it is traditional for men and women, even within the same family, to use separate facilities. While village builders are 'evolving by trial and error' double VIP latrines which meet this demand without losing in performance, Blair's studies of air flow in test latrines point to solutions very similar to those which are developing in the field. For best results, there must be two separate pits, each with its own vent-pipe.

Further development of the technology now seems to be safe in the hands of the users and builders. But we could well ask whether this stage could have been reached without the continuous efforts of the same Blair staff in assisting its development. Many good ideas produced by expatriates on short-term contracts fail to take root because the necessary follow-up depends on successors who do not stand to advance their own careers or reputations by developing somebody else's innovation. The ten years this latrine has needed to gather momentum does not seem too long for the originator to stick with the project if it stands on its own.

(*Waterlines* Vol. 1 No. 4 April 1983)

Why should a latrine look like a house?

BJORN BRANDBERG

Almost from the beginning of the IDWSSD, doubts have been raised about whether it is possible to implement its goals: Safe drinking-water and appropriate sanitation for all by 1990. These doubts have been particularly serious concerning the sanitation targets. At the same time, ventilated improved pit latrines (VIPs), have been advocated as the appropriate sanitation technology for the urban and rural poor.

In 1976, the First National Building Campaign was launched in Mozambique. In a few days, hundreds of thousands of latrines were built all over the country. In quantitative terms, the campaign was very successful: in Maputo today over 90 per cent of households have a latrine.

Few of the latrines built during the campaign looked like those in the manuals. They had no superstructure. The normal design turned out to be a pit covered with poles, scrap material and soil in a fenced-off corner of the housing plot. Unstable soil and high groundwater tables made the latrine building difficult or even impossible in large areas. Other technical difficulties also jeopardized possible health benefits:

O Materials and/or poor design often did not permit cleaning and created breeding places for parasites such as hookworm.
O Wooden structural components in contact with the soil were attacked by rot and termites, so that people were sometimes afraid to use the latrines lest they collapse.
O Non-existent or poorly fitting lids gave free access to flies and cockroaches.

To overcome these problems, especially in peri-urban ('slum') areas where health hazards are most serious, a research and development project was initiated in 1979.

Latrine research

The project started along several lines of enquiry at the same time:
O We surveyed hundreds of latrines to become familiar with existing design and building practices.
O We talked to everybody we could find who knew or had opinions about latrines (and they were many).
O We went through the literature to find suggestions for improvements (and we were impressed by the variety of solutions to solve the problems of how to keep people away from their faeces).
O We built experimental latrines in the actual areas and tried to evaluate them.

The Decade went forward and so did our project, but we found we were going in a different direction from most other countries. In the reports we saw, double pits and ventilated pits became BOTVIPs (in Botswana), ZIMVIPs (in Zimbabwe) and TANVIPs (in Tanzania), while we concentrated our efforts around developing a simple but effective latrine slab.

The VIP latrine design needs a dark 'house' and a screened vent-pipe to control the flies (and the smell inside the house). We had enormous difficulties simply finding building materials for houses for people to live in, let alone to build superstructures for their latrines. More and more reports came in from other countries of latrines with roofs and vent-pipes.

Again and again we asked ourselves the same question: Why should a

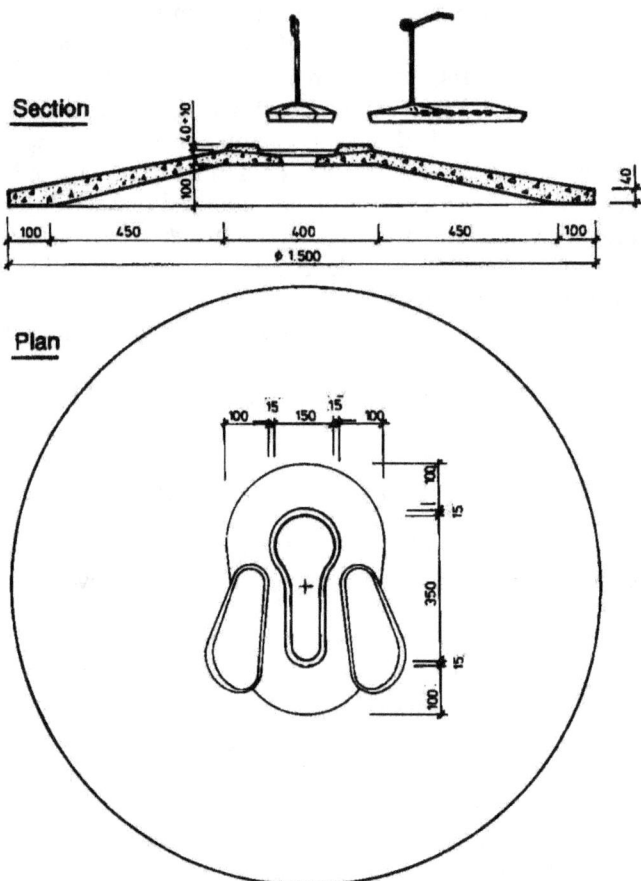

Engineering drawing (above) and technical data of the Mozanbican non-reinforced latrine slab. Dimensions in drawing in millimetres.

Diameter:	1.2-1.5m
Thickness:	40mm
Total height:	100-150mm*
Surface inclination:	1:5-1:6*
Weight:	100-200Kg*
Concrete mixture:	1 + 2 + 1.5 (volume parts of cement, clean river sand and 0.25in coarse stone)
Reinforcement:	None
Surface:	Concrete smoothed with a steel float
Strength:	Each slab is test-loaded with the weight of 6 persons after 7 days minimum curing time
Labour:	0.8 man-days/slab at continuous production
Price in Mozambique	1.5m diameter = 500 Metical (US $12.50)
	1.2m diameter = 400 Metical (US $10.00)

latrine look like a house? Until they built themselves latrines a few years ago, people would defecate anywhere that gave them a minimum of privacy. Fences are now always built to give a private area but it is seldom roofed. A report from Swaziland showed that Swazi peasants had refused latrines because they found it disgusting to defecate indoors.

Tight-fitting lid

Finally, it was the lack of building material that forced us to give up the idea of a roofed superstructure and a vent-pipe. The smell problem was solved by using a tight-fitting lid. There were also doubts about the life-time of the mesh which should top the vent-pipe. If the mesh was broken, it could provide easy access for flies, rather than reducing their numbers.

To control the flies we had introduced a light tight-fitting lid of high quality concrete, cast in the very hole of the slab where it was to fit. We found that this did not only stop the flies but also the smell, as long as it was properly fitted in the hole. And if it was not, the smell was a good reminder to do so.

In comparison with the VIPs, our tight-fitting latrine lid may actually have an advantage: it stops cockroaches. Cockroaches are permanent inhabitants of pit latrines, in large numbers. They normally leave the pit at night, so we doubt if they would be attracted by the light from the vent-pipe and trapped at the top as flies are. But we are sure that they cannot pass our lid, because it is so close-fitting.

Of course, there are developing countries where the urban poor want, and can afford, a latrine with a roof that will protect them from the rain. But we suspect there are many places where VIPs are only affordable if subsidized. Although governments may be prepared to offer subsidies in the context of aid-assisted projects in particular areas, most could never afford to offer them to their entire urban population. Our latrines are affordable and are even a source of income for the members of the co-operatives who make the slabs.

Acceptability tests

Before starting implementation on a large scale, we wanted to test the acceptability of our latrines. We tried with interviews, but got such positive replies that we were afraid to trust them. A more realistic test, we felt, would be to try to sell slabs and complete latrines at their real cost with a reasonable profit margin. Sales were slow in the beginning, but today we have sold 8,000 slabs and a few hundred complete latrines. We have 11 neighbourhood casting yards (9 of these are co-operatives) and the sales are growing more or less continuously. In the areas where our slabs are well known by the population, we sell all the slabs we are able to produce. It has even become normal to have a queue when we start selling the week's production, even if it is raining!

The slabs are adapted to suit the different types of pits in use in Mozambique. In unstable soil, pits may by wider and shallower than normal, lined or unlined, 'bottle' shaped or elevated in areas with a high water-table. Borehole latrines are used in sandy areas with a low water-table.

Manuals and drawings

A detailed description of the technical part of this project has been published by the International Development Research Centre,[68] which also financed a good part of the research and development work. The report includes drawings of the few moulds required and a manual with photographs which also shows step by step how the slabs are produced.

If you try to make our slabs, do not forget to keep the fresh slabs wet during the first week after casting (also over the week-end!). The strength of thin unreinforced concrete depends very much on this curing time.

(*Waterlines* Vol. 3 No.3, January 1985)

Sanitation for rural housing in Sri Lanka

ANDREW COTTON AND RICHARD FRANCEYS

In 1984, Sri Lanka's National Housing Development Authority (NHDA) established the 'Million Houses' project, a programme whereby the village-level community and individual householders become responsible for the provision of housing, with the NHDA assuming a purely supportive role. Individual householders are provided with loans from the NHDA for house-building on the condition that a latrine is constructed if the house does not already have one. Part of the loan may be used for this purpose.

Prior to 1984, household pit latrines were built to standard plans without giving due consideration to the characteristics of the site, an approach which caused many problems and raised important technical and social issues. These issues had to be considered when household sanitation was provided as part of the NHDA's support approach to housing.

Latrine selection

In Sri Lanka, people use water for anal cleansing, and latrines with water-seal bowls have been in use for decades. Basically, there are three types of water-seal latrine (Figure 1); direct and single offset-pit latrines are in

Figure 1. Pit latrine choices.

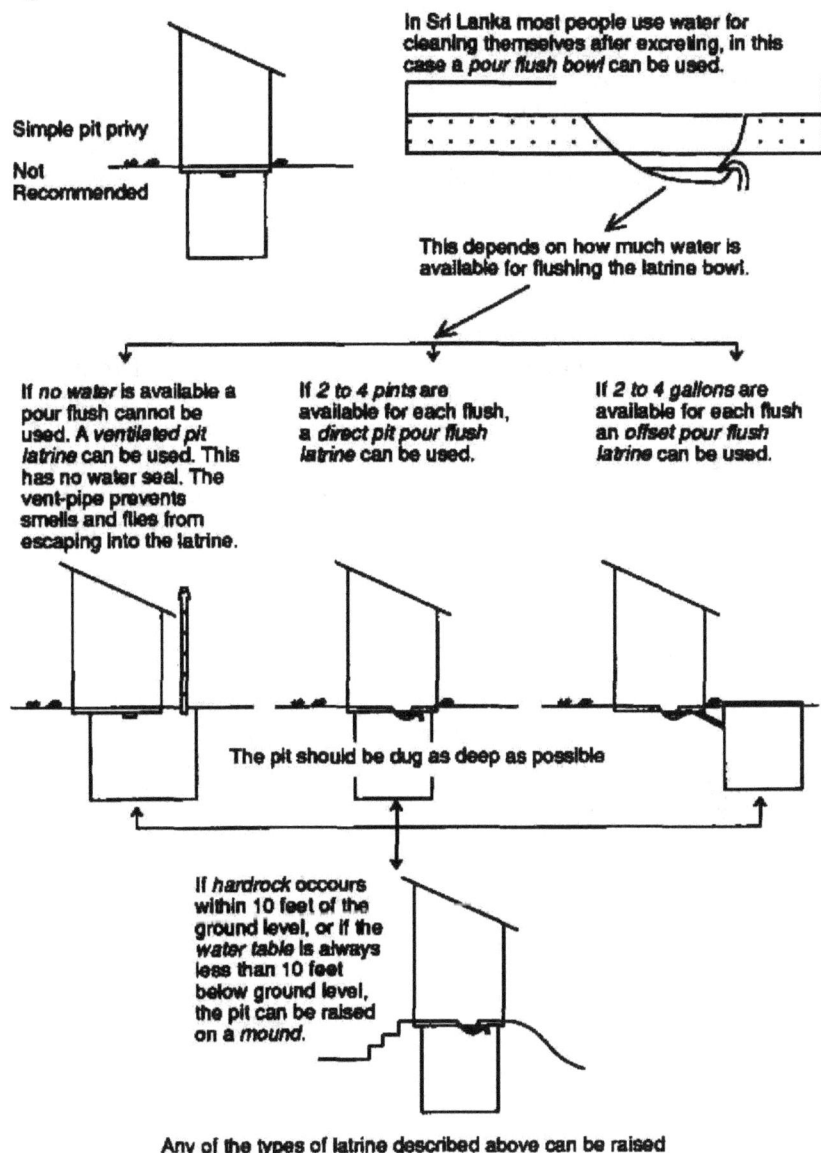

Simple pit privy

Not
Recommended

In Sri Lanka most people use water for
cleaning themselves after excreting, in this
case a *pour flush bowl* can be used.

This depends on how much water is
available for flushing the latrine bowl.

If *no water* is available a
pour flush cannot be
used. A *ventilated pit
latrine* can be used. This
has no water seal. The
vent-pipe prevents
smells and flies from
escaping into the latrine.

If *2 to 4 pints* are
available for each flush,
a *direct pit pour flush
latrine* can be used.

If *2 to 4 gallons* are
available for each flush
an *offset pour flush
latrine* can be used.

The pit should be dug as deep as possible

If *hardrock* occours
within 10 feet of the
ground level, or if the
water table is always
less than 10 feet
below ground level,
the pit can be raised
on a *mound*.

Any of the types of latrine described above can be raised

common use and often have deep pits with a long lifetime, while the
double-pit latrine is a relatively new idea.

With the direct pit, the pit is located directly below the squatting slab and
superstructure. This is probably the cheapest type, but it is difficult to empty
and not socially acceptable as people prefer not to squat directly over the
pit. In the single offset pit, the pit is offset from the slab and connected via a

length of sewer pipe. This is easier to empty when the pit is full, and has been a popular design in Sri Lanka for many years. The double-pit latrine has two offset pits connected to the slab via a 'Y' junction manhole (Figure 2). The sewer leading from the manhole to one of the pits is blocked off until the other pit has filled up; the entrance to the full pit is then closed off at the manhole to enable the empty pit to be used. By the time the second pit has been filled, the contents of the first pit will have decomposed and can be removed safely.

Water requirements

Householders use between one and two litres of water to flush the direct pit latrine. Yet eight to 16 litres are required with the offset-pit latrine as the solids have to be flushed down the length of sewer pipe connecting the bowl to the pit. A family of six might need at least 50 l/d to flush an offset pit, against just 6 l/d to flush a direct pit. It is thus critical to establish whether the local water supply is sufficient to service the proposed latrine, especially since offset-pit latrines have a certain status value in Sri Lanka and are generally preferred.

Figure 2. Double pit latrine (Kalbermatten, 1980)

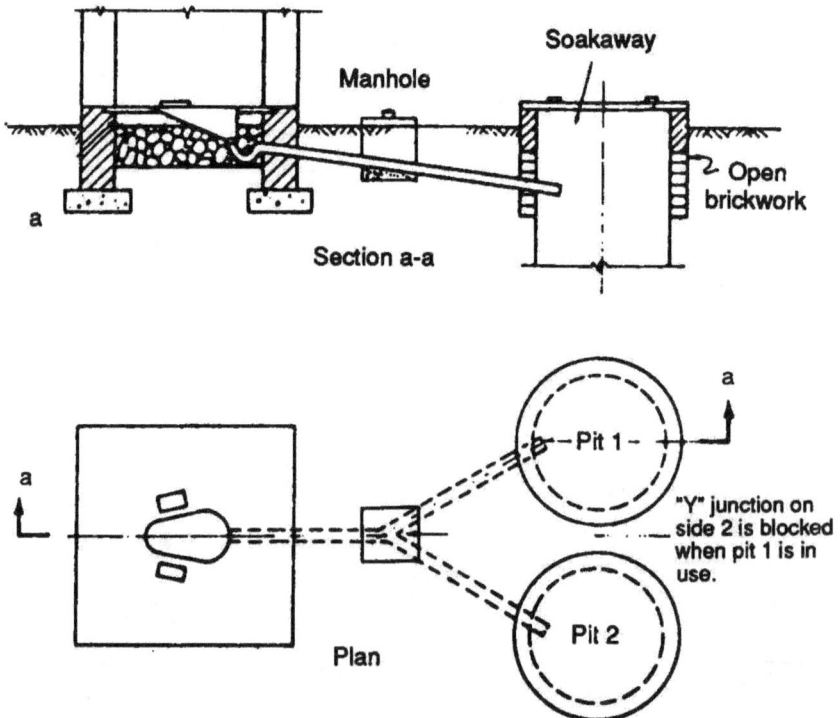

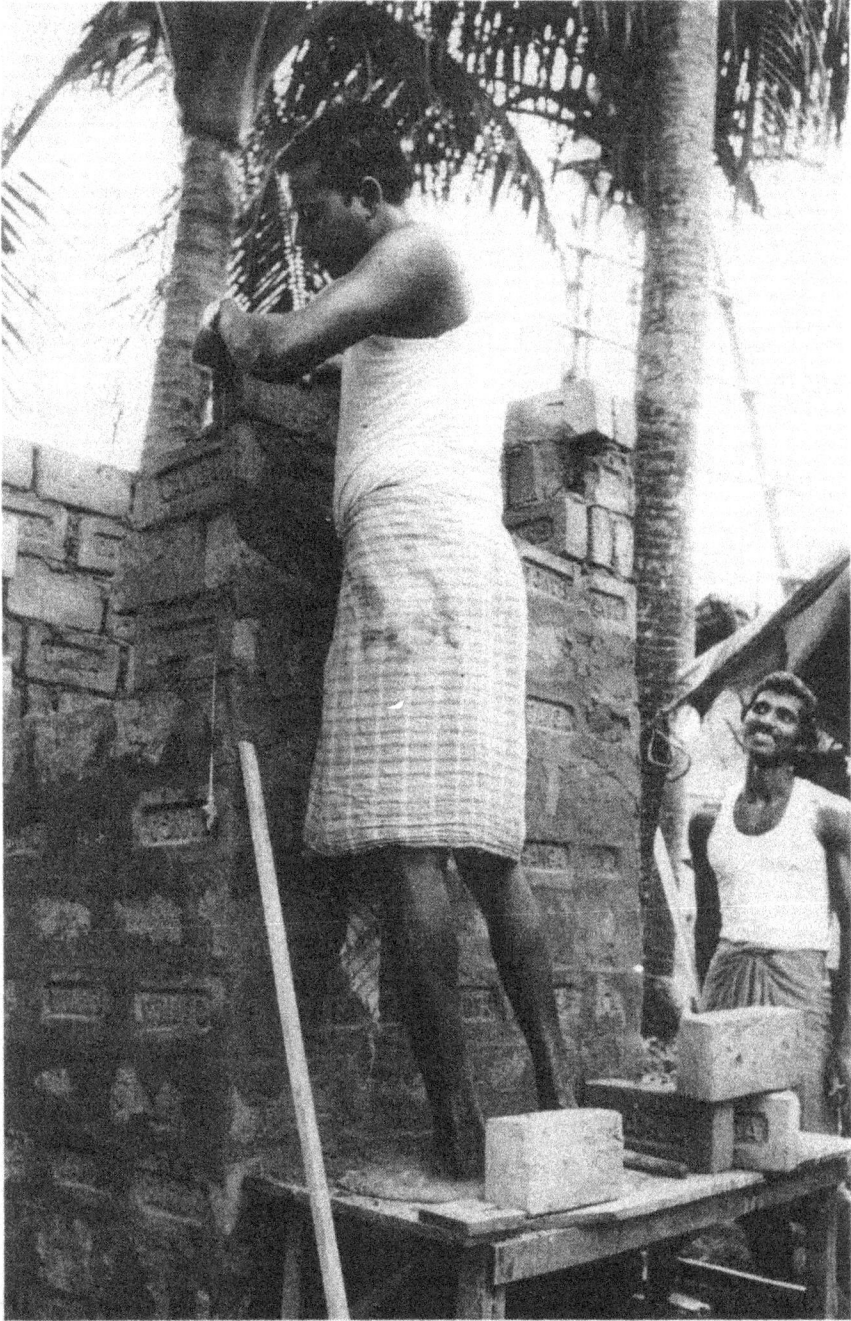

Building a latrine in a village near Calcutta. (WaterAid/Framework)

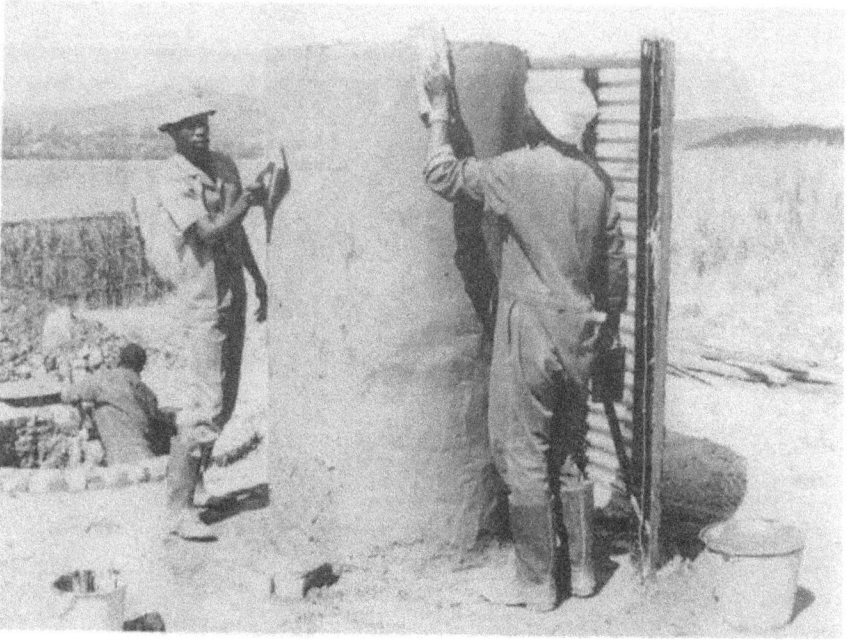

Finishing off a VIP latrine in Zimbabwe. (Blair/ P. Morgan)

A popular rural well in Kanem province, Chad. (UNICEF/Murray-Lee)

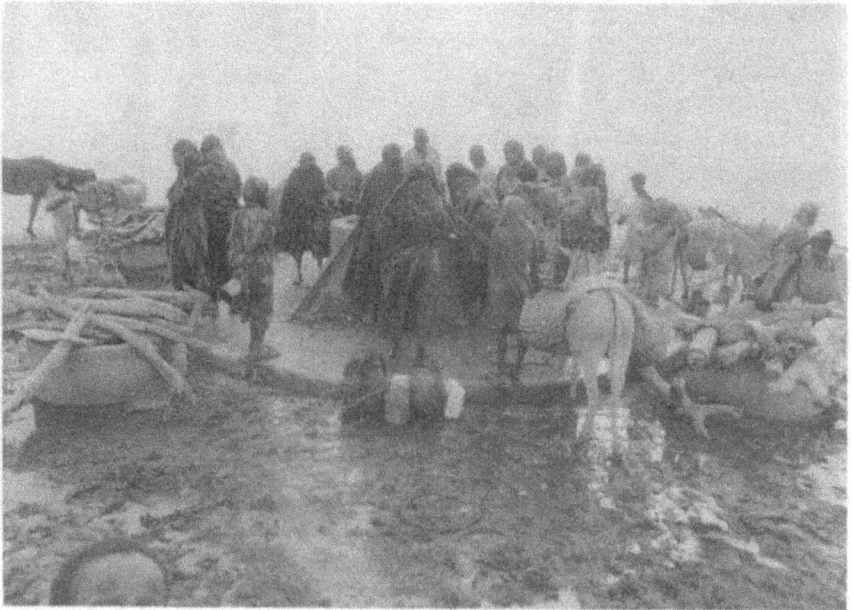

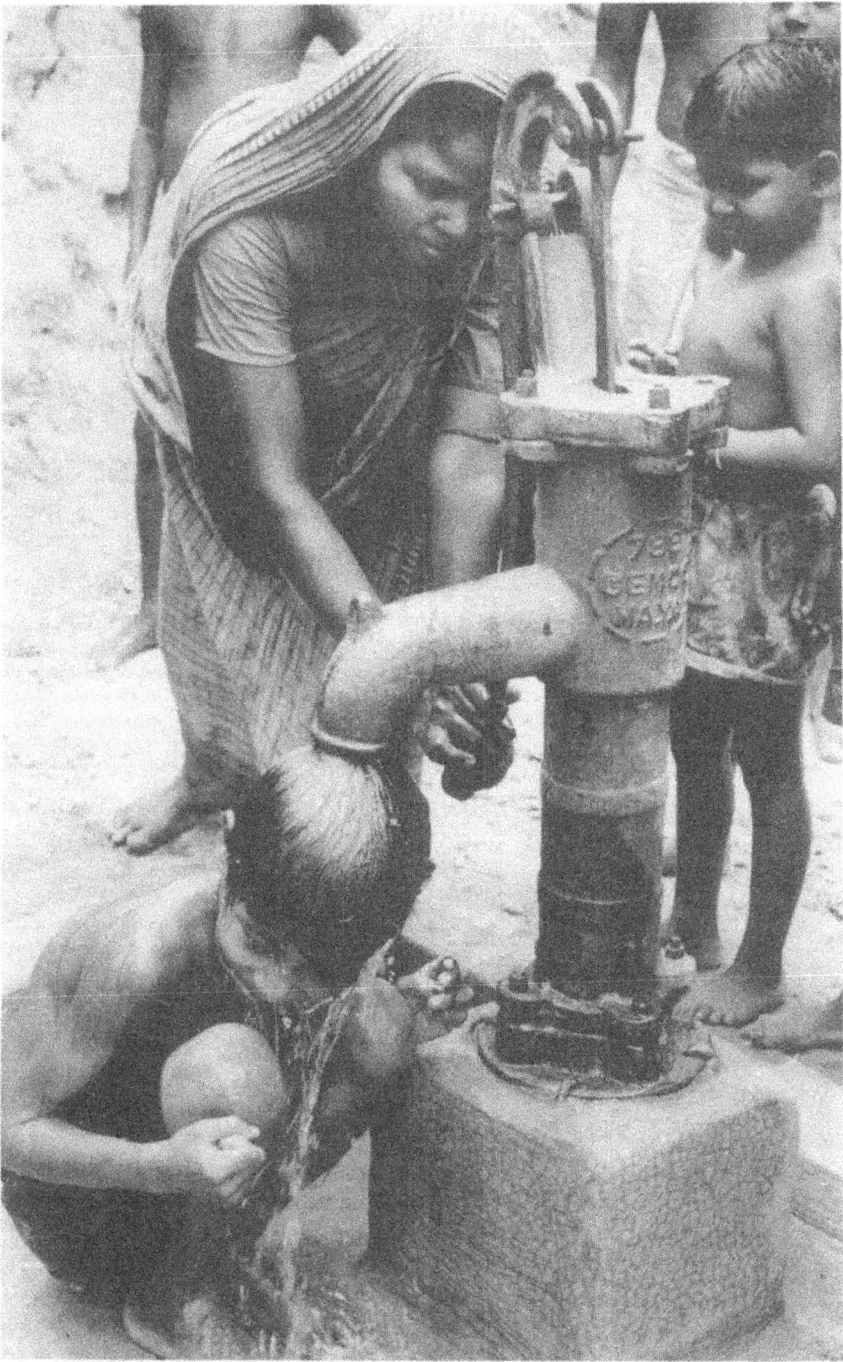

Bathing at the water source in West Bengal. (WaterAid/Framework)

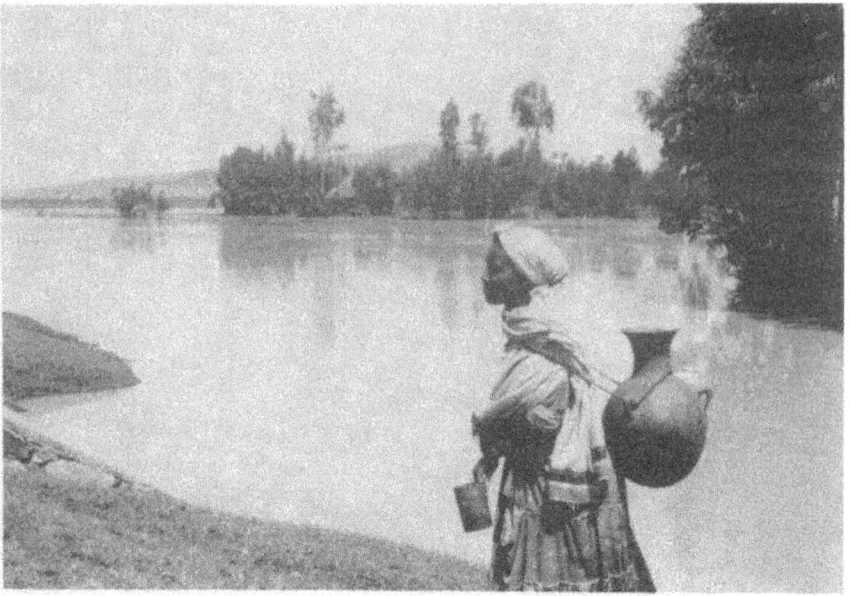

Carrying water in a jar from the dam in Ethiopia.
(WaterAid/Framework)

Kurdish women water-carriers using goatskin bags in Iraq. (WHO)

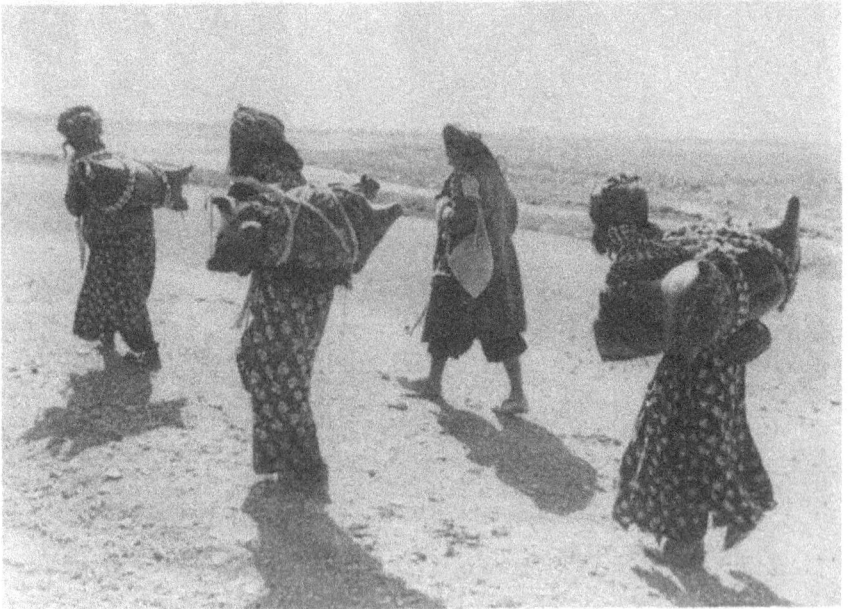

In the dry zones, where water is scarce in the dry season, there is unlikely to be enough available to flush even a direct-pit latrine. In such cases, a ventilated improved pit (VIP) latrine may be an appropriate alternative.[66] Sri Lanka's Ministry of Health advocates the construction of a direct-pit latrine with a removable water-seal bowl. This can be used as normal in the wet season, when water is available; if the latrine incorporates a ventilation pipe, the bowl can be removed during the dry season, allowing it to function as a VIP latrine.

Ground conditions

A deep pit cannot be dug if bed-rock exists near the ground surface or if the water table is permanently high. In such situations, the pit and superstructure can be raised to create a mound latrine. In wet conditions, the whole of the pit will need lining; the inside of the raised portion of the pit should always be rendered to prevent seepage. The double-pit latrine could be feasible in these circumstances, but local experience to date does not recommend it.

A raised shallow pit will need more frequent emptying than a deep pit. If it is assumed that a pit can be dug to a depth of 1.5m, raised a further 1.0m above ground level and is 0.9m square in plan, the expected pit life for five users is nine years in wet conditions, and six years in dry.[67]

In low-lying areas prone to flooding, some householders were uncertain whether the pit would work when full of water. The important factor is to ensure that the latrine slab is raised sufficiently above the expected flood level to permit the latrine to be flushed; water in the pit is necessary to aid the digestion of its contents.

Field experience and problems

Many of the householders with direct-pit or offset-pit latrines had dug pits to a depth of at least 5m. When asked why the pit was so deep, they invariably replied that it was to ensure that the latrine would last for as long as possible (typically 15 to 20 years) before having to be emptied or rebuilt.

The result of a survey of pit latrines on 39 housing sites is shown in

Table 1. Summarized survey data

	Number of sites	Sites with problems	Sites with no problems
Direct pit	9	4	5
Single offset pit	16	5	11
Double pit	11	9	2

No latrines on three sites: at least three houses were studied on each site.

Table 1; faults were found on nine out of 11 sites which had double-pit latrines. Some of the different construction faults included:

O The omission of the splitting manhole.
O The omission of benching in the manhole, causing excreta to be trapped.
O The incorrect use of 'honeycomb' brickwork for the pit walls.

More important perhaps was the widespread lack of understanding by the users of the way in which this type of latrine functions. The most common errors included:

O Not blocking off the entry to one of the pits in the manhole chamber, causing both pits to fill simultaneously.
O A total lack of appreciation of the need to empty the pits at intervals of approximately two years; householders exhibited no enthusiasm for emptying, and were not encouraged by the knowledge that the pit contents could be used as soil manure.

During water-supply and sanitation training workshops held for NHDA staff, it was found that few of the building inspectors understood the operation of the double-pit latrine; it is thus understandable that construction defects occurred. Householders need careful and precise instruction as to how to operate something which is new to them; the staff of NHDA were unable to provide this. If a new technical idea is introduced, it must be complemented by a thorough education programme for users.

The main problem with the offset-pit latrine was the lack of water for flushing; in one case, the direct-pit latrine failed for the same reason. This problem is not limited to the dry zone; the same situation cropped up in the wet zone with houses located high up on hillsides at some distance from a reliable water source down in the valley. People were not prepared to carry up the quantity of water needed to flush the offset-pit. This emphasizes the importance of considering water availablity when selecting latrine types. Other problems with offset- and direct-pits included:

O Too-long sewer lengths, allowing insufficient fall between the superstructure and the pit.
O Subsidence of the superstructure into an unlined pit and flooding in the wet season.

Lessons can be learned by observing existing solutions to well-known problems; the raised pit idea was used 20 years ago by one householder to overcome the problem of a high water-table. The support approach, which allows the householder to make the decision, will usually result in a choice of technology which is understood both by the individual and the local masons. This approach has resulted in far fewer problems with the more recently completed sanitation systems.

Comprehensive staff training

Whilst the introduction of the double-pit latrine was unsuccessful largely because of the lack of 'software' support, the support approach to housing and services requires comprehensive staff training. Thus NHDA staff must fully understand the sanitation options available, and must have access to comprehensive information both for their own use and to enable them to explain the problems and solutions to the householders.

In addition to regular district-level training workshops involving NHDA staff and community leaders, a range of documents has been prepared: a training manual, a check-list for pit-latrine selection and a series of leaflets aimed at householders to illustrate the types of pit latrine available. All this material is fully illustrated, concise, and attempts to avoid the use of jargon in explanations.

Conclusions

The introduction of double-pit latrines to Sri Lanka produced problems due to inadequate construction and the lack of a suitable user-education programme to support the introduction of a new technology. In order to implement sanitation within the context of a 'support approach' housing policy in which householders take the fundamental decisions, it it necessary to have a mechanism of information dissemination and training.

In general, the adoption of a 'support approach' to housing and services has been successful with respect to rural sanitation. Single deep-pit latrines are the preferred option in rural Sri Lanka; where these are not practical, the raised pit can be used. Water availability is critical to pit-latrine selection.

(*Waterlines* Vol. 5 No. 3, January 1987)

Further reading
A.P. Cotton, 'Training manuals for water supply and sanitation', WEDC/NHDA Reports, 1985.

The performance of aquaprivies in Thai refugee camps

ROBIN BIELLIK AND
PEGGY HENDERSON

A conventional aquaprivy consists of a squat plate with a drop-pipe making a water seal directly into a small septic tank underneath. Anaerobic digestion of the faecal material takes place in the tank, and excess effluent is drained off into a nearby seepaway (also called 'soakage pit'). To function properly, the septic tank must be water-tight, and the water seal where the pipe empties into the tank must be maintained. Variations include an aquaprivy which can accept household wastewater, and the sewered aquaprivy, where effluent flows directly into a sewage system

The sludge, which accumulates in the septic tank after partial breakdown of the faecal matter, must be periodically removed. During the normal use of a family-sized tank, desludging will be necessary only every few years.[69] When properly maintained, surface soil and water are protected from contamination, and there should be minimal nuisance from flies and odour.[70]

In practice, however, the aquaprivy has not always been successfully employed. In most cases this is because users have failed to maintain the water seal because not enough water is regularly flushed into the tank. This may have occurred where a water supply was not located close enough to the aquaprivy, or where there was reluctance, for cultural reasons, to carry water into the toilet.[71] When the water seal is not maintained, mosquitoes and flies breed in the privy creating a health hazard, and odour becomes a problem. In other cases, disposal of the liquid effluent into the soil failed, so that the seepaway required frequent mechanical emptying.[15] The drop-pipe may also become clogged, where solid materials are used for anal cleansing.

Aquaprivies were invented in India in the early 1900s.[72] They have subsequently been used in many countries in Asia, and their application appears to be successful in that continent.[15] Aquaprivies have been installed in several African countries, including Botswana, Nigeria, Tanzania and Zimbabwe, with mixed results.[71] Some aquaprivies were constructed in the West Indies in the 1950s and 1960s, with good public acceptance.[73] Aquaprivies appear to have been used most satisfactorily where water is used for anal cleansing, daily washing of the toilet bowl is practised, and the soil beneath is sufficiently permeable to absorb all effluent.

Aquaprivies were originally applied in Palestinian refugee camps in the Middle East as communal facilities,[70] and were subsequently adopted in Bengali refugee camps in India and for displaced persons in Bangladesh. While regarded as fairly successful in these situations,[74] their brick construction was too time-consuming to make them operational in large numbers.

Aquaprivies in Thailand

A new type of aquaprivy was adopted for use in the holding centres for Kampuchean refugees in Thailand established after October, 1979, following the Vietnamese overthrow of the Kampuchean government. The purpose of the present paper is to document the lessons learned concerning the Thai aquaprivies after over two years of field operation. To collect detailed information, the authors administered an extensive questionnaire to all sanitarians working in Khmer holding centres during March-April, 1982.

Khmer refugees were interned at several holding centres in eastern Thailand, where the combined population peaked at approximately 163,000 in early 1980. As well as providing a complex array of other services, the United Nations High Commissioner for Refugees (UNHCR) adopted the aquaprivy to take care of camp sanitation. A Thai manufacturer developed the 'Zeptik' glassfibre-reinforced plastic aquaprivy, and a total of 979 units were installed in five holding centres.

Zeptik unit design

Each Zeptik unit was designed for daily use by 80 persons. The units consisted of a centrally vented septic tank with a total volume of 4m^3, surmounted by four squat plates. Many aquaprivies were modified after installation to incorporate cheap, simple, external urinals to resolve the problems of corrosion and odours occasioned by males urinating on the exterior of the toilet sheds.

Individual seepaway systems incorporating submerged tanks made of concrete rings and four-cubicle toilet sheds were constructed. An integrated site plan was adopted for the five camps, consisting of self-contained, inward-facing quadrangles designed to encourage

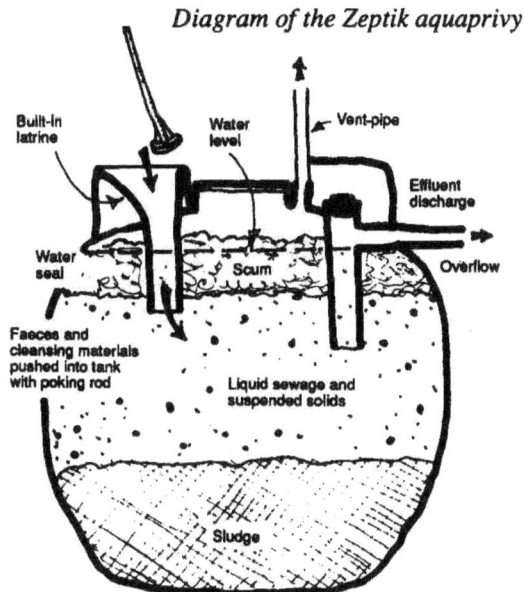

Diagram of the Zeptik aquaprivy

Built-in latrine

Water level

Vent-pipe

Effluent discharge

Water seal

Scum

Overflow

Faeces and cleansing materials pushed into tank with poking rod

Liquid sewage and suspended solids

Sludge

normal social interactions among refugee families. The distance to the toilets from the most distant houses never exceeded 50m. Each Zeptik unit, complete with seepaway and toilet shed, cost approximately US$1,300 to install in 1980.

On average, each aquaprivy required approximately 300 litres of water per day for maintaining the water seal and for cleaning. Such large quantities of water are available in most of Thailand and most other humid tropical zones throughout the developing countries.

However, these same regions tend to be associated with high rainfall, high water-tables, land with minimal slope, and low-permeability soils that flood easily. Eastern Thailand is no exception. Effluent disposal designs that function adequately under these conditions are available in the sanitary engineering literature.[69,70,74] Unfortunately, UNHCR underestimated the need to design the aquaprivy seepaways in accordance with the results of soil percolation tests. Many seepaways failed to drain adequately the 300-500 litres of aqueous effluent produced daily and subsequently overflowed, especially during the monsoon season.

UNHCR provided pump trucks with which to desludge aquaprivies mechanically in rotation about once every three months, and transferred the sludge into sedimentation-oxidation ponds located at a short distance from each camp. To counter the design failure in the short term, the pump trucks were assigned the additional task of emptying seepaways every three to five days. In some locations, sanitarians modified some seepaways with deeper gravel soakage pits, or linked others to a central lagoon collection system or raised filter beds. The accelerated pumping operation and additional engineering work incurred unexpected costs requiring additional UNHCR funding.

Acceptance and sustainability

The Khmers generally accepted the aquaprivies well, and largely observed the public education messages spread through health-sector relief agencies about normal maintenance and hygiene. Wherever the use of individual locks on toilet doors established family privacy, quadrangle residents were reported to maintain high standards of cleanliness inside the toilet sheds.

Surprisingly, public education promoting the maintenance of hygienic conditions and prevention of damage was not adequate in all camps. Some refugees used solid or non-degradable materials for anal cleansing and also to empty the down-pipe, including paper, plastic sticks, wire and stones. These materials occasionally combined to clog the squat plates and effluent discharge pipes, or to cause damage to the pumping equipment when the privies were emptied. Where adequate water was available, however, these problems occurred less frequently.

Dampness and urine rusted away the bottoms of many of the walls of the original toilet sheds. A number were later modified to ventilate the interior, but this in turn permitted easier access to flies and mosquitoes.

Sanitarians reported that, in at least one camp, acidic vented gases seriously corroded roofs in the vicinity of the vent-pipe. The vent-pipes incorporated a curve, which frequently clogged with scum and caused a great increase in gas production at the squat plates. Sanitarians also complained that the central man-hole was rendered inaccessible since the toilet sheds' four internal walls intersected immediately above it. Desludging therefore had to be conducted through one of the squat plates instead of the man-hole, as intended.

Conclusions

Under emergency conditions, the Zeptik aquaprivy performed well as a primary sewage treatment facility. Sanitarians agreed that the cultural acceptability of these toilets among Khmers was excellent; adults even used them to urinate, which is not always the case in south-east Asia. A few young children continued to defecate indiscriminately in the camps, but this group of offenders is habitual! The aquaprivies owed much of their acceptability to their close proximity to the users, in addition to good maintenance encouraged by private responsibility for the facilites.

Funding

The UNHCR relief operation for Khmer refugees in Thailand has been described as one of the most generously funded programmes of its kind ever mounted. [75,76] Resources were therefore available to permit the adoption of a relatively expensive sanitation system requiring high renewable inputs of water and maintenance. The glassfibre-reinforced plastic units had the advantage that they were transportable between construction site and installation, were durable and non-corrosive, and theoretically could be relocated if camps were moved at short notice.

The major deficiencies in the overall sanitation system related to engineering problems concerning the seepaways and toilet sheds. Most of these problems were resolved in situ by the introduction of practical modifications employing common designs available to the camp sanitarians.

Recently, authors have recommended against the aquaprivy as a viable sanitation option in most situations, since there are technically superior systems available now at lower cost. [69]

The authors of this article support the contention that aquaprivies are probably not suitable for permanent widespread use in developing countries on the grounds that they are expensive, and are accompanied by a high input of water and maintenance not required by many other systems.

•This article is an abbreviated version of one that appeared in Disasters 6(3):222-230; 1982. Reprints can be obtained form INTERTECT, PO Box 10502, Dallas, Texas 75207, USA.

(*Waterlines* Vol. 3 No. 1, July 1984)

Developing designs for toilets: the case of the Maldives

DEEPA NARAYAN-PARKER

Water-supply and sanitation problems for those living on small coral islands are unique. The Maldive Islands, south-west of Sri Lanka in the Indian Ocean, are a case in point. In the Maldives, human life is made possible by a thin lens-shaped body of fresh water derived entirely from accumulated rainfall, lying just below the surface of the island. Protecting this small reservoir against salt contamination from the sea and from organic pollution from above is of vital importance for continued human habitation.

Traditionally, Maldivians lived on the periphery of the islands, using the beach for defecation and drawing water for drinking and cooking from one or two public wells in the centre of the island. Increasing population pressure and the introduction of coral and lime masonry, however, brought about two changes which disrupted the precarious water supply situation.

Coral and lime masonry made it possible for individual households to build permanent shallow wells, within their compounds. This greatly increased fresh water consumption for all purposes. The fact that more people lived away from the beach also made it inconvenient to go there for defecation. Crowding on the islands also resulted in the beach space that could be set aside for defecation purposes being greatly diminished. These factors resulted in the emergence of two alternative excreta-disposal systems, both of which pollute and/or deplete the limited groundwater.

One was burying human waste within the walled washing area of the compound, knowns as the *gifili*. The waste is buried in the loose sand, and water for washing is obtained from the well in the compound. Due to the proximity of the groundwater to the surface and the porosity of the soil, pathogens rapidly percolate and contaminate the fresh water lens below the surface.

The second excreta-disposal system, used by wealthier households, was conventional flush toilets connected to either soakpits or sewers. Soakpits inject the waste directly into the ground water lens. Sewers generally work poorly, because the elevation of the island above the ocean is not sufficient to give a great enough gradient to move sewage in the pipes. Sewer leaks pollute the groundwater. But potentially worse, a system using waterborne sewerage rapidly depletes the aquifer by discharging wastewater directly into the sea.

Faced with these difficulties and financial constraints, the Government of Maldives undertook a programme to provide public toilets on each island. The programme was initiated in the mid-1970s with financial help fom the United Nations Capital Development Fund (UNCDF) and the United Nations Children's Fund (UNICEF), and with technical support from WHO.

Each public toilet consisted of a block of five cubicles with water-seal squat toilets, discharging waste directly into the sea. Water for washing and cleaning was obtained from a shallow well located in a compound outside the toilets. To overcome excreta-disposal problems, all the public toilets were located on the beach, so that the water used for flushing was saline and the fresh water lens was not affected. The short distance to the sea meant that the gradient was sufficient for a sewer to work. The toilets were to be constructed by the communities themselves using coral and lime masonry. All imported materials were provided by the Government.

Survey of attitudes

By 1983, it became evident to Government officials that the public toilets were not being used as planned. Still faced with the need to provide sanitary facilities, the Maldives Ministry of Health commissioned a three-month study in early 1984, to investigate the entire question of environmentally safe and socially acceptable toilets. The study was funded by the UNDP-WHO Water Decade Advisory Service Project.

Several different techniques were used to evaluate the project and to find out people's attitudes towards different excreta-disposal systems. They were:

O Interviews with 228 adults (114 men and 114 women) using questions that did not predetermine their answers.
O Meetings with local committees.
O Discussion of models of toilets with interchangeable parts in group meetings.
O Interviews with key informants.
O Observation of public toilets to see how much they were used and to rate their physical condition using two structured formats.

O Informal household visits.
O Review of written records and plans.

Field work was done during a two-week period, involving a visit by the study team to the five islands included in the survey. The team included six family and community health workers who were trained in data collection techniques, and a foreign social scientist who worked through an interpreter, myself.

All five islands surveyed were crowded, with little of the beach left for defecation purposes. The population ranged from 400 to 3,127 people. Each island had built two blocks of community toilets. Despite the lack of adequate beach space, 50 per cent of the population were still using the beach for defecation. Thirteen per cent used the *gifilis*. Private flush toilets were used by 18 per cent, while the community toilets were used by 16 per cent. The remaining 3 per cent used a variety of facilities including the sea and *divehi phakanas* (Maldivian toilets) which are built over the sea.

Assessing acceptability

The underlying philosophy guiding the case study was that, in order to understand the problems with the public toilets and to consider alternative designs for the future, it would be necessary to first understand people's satisfactions and dissatisfactions associated with all the existing sanitation options. Thus to be acceptable in the Maldivian context, toilets would have to incorporate features that provided satisfactions associated with using the beach and *gifili* and eliminate the dissatisfactions or problems associated with them.

People had no difficulty in describing specific, concrete advantages and disadvantages in using the beach for defecation. The major advantages of using the beach were that it was available at all times, it was close to water for washing (a reason given by 19 per cent of the sample), it was a pleasant environment to be in (15 per cent), and that they did not have to clean the beach as they did *gifilis* or toilets (11 per cent). As well as the 16 per cent who said that there were no advantages in using the beach, however, another 22 per cent said that they used the beach because no other alternative was available.

More importantly, all but 18 of 228 people interviewed spoke of problems in using the beach for defecation. Most of the problems were related to lack of privacy, space and safety (due to rocky shorelines). Other less frequently-mentioned problems were the unhygienic and unhealthy state of the defecation beaches and their distance from home.

Thus in the Maldives it is not true to say people avoided the public toilets because they had always used the beach for defecation.

The perceived advantages of *gifilis* for defecation were their privacy (21 per cent), and their convenience and proximity to the home, especially during illness and at night (13 per cent). However, *gifilis* were not used for defecation by most people if other facilities were available, and in fact were valued mainly for purposes other than defecation. People valued them for washing and bathing (35 per cent of sample), and for storing firewood or growing plants (13 per cent). The islands are crowded and *gifilis* are small. If they are used regularly for defecation, they quickly become dirty and smelly.

These findings have important implications for toilet design. If toilet designs are to incorporate the positive features of beaches and *gifilis* and eliminate the negative features, they should offer privacy, and be located close to people's homes. There should be a sufficient number of toilets, so that they are available when needed. They should be safe to use and result in sanitary disposal of faeces. Toilets should be attractive and easy to clean and use, with easy and private access to water for washing clothes and bathing.

Public toilets

Existing public toilets did not fulfil the above criteria. Most people were able to describe both advantages of and problems with the existing public toilets. The most frequently-mentioned advantage was the privacy offered by public toilets. The other major advantage was simply their availability in the absence of other options such as the beach, *gifili* and private toilets.

Thus, people seemed to be using the toilets not because they wanted to use them, but because they were the least undesirable of the options. People mentioned several disadvantages of the public toilets. The major problem was lack of cleanliness caused by there being too few toilets, or people's indifference to looking after them, lack of privacy in fetching the water from outside and lack of buckets in which to fetch the water. Other problems mentioned were distance from the home, the lack of doors or broken doors that tended to stick, lack of light, and waste pipes that were too short or broken. In addition, some people felt that the individual cubicles needed to be much larger and not completely enclosed.

Although some improvements could be made in the existing design to overcome the problems above, they would not be able to solve the main problem: lack of water inside the cubicle, and privacy. The ideal solution was to provide water inside individual cubicles, however this was impossible with the existing design without resorting to piping water from overhead storage tanks.

In addition, any public toilet was seen to have disadvantages compared with individual or private facilities. Thus, although inconvenience can be minimized by building a large number of toilets, it cannot be eliminated.

Problems such as cleanliness, maintenance and broken buckets still need to be tackled.

The Maldives have a strong tradition of community participation, including reclaiming land, building schools, mosques, island offices and jetties. Typically, this includes collecting coral and sand for construction, as most construction is based on coral masonry, all on the people's own initiative — until 10 years ago, the islands had very little contact with the outside world.

Although the public toilets programme was to have been implemented using a Community Education and Participation (CEP) approach, this had not been done when constructing the toilets. The communities had not participated in decision-making at any stage, although they did collect materials. Only one island, which had not been on the official list to receive toilets, had organized voluntary labour to complete toilet construction. On all the other islands, communities had been paid varying sums for skilled labour, eventually. However, the irregularity of the payments further compounded the construction problems and resulted in more delays and disagreements. These problems could be overcome by adopting a CEP approach tailored to fit the toilet programme in the Maldivian context.

Options for appropriate toilets

We came up with three main options for providing appropriate toilets in the atolls of the Maldives. These are: public toilets with a central well, improved toilets built over the sea, and dry private toilets.

Public toilets with a central well

In response to complaints about access to water, small cubicles, insufficient light and air and doors which stick, a small model of a new design developed by WHO was taken out to the atolls. This extends the traditional usage of wells in *gifilis* and consists of four large cubicles built around a central well on the beach, where the water is salty. Thus, each cubicle has private access to water but the fresh water lens is not depleted.

Everywhere people liked the basic design. The model was presented to people with optional doors, roofs and seats that could be manipulated in various ways. This allowed discussion of many options and resulted in clear preferences emerging for most options. For example, everywhere people wanted a roof. Some wanted the roof to be constructed in two parts, while others wanted a central hole or sky-light. On these small, crowded islands, it would be difficult to provide sufficient communal toilets of this type, because of the shortage of space on the beach.

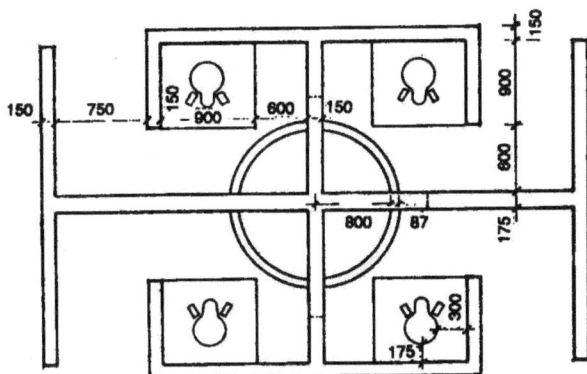

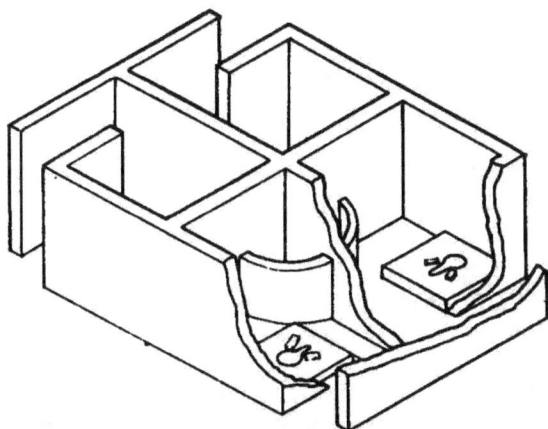

Partial or complete roof and addition of
doors to be determined by island
residents

*Sketch of a public toilet block with a central well; plan and cutaway
drawings.*

Improved *divehi phakhanas*

When Maldivians are asked if there is a traditional Maldivian toilet, the
answer is generally 'no'. However, there is one type of toilet called the
divehi or *jholi phakhana* that is nearly Maldivian. It is believed to have been
introduced to Male, the capital, by Indian traders in the 1940s and eventually found its way to the atolls.

It is built on a log pier extending 0.6-2.0m out into the sea. The end
consists of a log platform with a central hole for defecation. The walls are

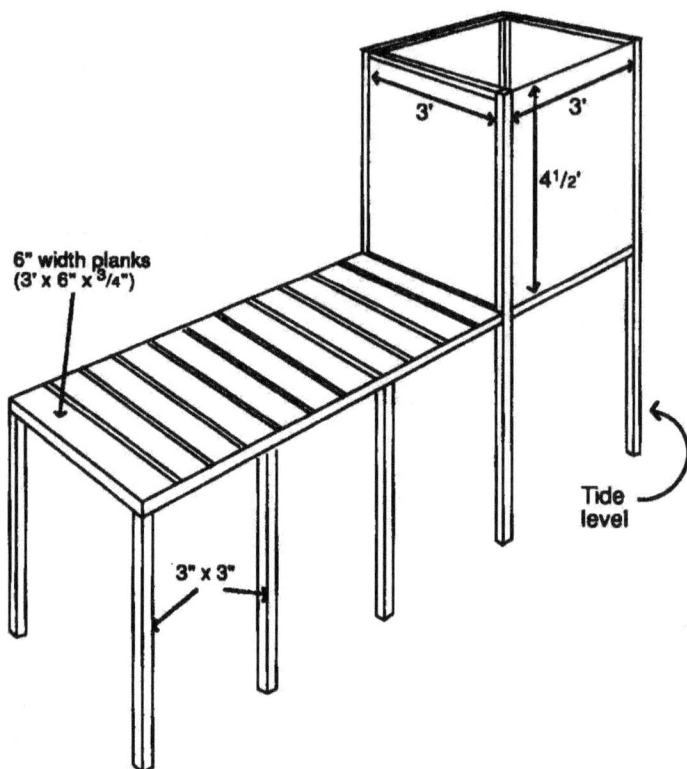

Sketch of a divehi phakhana toilet, *built on a pier over the sea so that excreta are washed away by the tide.*

waist high and there is no roof. Water for washing is obtained by lowering a rope tied to a bucket into the sea prior to defecation. The action of the tide carries the waste away.

This type of toilet was viewed as an acceptable solution to sanitation problems by communities in these crowded islands. It is practically maintenance-free, and easy and quick to build. It gets rid of waste without having to use pipes. On some islands, *divehi phakhanas* built by individuals are more heavily used than the public toilets.

Dry private toilets

While everyone appreciated the concept of public toilets, all strongly preferred private toilets. When asked why, only one person of the hundreds interviewed said that he wanted a toilet because it was 'modern' and therefore good. All the rest were able to give specific detailed reasons for wanting private toilets.

The reasons were similar to the advantages of community toilets

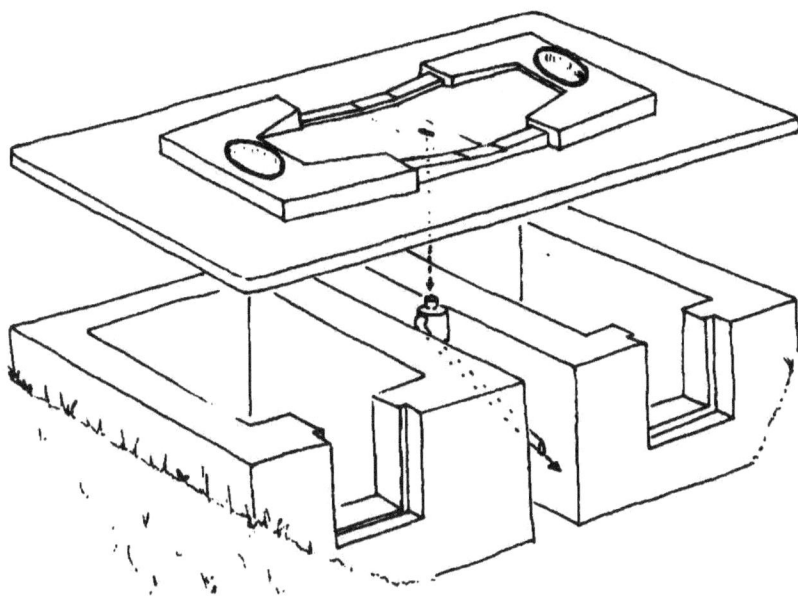

'Ash' toilet, a dry composting toilet. The two vaults are used alternately and urine is drained away.

compared with traditional arrangements. However, they emphasized the convenience, constant availability, privacy and safety factors. The biggest perceived advantage of private toilets was that they could be used during illness and diarrhoea in privacy. Additionally, it was felt that private toilets would not have so many problems with cleanliness and maintenance as the community toilets.

If people were so convinced about the desirability of private toilets, why did they not build more? We found that the major constraint was financial, not the lack of physical space. Conventional flush toilets cost more than most people could afford.

In the light of people's desire for a private toilet, the unsuitability of flush toilets and limited financial resources, there is a need for socially acceptable, technically sound, low-cost private toilets. Currently, two models have reached their final experimental stages.

One is a modified Vietnamese Ash toilet, developed by the International Human Assistance Programme (IHAP), and is known in the Maldives as the 'Ash' toilet. It is a double vault composter that requires daily addition of wood ash to the waste. The vaults are used alternately, one receiving faeces while the other filled vault is sealed off for composting. Each vault is designed to be cleaned out and reused every six months.

The second type of dry toilet is an extended term composter designed by

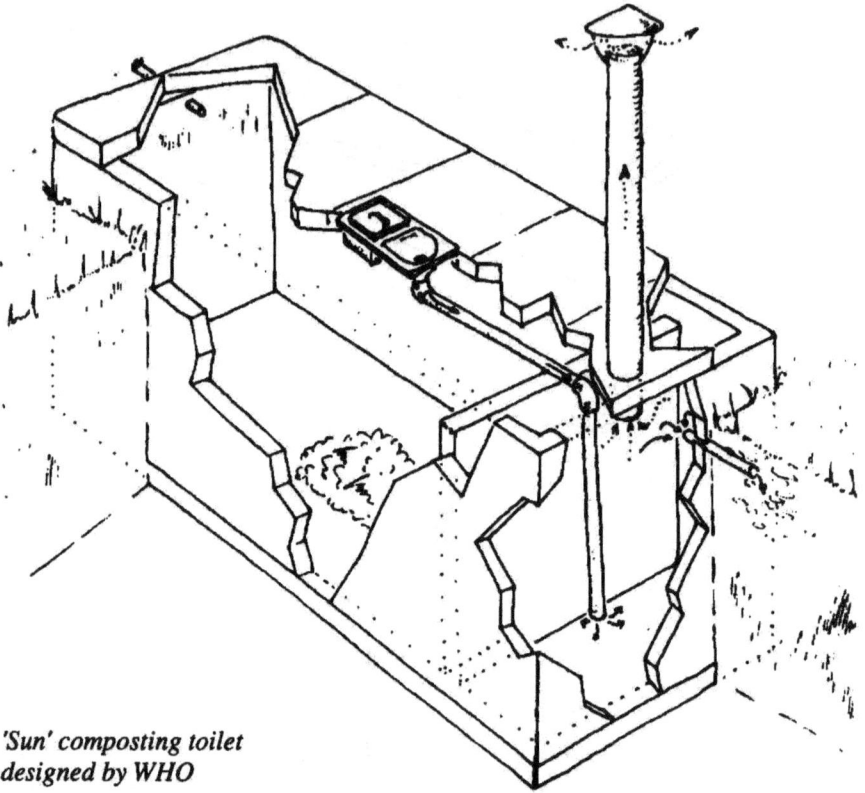

*'Sun' composting toilet
designed by WHO*

the WHO to last 15 to 20 years. After this, it is either cleaned out or abandoned. This toilet has come to be called the 'Sun' toilet locally. Both the 'Ash' and the 'Sun' toilets have sealed vaults to receive the solid material. In the case of the Ash toilet, the urine is drained to nearby vegetation. In the Sun toilet, it first passes through an anaerobic upflow filter, which assists in removing pathogens.

Conclusions

No engineering textbook will ever include toilet designs appropriate for every region in every country. Engineers in rural areas must work closely with the users in evolving toilet designs most appropriate in that particular environment. In the Maldives, the sanitation needs of all island people, rich and poor, can be satisfied by a mixture of improved public toilets and dry private toilets.

Further reading

Deepa Narayan-Parker, *Case study on community attitudes towards public and private latrines*, Maldives Water and Sanitation Authority, Ministry of Health, Government of Maldives, WHO Project: ICP CWS 003, May 1984.

(*Waterlines* Vol. 4 No. 2, October 1985)

CHAPTER 7

Other Sanitation

Sanitation comprises not only toilets but also waste disposal, drainage and public health (or hygiene) measures. The articles for this chapter have been selected to give some idea of different measures involved.

Jeremy Lumbers and Bob Andoh of London Imperial College comment on some myths behind the science of the design of waste-stabilization ponds. These ponds are widely used for wastewater treatment because they are simple to construct and require minimum maintenance, since little or no mechanical equipment is involved. They should be designed for the specific site conditions, and maintenance manuals should be provided.

John Ashworth brings out the problems of urban sullage in developing countries based on his experience in Tanzania and indicates some solutions, both engineering and sociological.

The question of using night-soil to produce biogas in digesters is discussed by Peter-John Meynell. This could offer not only safe disposal but also a valuable energy source. But he also highlights the pitfalls and complications, including social taboos, which have prevented widespread implementation outside China. In a subsequent article in Waterlines (April 1988) on the treatment of night-soil by biogas digesters in China, Zhao Xihui stated that, by August 1987, some 5 million family digesters had been built with a marked improvement in sanitary conditions in rural areas.

James Muir reports on the success of a community-based drain-building project in northern Pakistan, which produced some remarkable changes in the lives of villagers. This was a simple scheme requiring little finance.

The article from the Press Trust of India reports how the Vector Control Research Centre has virtually wiped out mosquito infestation in Pondicherry in just five years, thanks to a huge sanitation drive involving drain cleaning, chlorination and screening of septic tanks, and action on other breeding sites.

Bill Wood discusses simple sanitary construction to improve food storage and preparation techniques and other hygiene routines in remote African villages. This is based on his 20 years overseas experience. He was chief engineer for North Nigeria and chief of the Community Water Supply Unit of the WHO, based in Geneva.

Waste stabilization pond design: some myths behind the science

JEREMY LUMBERS AND BOB ANDOH

Waste stabilization ponds are one of the most simple forms of wastewater treatment requiring minimal maintenance, little or no mechanical equipment and basic construction techniques. They have found wide application in many countries and have been used in one form or another in most countries in the world.

Stabilization ponds are simply shallow lagoons in which the wastewater is held for a long period. Often a number of ponds in series are required to provide adequate treatment. Each pond in the series should be divided into at least two 'streams', so that treatment can continue during periodic desludging.

Ponds are best used in hot climates where wastewater needs shorter retention times. It is a fortunate coincidence of nature that it is in such climates that the problems of water/wastewater-related diseases are often the greatest and that ponds provide a better removal of pathogenic organisms than other more complex processes such as activated sludge and biological filtration, unless tertiary treatment and heavy chlorination is used as well.

The treatment mechanisms in ponds are well understood in principle. However, due to the complexity of the interactions of these mechanisms, design methods have not been able to take into account all the factors. This is not to argue against the use of ponds but rather to emphasize the need for caution when calculating the size of the ponds. The most common mistake is to build them too large.

It is not the objective of this article to make a detailed review of pond design, but to comment on some myths behind the science of facultative waste stabilization pond design. Pond design procedures are reviewed in references[77,78,79] and elsewhere. These common errors include:

O Basing the design on data from the coldest months of the year.
O Considering only the aerobic zone of the pond in design, and neglecting the bacterial activity in the sludge at the bottom of the pond.
O Believing that reducing the BOD (biochemical oxygen demand) of the effluent is the objective of treatment, whereas it is pathogen removal which is most important. BOD removal may not, in fact, be a very good indicator of pathogen removal.
O Using a regression analysis on graphs of BOD removal versus loading.
O Including counts of algae in the analysis of effluent BOD and suspended solids, when they have nothing to do with organic pollution.

Research at Imperial College, London, UK, is being directed at improving design methods for evaluating performance, taking into account the factors listed above, and their interaction. The techniques employed are sophisticated systems analysis methods such as recursive parameter estimation, but the final product will be an easy-to-use microcomputer software package.

Once a pond system has been designed and constructed, its subsequent performance relies largely on natural factors such as:

O Sunlight (solar radiation)
O Wind action (mixing and surface aeration)
O Temperature (aerobic and anaerobic biological activity)
O Rainfall and evaporation (affecting actual retentions time)

Other factors, such as limiting toxic industrial wastes in the wastewater to levels which do not inhibit treatment, can be controlled indirectly.

Being dependent on natural phenomena, which vary with the seasons of the year, it is clear that designs should consider the effect of seasonal factors and include them where necessary. Most workers have assumed that ponds perform worst at the coldest time of year.

Worst conditions?

The data plots in Figure I (bottom two lines on the graphs) clearly show that the worst performance in terms of BOD removal does not always occur in the coldest or warmest months. For example, looking at the bottom two lines of the plot on the left, the worst performance does correspond to the coldest periods, whereas for the one on the right there is no major variation in performance with the seasons.

Rather than using data from the coldest month when designing the pond, there are some phenomena which would argue for the hottest months to be considered the critical ones, as it is then that:

O The bacterial activity is fastest.
O The interchange between the sludge and the liquid layers is greatest.
O The dissolved oxygen in the pond is lowest.

Almost all approaches to design concentrate on the upper levels of the pond, where dissolved oxygen is present for only part of the day and where soluble materials are oxidized by the activity of heterotrophic bacteria. The rate of this reaction is often assumed to be proportional to the concentration of soluble waste present and also to be highly temperature-dependent. But this is only part of the story.

The activity of the bacteria in the sludge accumulated at the bottom of the pond is not generally considered in design. However, where temperatures in the bottom sludge exceed 15°C for at least part of the year, the activity and feed-back of end-products from the sludge zone plays a signifi-

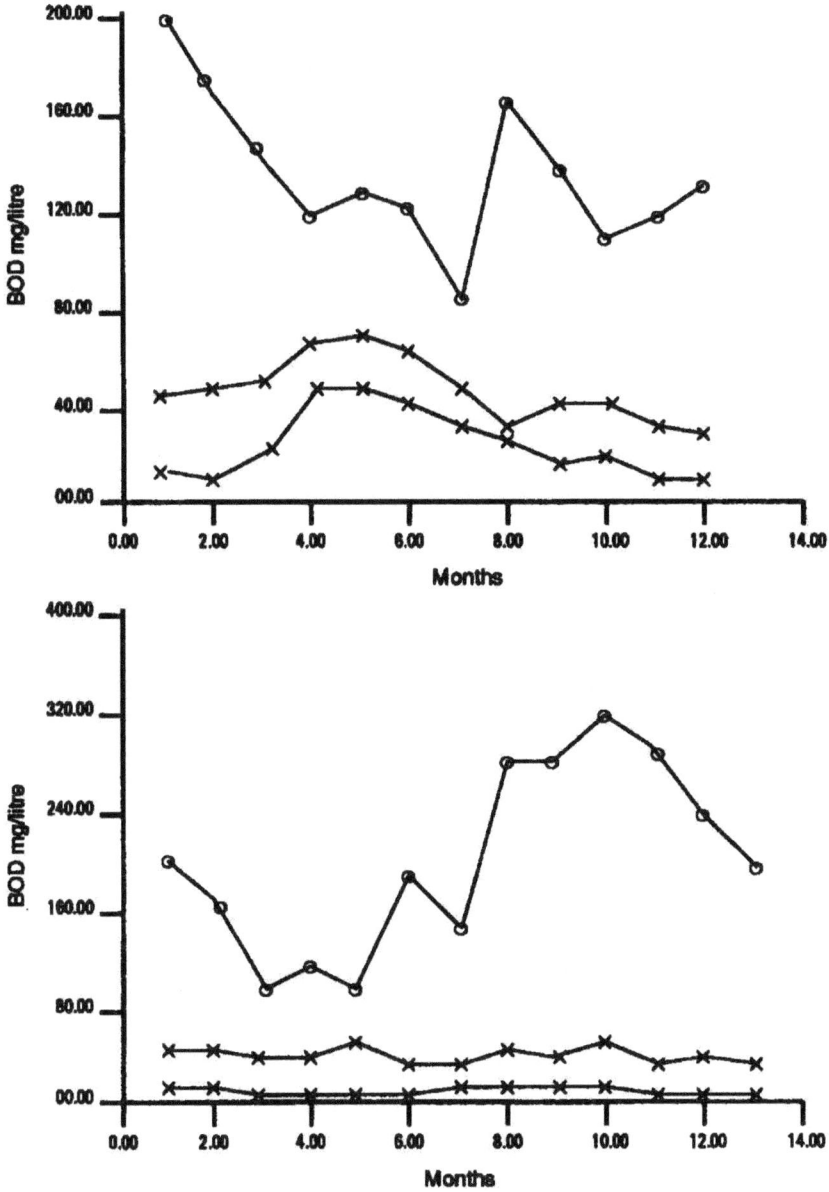

Figure 1. The plot on the top is from a pond system which does show a seasonal variation in efficiency (see bottom two lines), whereas the plot on the bottom is from a pond system with no marked seasonal variation

cant part in BOD removal. It should be noted that, most of the time, facultative ponds are largely anaerobic, as high concentrations of dissolved oxygen only exist in the upper layers during daylight hours. It is important to maintain adequate dissolved oxygen levels both in providing a zone where gas rising from the pond is absorbed, thus reducing the odour of the pond, and also for stabilizing soluble material from the inflowing wastewater and from the feedback from the sludge.

Wrong regression

A number of researchers have followed McGarry and Pescod's analysis to produce regression equations for pond systems.[82,83,84,85] These equations are used in design to predict expected BOD removals for a given BOD loading in the inflowing wastewater. Table 1 shows examples of regression equations developed to date giving the regression coefficient for cases where quoted. Such regression analyses are both invalid and misleading.

It is not surprising that a regression analysis performed for BOD removal versus BOD loading depicts a straight-line relationship with a high correlation, because 'loading' appears on both sides of the regression equation. Therefore the terms are functionally dependent, especially as output is small compared with loading. This misuse of the technique accounts for the spuriously high regression coefficients usually attained.[86]

Many designers currently use loading rates based on temperature. An example of this is given by McGarry and Pescod,[81] who developed an equation relating the maximum loading rate and ambient monthly mean temperature in the range 20 to 90°F.

$Lo = (1.054)T$
where Lo = BOD loading for the pond's area (pounds/acre/day)
$\quad\quad T$ = Mean monthly air temperature (°Fahrenheit)

This expression has been modified to incorporate subjective safety factors, for example:
$Lo = 20T - 120$ [8]
$Lo = 20T - 60$ [83]
where Lo = BOD loading for the pond's area (kg/hectare/day)
$\quad\quad T$ = Mean monthly air temperature (°Celsius)

We suggest that individual designers apply their safety factor to the original relationship according to the particular circumstances encountered, rather than adding safety factors to safety factors.

Table 1. Regression equations for pond systems

Equation	Units	Range of validity	Regression coefficient	Ref
$L_r = 0.725L_0 + 10.37$	kg/ha/d	34-560	0.995	81
$L_r = 0.73L_0 + 2$	kg/ha/d	50-150		82
$L_r = 0.73L_0 + 25$			0.965	83
$L_r = 0.81L_0 + 7.67$	kg/ha/d	200-1158	0.996	84
Concentration =				
$\qquad 0.61C_0 + 13$	mg/ltr/d		0.89	85
$L_r = 0.940L_0 - 1.04$	lb/acre/d		0.965	79

L_r = BOD removal rate
L_0 = BOD loading rate
C_0 = Influent concentration

(*Waterlines* Vol. 3 No. 4, April 1985)

Urban sullage in developing countries

JOHN ASHWORTH

Disease, directly attributable to poor sullage disposal, is often forgotten by engineers undertaking water and sanitation projects. This is partly due to lack of funds and the engineers' failure to include wastewater in plans for water supply and sewage disposal. The objective of any public health project is to reduce the very high incidence of water-related diseases, part of which is due to sullage.

In this context, sullage is defined as the wastewater from preparing food, cooking, washing kitchen utensils, clothes and personal hygiene. The problems of sullage disposal are often political: governments have limited funds or credit facilities, which they direct to the most pressing public problems or to prestigious projects. The provision of drinking-water supply and sewage-disposal systems to high-density urban areas may satisfy the public's demand and secure votes at the next elections. This will reduce major diseases like cholera and typhoid to some extent, but the incidence of diarrhoeal diseases in children may be unchanged if the problems of sullage control are not tackled as well.

Traditionally, engineers have provided only the richer sections of towns with drinking-water and sewerage, where return on investment is secure. The IDWSSD aims to persuade governments to accept the idea of providing these services to everyone, including urban squatters and slum dwellers. Through projects such as the World Bank-financed 'Sites and Services Scheme', where governments undertake to provide water supplies and sewage disposal and recognize the existence of squatters' homes by registering them, some areas have been 'legalized' with little destruction of housing to give access and services. But, after the basics have been installed, there is rarely direct government funding or encouragement to provide wastewater disposal facilities for every house.

Existing sullage disposal

Seventy to eighty per cent of town-dwellers in developing countries are low-income earners in high-density housing areas. Many of these people are squatters and, although some houses are reasonably durable, there may be up to 20 people living in a dwelling. There may be no roads and perhaps only a single stormwater ditch and a limited number of water standpipes. Some houses have a basic pit latrine and at least a curtained area for showering.

Cooking and laundry wastewater are usually thrown outside the house and may be channelled off to form pools of stagnant water. Water from the shower may also be discharged into these pools in quite large quantities. Small children play between the houses, surrounded by decaying refuse and pools of wastewater. During the rainy season, the rise in the groundwater table may cause the latrines to flood, particularly where latrines are also used for showering.

Some government housing projects have blockwork washing stands with wastewater discharging through a tap to soakpits below. Due to poor design and lack of maintenance, scraps of rice and vegetable peelings accumulate to prevent infiltration. Then the washing stand may overflow into roughly cut channels leading out of the compound.

Where governments or town councils have provided surface-water drainage but not sullage-disposal systems, problems soon occur. Sometimes illegal pipe connections are made to the storm channels for sullage disposal and even sewage disposal. Once the channels block, effluent forms ponds, where *Culex* mosquitoes can breed.

In the countryside, indiscriminate discharge of sullage brings less risk of disease than in high-density urban areas. In towns, the likelihood of transmitting water-borne diseases in these conditions is greatly increased because of the sheer numbers of people.

Water-transmitted diseases

Epidemic diseases such as typhoid and cholera are transmitted by water. Sullage can also be a breeding ground for *Culex* mosquitoes, carriers of the filaria worms which cause elephantiasis (*Bancroftian filariasis*). They block the body's lymph ducts and can cause massive swelling of connective tissue in any part of the body. If the wastewater is not stagnant or polluted the *Anopheles*, a malaria-carrying mosquito, can reproduce.

Gastroenteritis is transmitted from faeces to mouth, and young children are especially susceptible when they play in badly-drained areas. Hookworm is endemic in many areas where sewerage is inadequate, and enters the human body through the sole of the foot. Combined with measles it is a killer, although it does not directly increase child mortality. 'Water-washed, diseases such as trachoma, which leads to blindness when left untreated, and scabies, are hazards caused by not having enough water to wash hygienically.

Appropriate methods

Typically, about 20 per cent of houses in a Third World town are served by fully water-borne sewerage systems. The remaining 80 per cent would be improved by one of two lower-cost alternatives: small-bore sewerage systems or improved washing slabs.

The type of development which could most benefit from a small-bore sewerage system is a housing estate with about 200 people/ha which

Small-bore sewerage system for sullage disposal, showing (left) the sewered latrine and (right) the sewered washing slab which can be connected to it.

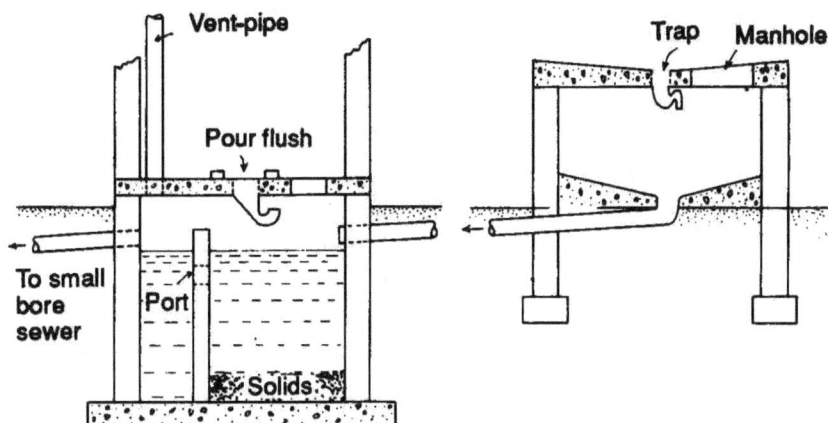

already has standpipes for water and a pit latrine in the yard of each house. However, pit latrines are commonly of poor design, not easily emptied by vacuum emptier.

A small-bore sewerage system is said to cost about 60 per cent as much as a full one. There, the pit latrine is replaced by a pour-flush lavatory discharging into a sump, which has a baffle to prevent solid excreta being carried into the sewer pipe. The accumulated sludge in the sump needs periodic emptying by a vacuum tanker. Water from washing or waste shower water should be discharged into the pit latrine sump to allow grit to settle rather than going direct into the sewer. Where a washing slab is used, the grit and organic-free effluent may be discharged to the small-bore sewer. A flow velocity of 0.3m/s should make the sewer self-cleansing, so it does not have to be laid at a gradient.

Improving washing slabs

An improved washing slab and soakaway might be suitable for lower-standard housing where standpipes are not available or the people cannot afford the monthly charges for both water and small-bore sewerage.

The soakage pit below the slab is designed to suit the soil's permeability, determined by a standard percolation test. [96] An access trap in the slab allows a vacuum tanker to draw off accumulated sludge, which would slow the rate at which the sullage water soaks away and shorten the life of the washing slab's soakage pit. More research and field trials are needed to obtain concrete figures on this.

If soil percolation tests show the soil to be impermeable, an evapo-transpiration bed — where sullage water is absorbed by the roots of plants over a wide area and given off as water vapour by the plant leaves — could be built. However, this has not been attempted for sullage to date, and unless it is feasible to install a series of sullage-containing vaults, small-bore sewerage is likely to be a better solution. Evapo-transpiration beds will probably only be suitable where less than 100 people live on each hectare.

In the past, the failure of engineers to use the skills of sociologists to discover the needs of local people is well-documented in sanitation projects. The final design must be

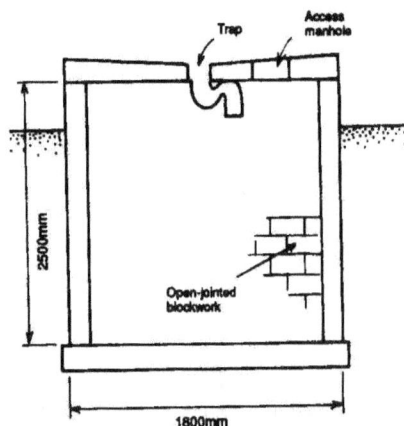

Improved washing slab with soakaway

tested before putting it into use. By constructing washing slabs at schools and in market-places as well as selected homes, many people can try out the design. If the design is at the right price and matches people's requirements, more demand will be generated for the washing slab, either with its own soakaway or connected to a small-bore sewerage system. House-to-house visits by council staff and village leaders might then be required to persuade households that improved sullage disposal facilities should be built.

Of the main choices for constructing a washing slab, contractor building is more likely to be successful than construction by government or the users themselves.

Less supervision is required by hard-worked council staff if the work is contracted out, and the builders must complete the work before they are paid. The contractor usually employs local labourers, and the more competent of these may be able to establish themselves as builders and provide a slab construction service to the area long after the contractor has departed. This develops skills within the community.

Improving cost recovery

Loan organizations are reluctant to release funds where they are not guaranteed to get their money back. Even for squatter communities, however, it is possible to improve the chances of cost recovery.

The loan could be made through a local leader, with assistance from council staff. In Africa, this would be the 'ward chief'. The community leader is usually responsible for assisting in income tax and house tax assessment and collection. In the case of absentee landlords, a council decree could recover the loan from the tenants' rents. Self-financing is possible even among squatters, and could perhaps be managed along the same lines as beer clubs in Uganda, which are run for periods of two weeks by a rota of people.

Educating the children

Health education campaigns, which are essential to improve the performance of the hardware installed, should be directed at children rather than adults, who are often very set in their ways and bound by tribal taboos. Most urban schools in developing countries have domestic science classes. The curricula do provide for personal hygiene lessons, although the syllabus and standard of teaching could often be improved.

During the domestic science period, primary school children could be encouraged to wash their hands after using the lavatory. They could also clean the latrines on a rota basis. Through parent/teacher meetings, cheap and effective footwear should be encouraged.

Secondary school children could study pathogenic bacteria with simple microscopes. Mosquitoes could be collected from drainage ditches or even pit latrines, and their larvae studied by the children.

The benefits of a school health-education programme will take several decades to become fully effective. Funds for this must be included in the engineering project.

Administration

Without enough qualified staff, a sullage disposal system plus health education will not achieve a large reduction in water-related diseases. USAID's Water & Sanitation for Health (WASH) Project offers a service for assisting engineers to re-evaluate their staff needs.

The staff needed to implement a sullage disposal project can often be drawn from the town council's health inspectorate department. The department is usually responsible for everything from food inspection to health education and septic tank design and construction. Engineers may be needed to strengthen such a department, but the temptation to expand too quickly must be resisted, if bureaucracy is to be avoided.

The responsibilities of the engineer should not be restricted to the design and construction of sullage, water supply or refuse-disposal works. He should also be responsible for sociological studies on the taboos and customs of the population, cost recovery, health education and organization to put plans into practice.

(*Waterlines* Vol. 1 No. 2, October 1982)

Why don't we use the night-soil to produce biogas?

PETER-JOHN MEYNELL

'Why don't we use the night-soil to produce biogas?' said the development worker. 'Night-soil should be looked on as a resource, not just thrown away, and the biogas can provide the village with cooking fuel rather than firewood.'

A good idea, and one which must have occurred to many workers in developing countries, but which has rarely been put into practice. It is worthwhile considering why sanitation and biogas have not really come together and to understand some of the problems which have to be solved.

Perhaps the main reason why human waste is not often treated by itself in a biogas plant is because sanitation and waste disposal is such a crucial and tricky development problem, that sanitation workers have not wanted to complicate the issue further by adding a biogas plant. These plants also have had a reputation for being temperamental. It may be, too, that biogas was considered as a secondary stage to be added at a later date, but, by that time, the planning process had hardened, and it was probably difficult to install a digester.

Role of the digester

The first thing which must be said is that human waste is just as good a feedstock for a digester as any other animal excreta. It digests well and produces roughly $0.28m^3$ of gas per person per day. Anaerobic digestion of sewage sludge is practised on sewage works throughout the world as a means of stabilizing the sludge before disposal to the land. The plants are usually sophisticated, heated and of massive concrete construction. They are traditionally only cost-effective when used on works serving large populations (over 100,000 typically), but recent developments in the design of prefabricated digesters have reduced the costs so that sludges from populations as small as 1,000 can be treated economically. The gas is often not used on sewage works since treatment is the prime objective.

In this context, digestion is not a complete treatment process, and the emphasis of a sewage works is the aerobic degradation of dissolved organic matter in the water. The primary solids have to be separated and diverted to the digester, where they are mixed with excess solids from the aerobic plant.

Biogas is never the prime aim in the digestion of sewage sludges, and indeed it is often flared off. It must be emphasized that the main aim of any sanitation scheme, sophisticated or not, must be the safe disposal of human excreta; and biogas is only a secondary benefit. Maximizing the cost-effectiveness of biogas production may well result in a lowering of treatment efficiency.

The design of a conventional sewage treatment works points to a fundamental design requirement for digesters, namely the need to work with a fairly thick sludge (4-7 per cent solids). Thus any waterborne method of waste disposal would require a separation stage to concentrate the sludge.

In systems where anaerobic digestion is to be the prime method of treatment, any superfluous water, such as rainwater and sullage, must be excluded. If necessary, a separate disposal system may have to be provided for sullage and any supernatant water on top of the solids.

Leaving aside conventional sewered systems, both septic tanks and aqua-privies do just this. They provide a chamber for the collection and build-up of sludge, which is emptied from time to time, while the supernatant is disposed of to a soakaway or small-bore sewer. One question often asked is whether a septic tank could be converted into a digester. Although a septic tank is anaerobic, it is designed as a separator, not as a digester. The liquid only has about 3 days retention time, and the sludge build-up is slow, so that not much gas would be produced from a comparatively large and expensive volume. If a much thicker sludge, eg unwatered night-soil, were put in, it would very quickly clog up.

Purpose-built digesters

A purpose-designed digester is considered to be better for the treatment of sludge and biogas production than a modified septic tank or aquaprivy. Of course the septic tank can be used for separation of sludges in waterborne waste disposal, but by the time sufficient quantity has been collected, much of it will have been digested. Thus, in the design of a waterborne collection system for biogas, the aquaprivy must be designed to concentrate the sludge better and to allow separate sludge removal from the bottom of the tank. A hopper-shaped tank with sides sloping at 60 degrees might be the

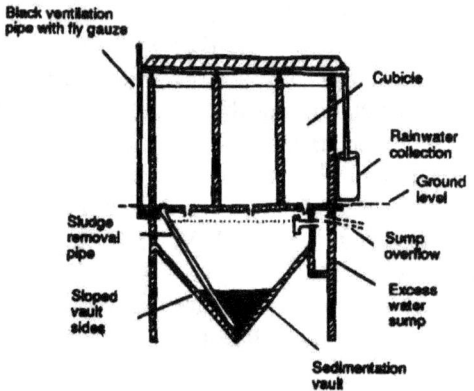

Figure 1. Pour-flush latrine with sedimentation vault.

answer. Sludge could be regularly removed by handpump or vacuum truck to a separate digester.[88] This approximates to the original Imhoff tank, which had two compartments, one for sludge separation and the other for digestion.

The dry method of collection of night-soil, for example by bucket and cartage or by vault and vacuum truck, has the advantage that no dirty water needs be separated off before digestion. There is, however, the disadvantage that it requires a regular collection service with its requirements of manpower and supervision. A waterborne, system, once installed, is less labour-intensive.

The water content of the sludge is not the only feedstock problem. Human excreta, including the urine, is very rich in nitrogen with a carbon:nitrogen ratio as low as 3:1. The optimum for digestion is often stated as 20-30:1. It is however better to have more rather than less nitrogen, but too much could produce toxic concentrations of ammonia in the digesting liquor, which would kill the methane-producing bacteria [89]

Digesters will work on a low C:N ratio provided they are acclimatized to it, but biogas production will be increased by the addition of more organic matter low in nitrogen: vegetable matter, for instance. Sewage sludge digesters work on a mixture of human excreta and other household wastes by which the C:N ratio is raised. The addition of human wastes to digesters treating cattle or pig manure is often advocated. Indeed many of the Chinese digesters serving a single household use a feedstock formula of 20 per cent human waste, 60 per cent animal manure and 20 per cent plant material.[90] Experiments in Nepal, India, Papua New Guinea and Korea all indicate that more biogas is produced if vegetable matter is mixed in. If such a mixed system is planned, the digester volume needs to be increased correspondingly to give the correct retention time.

Sizing the digester

Two examples illustrate how important it is to get the size of the digester right. In the first Oxfam, from experience with sanitation units in Bangladesh refugee camps, designed and built a fixed-roof digester large enough to supply two families with enough gas for cooking. It was to be fed with human waste from the two families, plus any dung and vegetable matter which could be collected. In the event, the additional material was not collected because, for the refugees, the time required for collecting the material was better spent in gathering firewood for sale.

The digester only ran on the smaller quantity of human waste, for which it was much too big, so not enough gas was produced for daily use. If biogas is going to be an option enough must be produced to give at least one family one hot meal a day.

Conversely, so successful were some women's latrines in a small town near Kathmandu which were connected to a digester, that they were oversubscribed. The digester was sized on the waste from 500 women. Double that number started to use the latrines so that the digester became overloaded and failed to produce the estimated quantity of biogas, because the retention time had been halved.[91]

The relatively small amount of gas which can be produced from a few people is not often appreciated. If a digester is sized to produce 5m³ of biogas per day (the most common size for one family's cooking needs) they would require 140kg of cattle dung from about 10 cows.[92]

If fueled by human excreta, a similar size digester would require the waste from just over 200 people. One family would not be able to provide anything like enough gas for its daily needs from its own waste products. If more than one family is involved, the question immediately arises of how to share the gas; the division of a scarce resource often leads to social problems, so that in the end both the incentive and the gas is lost.

Realistically, it would only be worthwhile planning a digester to run exclusively on human waste if more than 200 people were available to provide excreta on a daily basis.

In practice this means either a well-organized collection service for

night-soil as is the case in the largest night-soil digester in the world at
Foshan in China (which generates 90kW of electricity from the biogas
produced); or it means a digester attached to a public latrine serving a whole
community.

Even if a sizeable population can be served by such a scheme, the way is
not entirely clear, because it can never be worthwhile producing gas unless
there is a use for it. This may sound ridiculous, but it is essential thinking at
the planning stage. If one family cannot produce enough gas for its own
needs, and gas produced from a number of families cannot be shared, the
use must be communal or the gas sold to help maintain the system.

Examples of such uses might be the fuel for a local eating house or tea
shop, for a communal bakery, or for running refrigeration and lighting facilities in a rural clinic. Electricity generation has its problems, especially if
large continuous supplies of gas are required for the extra investment to be
worthwhile.

Problems of taboos

One of the social problems often held up as a reason for not digesting
human waste is the taboo against using a gas generated from excrement as a
fuel for cooking food. Although totally unfounded from a health viewpoint,
such a taboo can be a very real hazard to implementation. There has been no
problem in China, where the use of human waste is age-old, but in parts of
India only about 30 per cent of family digesters were connected to latrines.
In a community-scale biogas plant operated by Khadi & Village Industries
Commission (KVIC) in Dhaniv, the digester is designed in two stages with
the first stage using cattle manure only, so that villagers who object to gas
made from human waste can get 'pure' gobar-gas (produced from cow-
dung). In the second stage, the contents of eight public latrines are mixed
with the already digesting gobar. The Maya Farms in the Phillipines uses a
three-phase digestion system using night-soil from worker dormitories. [90]

There is often no better way of telling whether the community will object
to gas from human waste than asking it. If people do strongly object, then it
is probably best to consider a use which is not connected with the preparation of food, for example lighting, electricity generation, or a power source
for small workshops.

Basic designs

This is not really the place to consider different digester designs; however
the three basic designs are the fixed roof (Chinese) type, the floating roof
(Indian KVIC design) and the flexible bag type (for example the 'red mud'
digester or those marketed by Lockstoke Developments in the UK with two

bags connected in series for the rapid digestion of human wastes in hot, arid areas). The latter resemble the Oxfam emergency sanitation units.

All three types have their advantages and disadvantages and all can be used for treating human excreta. Probably the best guide for choosing the design is the ESCAP Guidebook on Biogas Development. [92] KVIC in India reports two operating problems which may influence the choice. One is the tendency of night-soil to separate within the digester into a heavier fraction which sinks to the bottom and a fatty scum which floats on the surface. The other is that in comparison to digesters working on gobar-cattle dung, the corrosion of steel gas holders seems to be more severe with night-soil due to the higher level of hydrogen sulphide produced with the biogas.[90]

Cause of failure

In all the failures of biogas schemes throughout the world — and there have been many — one of the commonest causes has been poor management.

Technically, well maintained biogas plants will continue to produce biogas, but, like any living organism, regular feeding and maintenance is essential. When feeding is intermittent or the feed too weak or watery, gas production will fall. With falling gas production, disenchantment with the system may set in and feeding becomes even less frequent until production ceases altogether. Management of public latrines is also very difficult and a similar disenchantment sets in as the latrine area becomes more and more sordid. When the two systems are combined without proper provision for people to clean the site and to look after the digester and to be paid for doing so, then disaster will overtake the system quickly. The situations in which some sort of control and discipline can be exercised effectively are in a school, religious community or prison.

Perhaps one of the best known digesters running on night-soil is the project set up by NEERI (National Envrionmental Engineering Institute) at Nagpur Central Jail, India. The 1,000 inmates provide the night-soil for three digesters with a total capacity of 43m³. Other examples include a 14m³ plant using the night-soil from 187 inmates of a leprosy home near Pune, two (10m³ and 4m³) units at a women's college in Tamil Nadu and a 5.5m³ digester at a bus station in Maharashtra. [93]

In particular, the Gandhi Samarak Nidhi Institution advocates night-soil-based plants, and there is some indication that the idea of the paying public latrine may be catching on. In some public latrines in India, people are prepared to pay a small amount provided they are well maintained. The income generated helps to pay for the service and, in this sort of situation, where substantial numbers of people use the facility, a logical extension to the system would be to produce biogas from the waste to increase its economic viability or even profitability.

Pathogen destruction

At the beginning of this article, I suggested that the prime aim of any sanitation scheme was to dispose of the waste safely. There is no point in having a sanitation/biogas system if it does not provide adequate treatment. Digestion will reduce the volume of sludge to be disposed of without reducing its nutrient value, but the total volume of liquor will remain the same. The sludge can be laid out on drying beds before discharge to the land, but it is worthwhile looking at the treatment capability of digesters before discharging liquid effluent to land.

Under anaerobic conditions, the rate of pathogen kill is dependent upon the temperature and the retention time. Table 1 shows the survival of different pathogens under tropical anaerobic conditions. Since it is unlikely that the simple digesters considered here will be heated, it is suggested that a longer retention time (between 1 and 2 months) be used than might normally be considered for optimum biogas production. The only pathogens remaining after this time inside a digester are the ova of round worm (*Ascaris*), whipworm (*Trichuris*) and tapeworm (*Taenia*). Nevertheless the Chinese do claim satisfactory reductions in *Ascaris* in sludge digested for two months.[94]

If the digester temperature is raised, then the retention time for adequate pathogen control can be reduced. Normal 'mesophilic' sewage sludge

Table 1. Pathogen concentration estimated in final product of anaerobic composting toilets operating at ambient temperatures in warm climates.

Pathogen	Retention time (months)						
	1	2	3	4	6	8	10
Enteric viruses	+	+	0	0	0	0	0
Salmonellae	+	+	0	0	0	0	0
Shigellae	+	+	0	0	0	0	0
Vibrio cholerae	+	0	0	0	0	0	0
Path. *E. coli*	+	+	0	0	0	0	0
Leptospira	0	0	0	0	0	0	0
Entamoeba	0	0	0	0	0	0	0
Giardia	+	+	0	0	0	0	0
Balantidium	+	0	0	0	0	0	0
Ascaris	++	++	++	++	+	+	+
Trichuris	++	++	+	+	+	+	0
Hookworms	+	+	0	0	0	0	0
Schistosoma	0	0	0	0	0	0	0
Taenia	++	++	++	++	+	+	+

0 Probable complete elimination
+ Probable low concentration
++ Probable high concentration

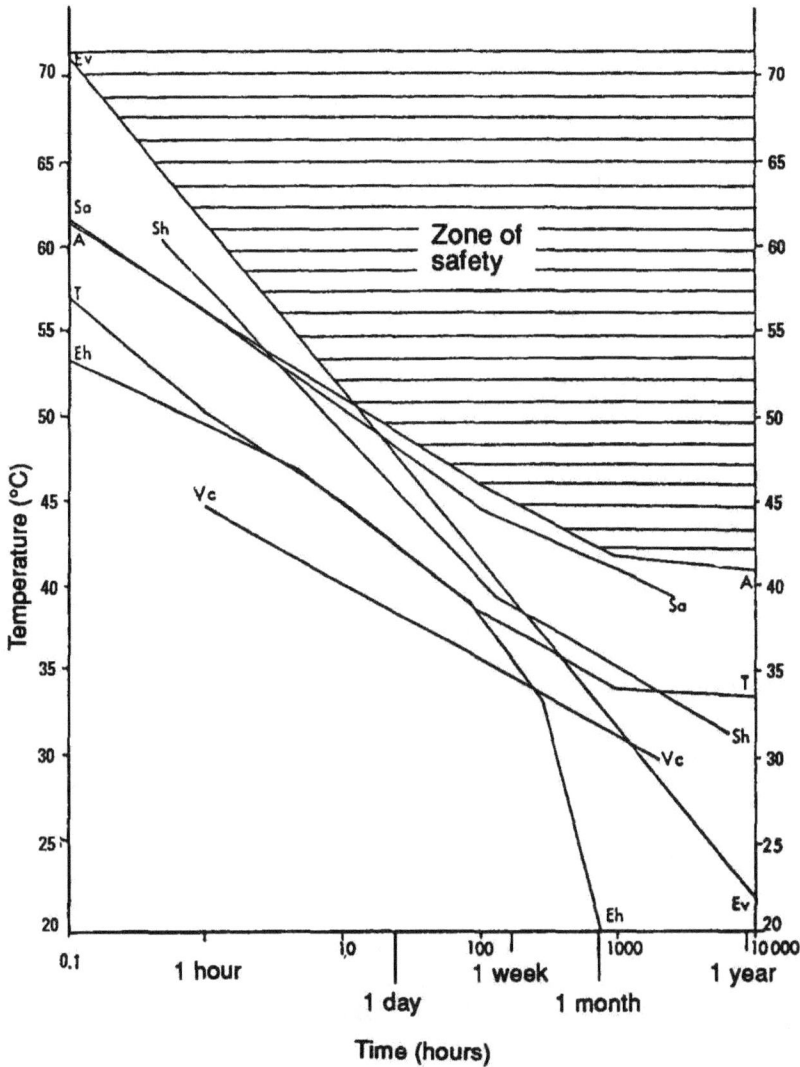

Figure 2. The influence of time and temperatures on a variety of excreted pathogens: the lines represent conservative estimates of the highest temperatures at which the parasites would die.

Key:
Ev Enteric viruses (excluding Hepatitis A)
Sa *Salmonella* (gastroenteritis)
Sh *Shigella*
Vc *Vibrio cholerae* (cholera)

Eh *Entamoeba hystolytica* (dysentery)
A *Ascaris* (roundworm)
T *Taenia* (tapeworm)

digesters at 35°C operate on a 15-30 day retention time, and this considerably reduces the capacity required in these large digesters. Thermophilic digestion (at around 50°C) would reduce the safe digestion time to about 1 day, although for optimum biogas production it would have to be longer. Thermophilic digestion is a sensitive process which has not really been developed in working situations yet, let alone in simple sanitation schemes.

Partial digestion

Another variation which might be considered if the size of the digester must be limited, is to partially digest the night-soil for optimum biogas production and then to compost the digested sludge with domestic refuse and vegetable matter. Composting is an aerobic process in which the temperature may get as high as 50-60°C over a period of time. This would kill roundworm (*Ascaris*) ova, the most persistent pathogens, within a day. Figure 2 shows the influence of time and temperature on excreted pathogens; a process, aerobic or anaerobic, with time/temperature characteristics lying within the zone of safety should guarantee the inactivation of all excreted pathogens. [95]

Any sanitation scheme is always a compromise, and it is rare that they are completely effective in killing off all the pathogens. The aim, however, is to make a substantial improvement in the health of the population by reducing the risks of pathogen spread to an acceptable level in comparison with the situation beforehand. Digestion offers a method which is at least as good technically as other methods of treatment; it is in the area of social practice where further experience needs to be gained.

So, for any biogas/sanitation scheme three main points must be considered:
O The safe collection and treatment of both liquids and solids.
O The safe disposal of solids, possibly as a composted fertilizer.
O The production of biogas and its use, and the management of all three.

It is essential that all three aspects are thought through to final use or disposal, for a hold-up in any one aspect could jeopardize the whole, and a sanitation scheme which might have worked would fail. If the sale of gas and fertilizer is successfully planned and put into practice, it can provide the incentive and the resource for a community to continue good sanitation practice.

Rural health in northern Pakistan

JAMES MUIR

Several years ago a Norwegian missionary, Father Wendy, after spending many years working in villages in India remarked, 'Development can only occur where there is hope and dignity.' To illustrate the truth behind this principle, the construction of a surface drainage system in a group of villages in Pakistan served as the key that unlocked the door to a surge of creative activity, which considerably raised the standards of living, health and hygiene.

The Punjab is the second largest of the four provinces of Pakistan and contains 57 per cent of the population. It is flat and fertile, and produces most of the wheat and rice that feed the people. About 72 per cent of Punjabis live in 25,000 villages, and the density of the population is more than twice the national average.

In the north-eastern corner of the Punjab lies the city of Sialkot with a population of about 200,000. Near the centre of this big, sprawling city lies The Memorial Christian Hospital, run by the American Presbyterian Church, which has a small but effective public health team led by one of the three doctors on the staff, Dr. Zaffar-Ul-Haq, who is assisted by two male orderlies and three nurses. The team travels extensively around the villages near Sialkot, working as a travelling clinic and immunizing against measles, polio, typhoid, cholera and diptheria. The team also has an extensive educational role, teaching the villagers elementary facts about basic hygiene, such as how to prepare food, how to feed babies and how to avoid parasites.

Need for better drainage

In 1980, the team decided to embark upon a drain-building project, for a number of reasons. First, during the monsoon season in the month of July alone, up to 12in (30mm) of rain falls. Since most of the houses, streets and walls are made of dried mud, villages rapidly turn into quagmires in the absence of good drainage. Second, even during the dry season there is a drainage problem caused by the replacement of the traditional village well by handpumps for each household. This has greatly increased the volume of water that is pumped out into the village streets. This water accumulates, along with human and cattle refuse. It is churned into mud by buffaloes and cows, making the streets completely impassable in places. These sewage pools are ideal breeding grounds for flies and various parasites, and since they are in close proximity to the houses, children playing outside rapidly become infected. The infant mortality in the villages is said by Dr Zaffar to be as high as 30 to 50 per cent.

A survey carried out on the children in the area in 1979 (by P. Johnson, *et al*) found that up to 93 per cent of the children had parasites in their stools, and an average of 63 per cent were found to have *Giardia* lamblia. Since no effective chemicals are available to kill the cysts of these parasites, and since re-infection would always recur shortly after worming, sanitation and hygiene were considered to be of the utmost importance; hence it was decided to embark upon a drain-building project. The financial burden of the project was (and still continues to be) shared equally between the villagers themselves and the American Presbyterian Missionary Society, which matched money raised from the villagers rupee for rupee.

Organizing the project

It soon became apparent that drainage systems should not be imposed on a village. Even if three or four seniors were asking for drains, attempts were not made to build them unless:

O The village was found to need drainage badly.

O The entire village was prepared to work together to build the drains.

O The village was prepared to undertake responsibility for maintenance of the drains once they were built.

A good indication of the probable success of the project was found to be the strength of the village leadership. In villages where there was strong leadership, and where villagers were willing to co-operate with the leaders, the chances of success were high. Since the project depended on the villagers themselves for finance, labour and hospitality, it could not work without their full support and commitment.

The first step was to draw a map of the village, marking all the streets, the length of the drains required, the direction of the flow of water, and the ponds into which the water was to drain. A starting date was set, and the village leaders were asked to collect money (for example, Rs100 per family), buy bricks, obtain sand and organize labour.

Sand was important as it was needed to mix with cement in a 4:1 ratio, and it was also used as a foundation for the drain in marshy areas. Base bricks were never laid on ground which was not solid underfoot. If the ground at the bottom of the trench felt spongy, the earth was removed to a depth of at least a foot, or until solid ground was reached, then filled in with sand and compacted with a pounder.

Labourers were needed to dig the trenches, fill them in with sand where necessary, carry bricks and lay them alongside the trench, soak them in water and hand them to the masons. Eight labourers were required at any one time; and it was a good idea for all the labourers to work together along the length of drain allotted to them, rather than having individual house-holders working only outside their house. Children were found to be

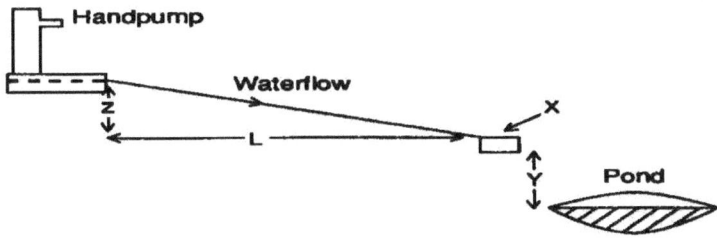

Figure 1. 'Y' marks the safety of 8 to 12in. beyond which backflow will result.

extremely good at transporting bricks. A team of six masons was employed to build the drains; this team continued working throughout the seasons, moving from village to village.

Construction method

The difference in height was surveyed between the upper courtyard and a brick which was placed 8 to 12in. (20-30mm) above the surface of the pond to indicate the drain outlet-level. In Figure 1, the top surface of the brick 'X' marks the position that the base of the drain would occupy. 'Y' is a safety margin of about 8 to 12in., so that in the monsoon the level of the pond could rise without causing backflow up the drains. 'Z' is the height difference between the inlet and outlet and 'L' is the total length of the drain.

The gradient of the drain was calculated from 'Z' and 'L', as the ratio of 'Z':'L' (for example, 0.45:80, which simplified is 1:178). Officially, 9in. drains should have a minimum gradient of 1:150, but Punjabi villages are usually too flat to allow this gradient; a more realistic minimum was used: 1:300. If this gradient could not be obtained naturally, it could be achieved artificially by raising the street and courtyard level at the top end of the drain . The shaded area was raised by filling with earth and the dotted area was levelled by removing the earth. After this, ranging poles were placed in position, and connected with string to mark the line along which the drain was to run. Although the final decision lay with the villagers, it was found best to place the line down the centre of the street for two reasons:
O It was usually the deepest part, so water tended to collect there. If the drain was built along the (higher) sides then the problem remained of filling in the centre of the street with earth;
O Many villagers seemed to regard the drains not so much as a system of carrying water, than as a system of indicating the division of property.

Once a provisional line down the centre of the street was marked, the villagers were left to determine the exact line. The drain-building was only started when all the villagers and village leaders agreed about the line.

Laying the bricks

Laying the bricks was the next stage. The level bricks were set with a spirit level at strategic intervals, such as every 50ft (15m), along the length of the drain. Ideally (unless hampered by a minimum gradient) these bricks were set sufficiently deep for all the water from the surrounding street and court-yards to drain on to their top surface. The ideal level brick would be placed so that its top surface was one brick's width below the lowest point in the street, so that the sides of the finished drain would be below the surface.

Unless the water on either side of the street could flow down into the drain, it would form puddles and the street would become impassable. Since the villagers were not good at filling in the sides of the streets with earth, it was better to build a deep drain in the first place. T-bones were used to place more level bricks at intervals of 3 or 4 metres . Keeping T-bones fixed in positions 1 and 5, the points in-between (bricks 2, 3 and 4) could be levelled by eye, using a third T-bone. Following this, the village labourers dug a trench to the same depth as the bottom of the level bricks, the width depending on the estimated width of the future drain. Usually, a 9in. drain was adequate .

Six-inch drains were used in small tributaries, where only three or four houses were to be drained into a larger system. Twelve or 18in. drains were used for the main system, in a situation where, say, a third of a village was being drained into a pond. Where a drain had to be built with a small gradi-ent or gradual fall of less than 1:300, it was found necessary to make the drains extra wide or with high sides: for example a 12in. drain instead of a 9in. drain. The water would not drain into the pond more rapidly, but it could remain within the drain, while it slowly flowed away.

Once the trench had been dug, the mason placed a string tautly across the level bricks, and laid the base bricks where its position indicated. When the base bricks were laid, the masons built the sides of the drain, their height depending on the distance below the ground that the drains had to go. Usually, the construction of deep drains could be avoided by digging away the earth at either side, but sometimes this was impossible to do, for fear of undermining a nearby wall or house. When a drain had to be laid more than about 2 feet below ground level, then the use of a pipe was considered. A 9in. drain was led into a 12in. pipe, the only complication arising when a pipe had to be laid through a bend, in which case a manhole was constructed at the bend in order to allow the pipes to be cleaned.

Finally, the masons 'benched' or plastered the drain — a simple, but time-consuming, procedure. The villagers were told not to use the drain until the plaster had dried completely. It was advisable to cover the drains with branches or thorns while the plaster was setting, to dissuade people or animals from walking on it. Using this method of drain building, about 2,000 feet of drain could be built in a week in good conditions.

Maintenance

Since surface drains are continually exposed to the wear and tear caused by buffaloes, horses and tractors, it was found necessary to make various provisions for their protection and maintenance.

O Pavements 22in. wide were made on each side of the drains to strengthen and protect them.

O Tractor routes were planned through each village and the drains along these routes were reinforced and bridged where necessary. Streets and alleys not on the tractor routes were blocked off by bollards to protect the non-reinforced drains from vehicle damage.

O An annual levy of Rs15 per household was imposed (agreed before the drain-building began), to pay for the running costs of drain maintenance.

Hope and dignity

Village streets that were once little more than sewage pits were made at least passable, and at best clean, thereby reducing the risks from parasites. Although the public health team withdrew much of their efforts once the drains were built, the villagers continued their self-improvement efforts; the drains seeming to have acted as a springboard, stimulating them to greater achievement. Why was this? The answer is indicated in Father Wendy's observation: the villagers had been given hope and dignity with the result that development was occurring.

In rural Pakistan, the average family has seven to eight children, and the average house consists of one room only. Most villagers do not own the land on which they work, and often they do not own the house in which they live: until recently 50 per cent of the area of Pakistan was owned by only 26 families. The villagers earn enough to keep themselves and their families alive. Their lives are governed by a resigned fatalism, expressed in the phrase 'It is the will of Allah'.

The construction of drains seemed to give the villagers hope. They had banded together and with only a minimum of organization and financial help from outside, they had achieved a major improvement in their community. In the months following the drain building some remarkable changes took place. Spurred on by their new-found confidence, and using the clean streets as a basis on which to work, the villages underwent a transformation.

First, they started to clean up and rebuild their houses. Mud huts were replaced by brick houses. One village hired a bulldozer to reclaim some marshy wasteland, so that it could be transformed into farmland. The same village cleared out the village pond and turned in into a fish farm. Another village built a poultry farm. The true culmination of the work, however, occurred when one villager decided to build a latrine, complete with a septic tank. This was the first water latrine to be built in any village in the Sialkot area, and it marked the beginning of proper sanitation, a most significant answer to the desperate health problems in the area.

Thousands of people in the Third World are dying every day because of the squalid conditions in which they live. The West has responded by pouring millions of pounds of aid into these countries. Is that aid being used in the best way? Is giving money, tractors, food, clothes or advanced tehnology going to be of any lasting benefit, when the recipients are too resigned and too subservient to be motivated to change, or believe that they can change? The author considers that the people of the Third World must first be given hope and dignity, by simple schemes such as the one described; and with little finance from outside, development will occur.

(*Waterlines* Vol. 5 No. 2, October 1986.)

Better sanitation to beat mosquito breeding

PRESS TRUST OF INDIA

Five years ago, the people of Pondicherry were reeling under the menace of mosquitoes. One in every five pople in the town suffered from filariasis. But today, thanks to the Vector Control Research Centre (VCRC) in Pondicherry, which launched a massive project to eradicate mosquitoes, the incidence of fresh infection has become virtually nil. The first urban centre in India to rid itself of mosquitoes entirely, Pondicherry has set an example for other mosquito-infested towns and villages. The VCRC scientists made this possible not by the use of insecticides but by improving the environment. The strategy was simple: environmental management through community participation.

Success in Pondicherry

When the VCRC began the project in 1981 under the Indian Council of Medical Research, it concluded that the filariasis problem in Pondicherry was due to years of unplanned and uncontrolled urbanization. This had led to the creation of numerous breeding sites for mosquitoes. Consequently, environmental management, particularly reducing the number of breeding sites, was selected as the basis of cost-effective control operations with a lasting effect. The environmental management activities consisted of filling, channelling, draining, weeding and desilting.

In fact, what the VCRC did in co-operation with the town's civic authorities, was to unleash a big sanitation drive actively supported by the people.

Seawater carried by tankers flushed out the town's drains previously clogged with garbage and waste. The drains not only became operational but the salty water killed the mosquito eggs. The numerous *kuchcha* roadside drains were desilted, deweeded and narrowed. Thousands of septic tanks in the town were chlorinated and their vent-pipes screened with cloth to prevent the entry of mosquitoes. Pits on roadsides were systematically filled with sand. Lids were put on cement tanks used for storing water outside building sites, and larvae-eating fish were dropped into unused wells.

The surface water area eliminated in Pondicherry by filling operations alone almost doubled from 7,633m² in 1981 to 14,573m² in 1984. Equally significant is the fact that more than Rs80,000 was saved on insecticide purchases during the four-year period because of the reduction in the number of sources, even after deducting the cost of the environmental works.

The VCRC, government departments and municipal authorities worked together to flush out the disease-carrying mosquitoes. Another key to the success was community participation following massive campaigns by the VCRC to educate and motivate people on the prevention of mosquito breeding. Besides its own staff, the VCRC employed people who were physically handicapped as a result of chronic filariasis, for house-to-house visits. Their message that filariasis can be prevented by maintaining a cleaner environment had a strong impact.

Spurred by the success of the mosquito-control strategy in Pondicherry, the VCRC extended the project to 21 nearby villages with a total population of 20,000 people. Here the strategy adopted was to integrate mosquito control with primary health care and government welfare programmes. The first step was to win the confidence of villagers so VCRC took up welfare measures which had nothing to do with mosquito control. For instance, in Pudukuppam village, where there was no provision for drinking-water, the VCRC installed a bore-well and pump set.

Adoption in Kheda

The VCRC strategy has also been adopted by the Malaria Reseach Centre, another ICMR institute for controlling malarial mosquitoes in Kheda, Gujarat. Work was taken up in January 1984 in eight villages with a total population of 30,000 people. Many small pits, ditches and temporary water ponds were levelled. Some poorly maintained drains were eliminated; instead, small pits were dug which were emptied every week to prevent mosquito breeding. All leaking taps were repaired. In one village, waste land was converted into playgrounds. Health committees were formed in all villages.

As a result, mosquito breeding in the ponds was considerably reduced and in many ponds completely eliminated. The irrigation department developed a better drainage system to prevent water-logging. *Panchayats* also unanimously agreed to take up social forestry, and the forestry department consented to plant trees that would eliminate many marshy areas, improve the environment and add to the income of *panchayats*. In just seven months, malaria cases were down from 97 to 24 and four out of the eight villages were free from malaria by April 1984. The mosquito density in seven out of eight villages was reduced to a level at which malaria transmission cannot occur.

Bangalore filariasis control

The Karnataka government, too, has invited the VCRC to assist it in implementing a similar programme for controlling filariasis in the city of Bangalore. The VCRC scientists say that the breeding grounds for mosquitoes in Bangalore, which has an area of 400km^2 and a population of four million, are open *nullahs*, storm water drains, some 50 small and big tanks, 12,000 wells, a dozen quarries, wet cultivation and an assortment of man-made breeding places such as fountains, cesspools, septic tanks and brick pits. The VCRC aims to prepare a master plan for mosquito control, and to set up a station in Bangalore for guiding the operation.

Kerala coastal programme

The VCRC will also launch a major programme in coastal Kerala, which is the largest single tract in India endemic in Malayan filariasis. This disease is caused by a parasite called *brugia malayi*, transmitted by *monsonia* mosquitoes that breed in ponds maintained in each house. The water in the ponds is used for bathing, drinking and, most of all, for rotting coconut husks since coir-making is a cottage industry in Kerala. The residents grow a vegetation called *pistia* in these ponds and use it as manure for the coconut trees and other tuber cultivations. The larvae of the *monsonia* mosquitoes are to be found in the roots of the plant.

In Shertallai *taluk* alone, there are over 75,000 ponds, but it is hoped that the filariasis problem can be totally controlled in Shertallai through the environmental approach because the breeding places are well-defined. Among the approaches considered are environmental management, introduction of larvae-eating fish in the ponds, and economic exploitation of the aquatic plants like *pistia* and *eichorina* for fertilizer and other industrial products.

The VCRC's environmental control programme could be a boon to the health ministry as millions of rupees are currently being spent in order to control filariasis. All the developed countries have eradicated mosquitoes not with the use of insecticides but through sanitation and environmental management.

(*Waterlines* Vol. 5 No. 1, July 1986)

Hygienic construction in remote African villages

BILL WOOD

When we speak of 'rural sanitation', we normally refer to village water supplies and domestic latrines. These two items are generally regarded as the most important constituents of rural sanitary programmes, but they are not the only factors in improving the health of the villagers.

Water is probably the route by which most epidemics are spread, but insects and rodents carry disease, unhygienic practices in the storage and preparation of food play their part, and soil contamination with helminths such as hookworm can account for much misery and sickness.

The rural engineer may therefore be called upon to provide a number of public health amenities in addition to safe water and sanitary disposal of excreta. Examples of these are: hygienic food market stalls; village clinics; communal grain stores; market and street drainage; incinerators for market and medical wastes; proofing of buildings against rats, flies, mosquitoes, bats and termites; communal bathing and clothes-washing facilities (especially in areas where schistosomiasis is prevalent); protection (fencing or concrete aprons) around watering points; market latrines; and other minor sanitary works to fill particular local needs.

Rarely do any of these call for special design or highly skilled construction; indeed simplicity is the virtue to be cultivated at all stages. It is the fact that a multiplicity of little jobs have to be undertaken simultaneously in remote areas, far from stores, supervision and other 'back-up', that calls for ingenuity and the development of unorthodox methods that would be quite unacceptable under more favourable conditons.

It goes without saying that there is never enough money to carry out a programme properly. There are, however, other constraints that may be more difficult to overcome than lack of funds, a point rarely appreciated by those planners and politicians who consider that a paper transfer of an allocation into a departmental vote is sufficient to remove all obstacles to a speedy implementation of their proposals.

Small projects do not readily lend themselves to contract procedures, even where local contractors are available. The preparatory stages, including formal designs, contract documents, tendering, accounting, and the supervision and acceptance of the completed job are often out of all proportion to the value of the works to be carried out. Direct labour by skilled craftsmen (who are usually in short supply) presents its own difficulties of organization, not least being the reluctance of staff to travel to remote areas, especially when this involves living under conditions that are more primi-tive than those to which they are accustomed. This reluctance is increased when they are married men with families.

It is tempting to rely heavily on the participation of the villagers themselves, but this requires careful preparation and organization of a different kind. Experience suggests that local participation can only be successful when the contribution expected is capable of being broken down into precisely specified tasks; even then there is little control over volunteer labour, and such matters as the loan of tools and the technical guidance of willing but inexperienced workers are time-consuming and must be arranged in advance. Again, for minor works, the time that must be spent in supervision may be unjustifiable in the light of the results obtained.

Relaxation of standards

Against these considerations must be set the unpalatable fact that if the work is to be carried out to a high standard of quality and efficiency it will probably never get done at all. Standards have to be relaxed and supervision reduced to the bare minimum, otherwise results will be confined to a few accessible communities where normal construction methods can be observed. Short-cuts and makeshift procedures can, however, be devised, provided that thought and ingenuity go into their planning and preparation.

The following example of an actual programme is intended to show how such makeshifts can be made to work in practice. There was nothing remarkable about the work itself, which was extremely simple. It is described here, not for the technical details of construction, but to show the method of approach and how the co-operation of the villagers was enlisted. It might not be considered one of the more usual projects of water supply or rural sanitation, but the experience gained was later used in rather more ambitious sanitary improvements.

The problem

A new medical officer had been appointed to a rural province in an African country. The provincial works department was responsible for all health construction and maintenance (including water supplies, community sewerage and hospitals) as well as the normal local road construction and maintenance, schools and other buildings, and work for other departments. It was perpetually understaffed, short of funds, and continually being pressed to increase its activities within the staff and funds already available.

The new medical officer took a keen interest in food hygiene, and was particularly horrified at the conditions under which animals were slaughtered for human consumption in the villages. The animals concerned were mainly goats, some sheep, and very occasionally cattle. Slaughtering was carried out outside each village, the beasts being butchered, skinned and cut up on bare ground, all bones, stomach contents and unsaleable portions being left for scavengers such as vultures and hyenas. The whole area soon became surrounded with stinking animal refuse of all kinds, the ground impregnated with blood and urine, and it was infested with rats and flies which obviously spread their activities throughout the village.

A simple remedy, the health department suggested, would be to provide a slaughter slab of concrete, a well nearby for washing down and for ablutions of the butchers, and a soakaway to take the liquid refuse from the slab. A large number of villages would require slabs, 50 being considered the most urgent.

The reaction of the works department was predictable. There was no provision in the budget, the year's allocation for minor works was already overstretched, all mobile teams of craftsmen were fully committed, and a great deal of preparatory work at village level would be necessary. It might just be possible to include (literally) two or three slabs in villages where other work was taking place, but a programme of the magnitude suggested was out of the question in the foreseeable future. The health department countered with the offer of (a little) money and the services of their local sanitarians to assist in preparation and supervision. But these men — competent in their own field — had neither experience in construction nor authority to supervise the work of another department's employees.

After several rather heated discussions the compromise described below was agreed upon as an experiment, using semi-skilled 'craftsmen', village labour, and back-up from provincial headquarters. It should be explained that the usual approach to minor village works was that villagers provided unskilled labour and locally available materials from their own resources, while skilled labour, supervision, imported materials, transport, and the loan of tools and equipment were supplied from provincial funds. Such works could only be carried out on direct application by the villagers themselves, so it would be necessary to 'sell' the proposals to the village councils before anything could be done. The health department, through their corps of sanitarians, would have to persuade the local people to apply for a slab and, possibly more difficult, to persuade the butchers to break their age-old habits and make use of the facilities when provided. Well-sinking was normally the responsibility of the village councils, using their own teams that had been trained and equipped for the purpose, so it would also be necessary to arrange with them to give priority to a suitably sited well within their own programmes.

The programme as planned

The agreed design of the proposed slab was the simplest possible. It would consist of concrete, roughly 4m by 2.5m and 10cm thick, surrrounded by precast concrete blocks that would act as edging for the slab and project upward some 10cm to act as a kerb. The slab surface would slope at 1 in 100 to one corner where a soakaway would be sunk. At the opposite end would be fixed a hanging rail 1.5m high, prefabricated of galvanized iron piping, to which carcasses would be hooked to make dressing easier and to keep meat off the ground during skinning and cutting up. Once agreed, this pattern was to be maintained throughout and no variation in dimensions was contemplated. In the case of larger villages, where the size of the slab would be inadequate, two slabs, similar but separate, would be constructed.

The volume of concrete in the slab itself would be 1m³; some additional concrete would be necessary around the legs supporting the hanging rail and as backing to the edging blocks. The villagers would be required to supply 1.5m³ of mixed gravel plus 0.5m³ of sand for mortar to set and point the edging blocks. Most of the villagers were used to the selection and collection of suitable aggregate, since this was a common form of contribution to such communal projects as road culverts, and a small stock of picks, shovels, sand sieves and the like was held by each village council for the purpose. A total of six 50kg bags of cement would be needed, and the whole job should be completed in a little over one week except during the height of the rainy season.

In addition to the sand and gravel, the village would be expected to provide the services of six labourers for ground preparation, concrete mixing and placement; accommodation for two men from headquarters; covered storage for cement and tools (with a night watchman should this be considered desirable); and water for concrete mixing. The actual site would be agreed and identified in advance by the sanitarian, who would arrange for it to be cleared of refuse before any work was started.

Operation

The man chosen as 'headman' for the programme had been working as a kerb layer with the road repair section of the provincial works department. He had been with the department for many years and had experience of road drainage, concreting and similar jobs. He was an elderly widower, locally born, and was highly respected socially as a distant relative of the religious leader in the district. These considerations may appear trivial, but in retrospect it can be seen that the smooth working of the project depended greatly on these very points. The key to cooperation with the villagers lay in his being no stranger to them and their ways; it happened that nearly all the skilled craftsmen working in the department came from outside the province and were of another tribe. Although theoretically this should have had no significance, in practice the differences of speech, customs, religion — even food — would have been likely to be causes of friction. Added to this the reluctance of 'strangers' to adapt to village life, the fact of their being continually on the move and parted from their families and compatriots could have led to lack of enthusiasm and dissatisfaction with the job.

In the event, the headman chosen proved very popular and his stay in the various villages something of a social occasion. He selected his own assistant (his nephew!) to travel with him, who would in due course be promoted headman and take over a parallel programme of his own. However, both suffered from being virtually illiterate, unable to read a plan or use a measuring tape.

Accordingly, a simple device of knotted cords (usually referred to as the 'cat's cradle') was produced in the dimension of the slab, with diagonals and a metal ring at each corner (see Figure 1). When this was stretched tightly by four labourers, a peg driven into the ground through each ring, and the cat's cradle removed, the corners of the slab were identified and another cord round the pegs marked the limits of the work. The prefabricated edging blocks were positioned with the help of a straightedge and a 'drainage level'.

This latter (see Figure 2) was a locally made triangular plumb bob level, its special feature being that, in addition to the level indicator beneath the bob, two additional indicators showed when the lower member was sloping

Figure 1. 'Cat's cradle' of knotted cords used in slab construction.

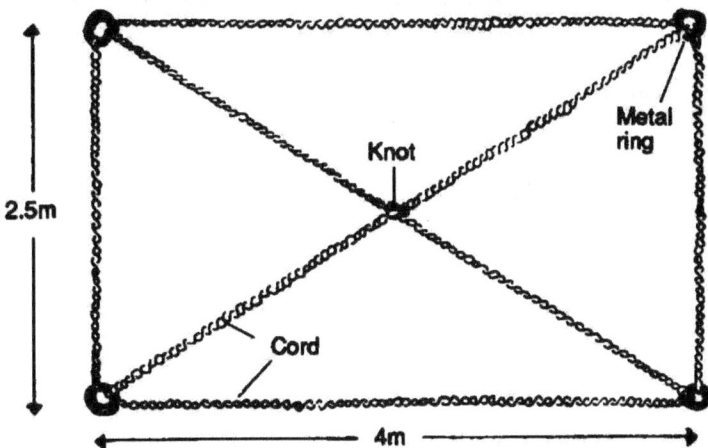

at 1 in 100 in either direction. The edging blocks, the ground prepared for concreting, and the slab surface were all adjusted to the same slope with the help of this device.

The hanging rail was also prefabricated at headquarters, the ends to be concreted into the ground being split to form a key, with a dab of paint on each leg showing the level to which each was to be buried (Figure 3).

The first few slabs were constructed under strict supervision to iron out any difficulties. Thereafter the procedure was on the following lines.

On Saturday morning (Friday being the rest day) a truck from provincial headquarters would leave for the next village on the priority list carrying the headman and his assistant; 26 edging blocks; 6 bags of cement; the hanging rail assembly; mixing shovels and other tools for labourers and for the headman; the drainage level, cat's cradle, straightedges and other bits and pieces.

Figure 2. Drainage level, showing the position of two extra panel pins to indicate inclines of 1 in 100.

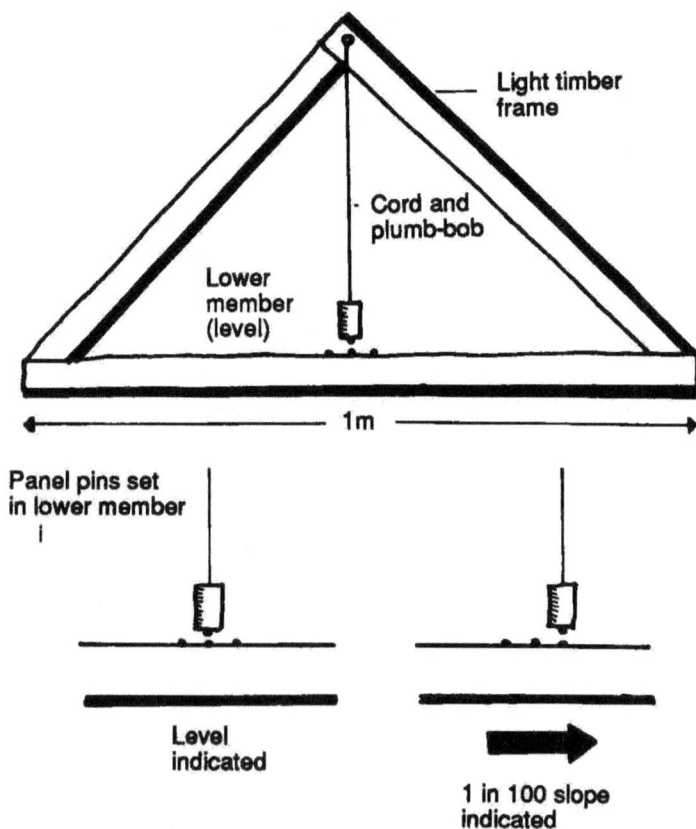

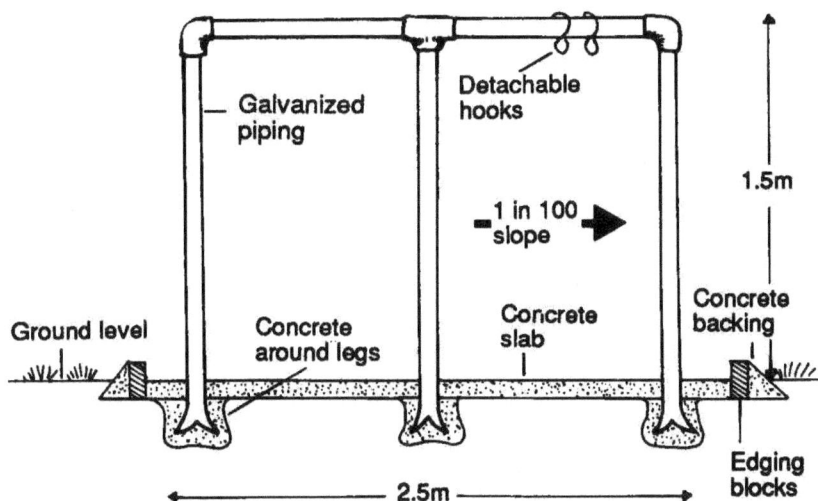

Figure 3. Prefabricated butchering rail.

On arrival at the village they would be met by the village council representative and (usually) by the sanitarian. With them the headman would check that the site was identified and clear, the labourers available, and the concrete aggregate collected and stacked ready for use. In the early stages of the programme, it was sometimes found that these preparations had not, in fact, been made. The driver had instructions not to unload in such cases, but to proceed immediately to the next village on the list. After this had happened once or twice, the word got round, and everything was usually ready on arrival.

The truck was then unloaded and left for provincial headquarters, returning in 12 days' time (a Thursday) to pick up the headman, assistant, and tools and take them back to headquarters. If the work was not completed by then, it was left unfinished and, again, this only needed to happen on a couple of occasions to ensure that future slabs were completed on time. In practice, the work was usually finished early in the second week, so that the headman enjoyed a day or two's idleness as his 'perks'. Thus steady progress of one completed slab per fortnight, later to be increased to two per fortnight when the second team was working, was regularly maintained.

Conclusion

As a model for repetitive minor construction jobs in remote villages, the programme was considered reasonably successful, and the following conditions were identified as contributing to that success:

○ The headman must be compatible with the communities among whom he has to live.
○ The work must be simple, as must be the tools and methods used. Once a pattern has been established as a routine, this should not be varied from one place to another.
○ As much work as possible (in this case blocks and hanging rails) should be prefabricated elsewhere under supervision.
○ The whole procedure must be worked out in the fullest possible detail before the programme starts, and there must be one or two trials under close supervision so that the headman knows exactly what he is doing and what snags may arise in practice. The points on which decisions have to be made on site should be kept to a minimum.
○ The programme must be 'sold' in advance so that each community genuinely wants the work done and has applied for it. Without this, the people would feel that the project had been imposed on them from outside, leading to a reluctance to co-operate that would doom the whole programme as a time-wasting exercise.
○ Undoubtedly a number of slabs were less than perfect — with sides out of alignment, hanging rails not level or concrete surfaces irregular. While the attention of the headman should be (and was) called to such defects with a view to future improvement, it is felt that too much emphasis should not be given to them.
○ While there was no supervision in a formal sense, an official interest in the programme was maintained whenever possible. An occasional visit by engineering or medical staff when in the neighbourhood, and a word of encouragement from time to time, were considred to be helpful in promoting enthusiasm among villagers and headmen alike.

(*Waterlines* Vol. 1 No. 3, January 1983)

CHAPTER 8

Training for Health

Chapters 8 and 9 are complementary, as training, education, communication and participation are closely intertwined. This chapter deals essentially with the training of the teachers or health promoters, while chapter 9 looks at education and community participation, but inevitably there is overlap.

The WASH experience and methods are described by Ray Isely and Fred Rosenweig. The WASH approach is intended to turn non-technical workers into developers and implementers of village water and sanitation projects. To this end, WASH has developed training guides containing all the information a trainee needs to conduct a workshop, lasting about a fortnight, based on a specific community project.

Kristian Laubjerg describes an experiment in Tanzania to train village women as health promoters. The women were chosen by their peers; few held any influence through their own or their husband's position, but were apparently chosen because they were known to be outspoken on issues of public concern and to take good care of their families and houses. These health promoters held group meetings in which they led and guided discussions and encouraged participation through the contribution of ideas. The study showed that it is possible to use untrained village women as health promoters.

In Nepal, sanitation was introduced into the water-supply programme. Vanessa Tobin describes the organization together with the training of Nepali technicians to demonstrate, motivate and supervise the construction of pit latrines. Slow progress is being made in this formidable programme.

DMB Jagne describes a sanitation project supervised by the School of Public Health of Gambia College financed by IDRC. The work is done through village health educators, and one of its main objectives is to introduce suitable sanitary structures that could be replicated in other areas.

Women's organizations and programmes have great potential to mobilize women to improve their own water supply and sanitation, if they are not served by other programmes. Christine van Wijk-Sijbesma in this article, extracted from an IRC publication,[97] outlines a few examples and recommends that these efforts be incorporated and supported in national programmes by donor agencies.

Training non-technical workers for rural water and sanitation projects

RAY ISELY AND FRED ROSENSWEIG

In many countries, constraints such as limited budgets and lack of transportation make it difficult for water-supply agencies to hire new staff to work with communities .

For the immediate future, a better solution would be to employ the cadres already working at the community level. This nucleus of personnel, including nurses assigned to rural health posts, health assistants, health promoters, social affairs agents, and rural development workers, for the most part lack technical skills in water supply and sanitation. They tend to have broad-based responsibilities in either health or community development. Although they are well aware of the water and sanitation problems faced by communities, they often do not have the technical expertise to assist them to overcome such problems.

Some have been exposed to water-supply and sanitation issues in their training, but have generally had little practical experience. What is required, therefore, is the retraining of these workers so that they have the necessary skills and knowledge. They should work with community leaders, local skilled tradesmen and government technical personnel to promote low cost technologies.

The problem of staffing

There are serious personnel deficiencies in the water-supply agencies charged with carrying out IDWSSD plans and programmes. Because many of the agencies have focused their energies and resources on urban areas and high technology, they lack the staff to serve the essentially unsophisticated technological needs of rural people. Even where rural water supply is assigned to a special agency, only a few staff are usually available to cover wide areas of the countryside. Furthermore, sanitation is almost never a part of the programmme, because the responsibility for this area usually lies with the Ministry of Health. Instances of effective collaboration between water-supply agencies and Ministries of Health, while increasing, are still the exception rather than the rule. Decade goals, therefore, may not be reached in many countries unless a solution to the shortage of qualified personnel can be found.

In most countries, the field staff of the ministries closest to rural communities are usually primary school teachers and agricultural-extension, rural-development and health workers. These workers are frequently at the periphery of projects during the installation of water supplies or latrines, but become intimately involved when facilities break down, or are not used properly. All too often they see the problems, but, lacking technical skills, are unable to help communities find solutions. Moreover, they are often acutely aware of communities needing improved water-supply and sanitation facilities, but are unable to help these communities initiate local projects.

Suggested areas for training

While each of these types of people has special skills and knowledge, health personnel, by virtue of their interest and training in sanitation, hygiene, and health education, may have the most to offer. They cannot, however, be expected to acquire all the technical skills related to water-supply and sanitation systems, such as those requiring motorized pumping, conventional water treatment, or lay-out of a piped distribution system. Nevertheless, a grounding in these subjects can be taught to non-technical personnel. Suggested technical areas in which non-technical personnel can be trained include:

1. Maintenance and repair of handpumps
O Fundamental steps for maintaining the handpump models being used in the area, including the ability to train local caretakers in the same skills.
O Recognition of breakdowns, simple repairs, and knowledge of where to refer problems to more technically qualified personnel.

2. Development of water sources: springs, shallow wells and cisterns for rain catchment
O Concrete-making skills.
O Steps to assess a spring for possible capping.
O Steps in spring-capping.
O Steps in digging a shallow well, including an assessment of when to ask for assistance from a technical agency (for example, when soft soil is encountered).
O How to construct a cistern of the right size for the numbers of users.
O How to assemble a roof-catchment system.

3. Protection of wells
O Parapet construction.
O Well lining.
O Apron and drain construction.

O Animal watering-trough construction.
O Protection of well surroundings from domestic animals.

4. Construction of latrines, both simple and improved.
O Digging the pit, including lining when necessary.
O Making and installing the slab.
O Building the superstructures.

5. Protection of water during transport and storage
O Protection of vessels.
O Disinfection.

6. Solid waste disposal
O Individual.
O Collective.

7. Sullage
O Drainage.
O Use of sullage for gardens.

The WASH approach

Since its inception in 1980, the WASH Project has accumulated field experience in training non-technical workers in some of these areas.

The WASH approach is based on a realistic assessment of the role and job responsibilities of non-technical workers.

First, these workers have responsibilities other than in the areas of either water or sanitation. Because they are the focal point of services at the rural level for their ministries or agencies, these individuals are usually overworked, and, therefore, have little time for new responsibilities.

Second, because it is unrealistic to expect to turn them into trained water and sanitation technicians, it is most effective to provide them with skills for planning and community organization as well as basic technical skills for village-level projects. Because most community workers work with between 10 to 20 communities, it is important to use an approach that puts them in planning and supervisory roles.

WASH emphasizes a project-oriented approach during its training courses. The two-week workshops lead the participants through a series of activities related to each stage of the project cycle, that is, pre-planning and assessment, planning and design, construction, maintenance and repair and evaluation: a balance of technical and organizational skills.

It is expected that the non-technical worker will ensure that the community is interested, carry out the detailed planning tasks, and supervise - but not carry out - the construction. The construction is usually completed by local masons or other skilled village tradesmen, who are assisted by community labour. The fieldworkers supervise and monitor progress. They are prepared for this by constructing a system during the workshop.

The approach in action

In short, the WASH approach is intended to turn the non-technical worker into a developer and implementer of village water and sanitation projects. This 'hands-on' approach was used to train social affairs agents in Togo in spring-capping and rainwater roof catchment. These agents are the fieldworkers with primary responsibility for implementing a rural water-supply project funded by the US Agency for International Development (USAID).

The original technology chosen for the project was drilled wells with handpumps. But because a high percentage of the wells were dry, the project decided to expand the low-cost technologies at its disposal. The social afffairs agents had three years diploma training after high school but little technical background. As a result, WASH sponsored two workshops, one for each technology. During the workshops, a spring was capped using a retaining wall system and a roof catchment cistern with a capacity of 19.2 m³ was built.

In Bakel, Senegal, 16 nurses assigned to rural health posts were trained in latrine construction, solid waste disposal and sullage disposal. Because they had all been trained as clinical nurses in a two- to three-year programme after secondary school, they were aware of disease cycles and the need for excreta disposal and safe water supplies. Most, however, had no technical skills. As the chief primary health-care workers at the village level, however, the nurses held the only solution to expanding water and sanitation coverage. During the workshop, five latrines were built, using a type of latrine and a method of construction appropriate and familiar to that area of Senegal.

Also under the auspices of the WASH Project, two workshops were held in the Dominican Republic on latrine construction. The participants, community organizers, were high school graduates and a few had a university education. None had a technical background. They were working for the Ministry of Health in a USAID-funded rural water-supply and sanitation project with three main components: handpumps, latrines, and health education. Their role was to do the preliminary work with the communities before the drilling rig and handpump installation teams arrived and to promote the construction and use of latrines. As such, the workshops were designed to prepare the community organizers to work with the communities more effectively and to monitor the construction of the latrines. Six latrines were constructed in a community during the workshop, using the latrine design adopted by the project.

Training guides

To make the training of non-technical workers a less formidable task, WASH has developed four training guides on low-cost water-supply and sanitation technologies. These training guides contain all the information a trainer needs to plan and conduct a comprehensive workshop, including training designs, trainer guidelines, participant handouts, and trainer reference materials. Each workshop is approximately two weeks long.

The guides use highly participatory training methods based on the principles of adult learning. They contain a variety of training techniques, including demonstrations, small group tasks, role playing, case studies, and 'hands-on' field tasks. Training takes place in a rural setting similar to the participants' normal work situation and uses village labour and local masons, just as in an actual project. In addition to the four training guides currently available, others are planned for the future on hand-dug wells, domestic sanitation (excluding excreta disposal), and community participation. They are available from WASH.

Preliminary recommendations

Although the major purpose of the work reported was to pre-test and revise the training guides in the technical areas mentioned, it is possible to make some preliminary recommendations, based on lessons learned, regarding the feasibility of training non-technical workers in water-supply and sanitation technologies.

First, there is the obvious conclusion that health, social, and other non-technical workers are able to acquire skills needed to play significant roles in water supply and sanitation, with the provision that such skills be restricted to those required in a certain minimal package needed for community-level projects. We did not teach skills related to motorized pumps, multi-branched gravity flow water systems, and other complex installations.

Skills are best learned if they are acquired within the context of planning a community project, that is, mobilizing the community, planning for construction, organizing a village labour force, planning for maintenance and repair, and the education of the population in the proper use of the water and sanitation installations.

Lastly and most importantly, these skills should be taught to non-technical staff only if there is an opportunity in which to use them. In Togo, the acquisition of spring-capping or rainwater catchment skills was linked to project planning by villagers in the project area, so that a village could receive a grant of $8,000 for a local project if its plan was approved. Some of these projects would undoubtedly involve spring-capping or rainwater catchment, but when the trainees finished their workshops, no village had yet started one. Further, it was decided to delay the initiation of subsidiary projects related to water supply until after the arrival of a project engineer in mid-1984. Thus, nearly a year was expected to pass until workers could put their new skills into operation. The workshop, while useful for pre-testing the training guide, was poorly co-ordinated with project operations.

(Waterlines Vol. 3 No. 2, October 1984)

Training village women as health promoters in Tanzania

KRISTIAN LAUBJERG

During the preparation of the Water Master Plan for Mbeya Region in the south-western highlands of Tanzania between 1980 and 1983, UNICEF experimented with village participation at Utengule. One of the experiments involved recruiting volunteer village women as health promoters in a village.

The experiments resulted in a field manual to be used by the technical staff from the water department, the health staff, and the community development staff. The manual explains in detail how the health education component is to be integrated with the overall water project, giving the 'hows', the 'whos' and the 'whens'. The manual has in principle been accepted by the Ministry of Water & Natural Resources in Tanzania.[98]

While the overall purpose of the experiment was to plan future health education projects in combination with water projects, the specific objectives for recruiting women as health promoters were:

O To increase villagers' awareness of diseases which may be related to water, poor hygiene or poor sanitation.

O To encourage individuals and groups to improve or change their environment in such a way that it can facilitate and reinforce behaviour which is in agreement with principles for proper health, hygiene and sanitation.

We assumed that behaviour modifications can only occur when health education is accompanied by changes in the physical environment of the villagers.

Before the contents of the health education component were decided, baseline studies were undertaken to examine how much contamination took place between when the water was collected and when it was consumed, and to examine hygiene and sanitary habits among the villagers. In addition, to permit evaluation of the previous health education intervention, a small household survey was undertaken.

Putting participation into practice

Bearing in mind the constraints presented by the shortage of health workers in the rural areas of Tanzania, it was decided to carry out the health-education experiment in as participatory a manner as possible. We aimed at training a cadre of villagers who, in turn, would teach other villagers. The district health authorities were involved in all aspects of the planning of the project, but due to a cholera outbreak elsewhere, they were not involved in the actual implementation.

Originally, it had been planned to involve dispensary staff and the primary school teachers. But the teachers' tight working schedule combined with the final exams for their standard-seven pupils made this impossible. The dispensary staff could not participate fully either because the times of the meetings chosen by the women participants (see below) were not compatible with their working hours. Most project activities took place in the morning when the dispensary staff were busy attending to patients; consequently they too could not be fully involved. For these reasons, it was decided that project staff would be in charge of the experiment throughout. The project staff consisted of two female assistants with no previous experience of health or education projects.

Often, actual changes in the physical environment are needed to prompt the desired behaviour modification. Since attitudes are formed in the process of interacting with other people, group discussions were considered to be the best method for modifying attitudes and behaviour.

Mothers, infants and young children belong to the highest risk groups. Traditionally, women are responsible for the collection of water. Therefore, the aim of the experiment was to improve the health of mothers and children and thus indirectly that of the whole family. The project had decided that it would attempt to use village women as health educators.

The main subjects to be covered during the training of the village health promoters were suggested by the project group based on the baseline studies. It had specified the desired behaviour to be achieved in relation to each main subject. The actual training content was prepared by the District Health Officer. There were five topics:

O Water use at home.
O Water use at the tap.
O Water use at traditional sources.
O Sanitation and personal hygiene.
O Cattle keeping.

This was of relevance because villagers tended to water the milk with contaminated water to make it go further.

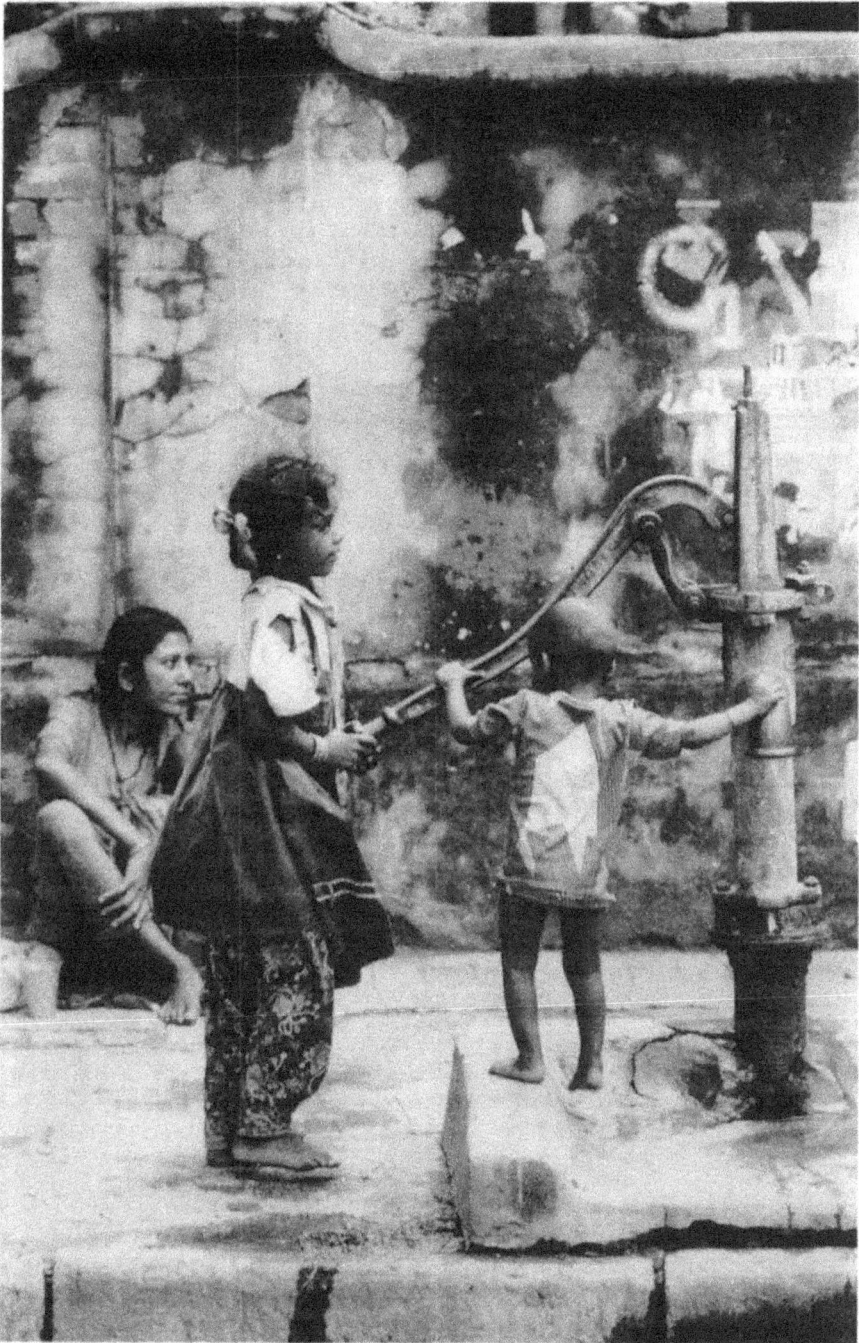

An old handpump installation in need of maintenance.
(WaterAid/Framework)

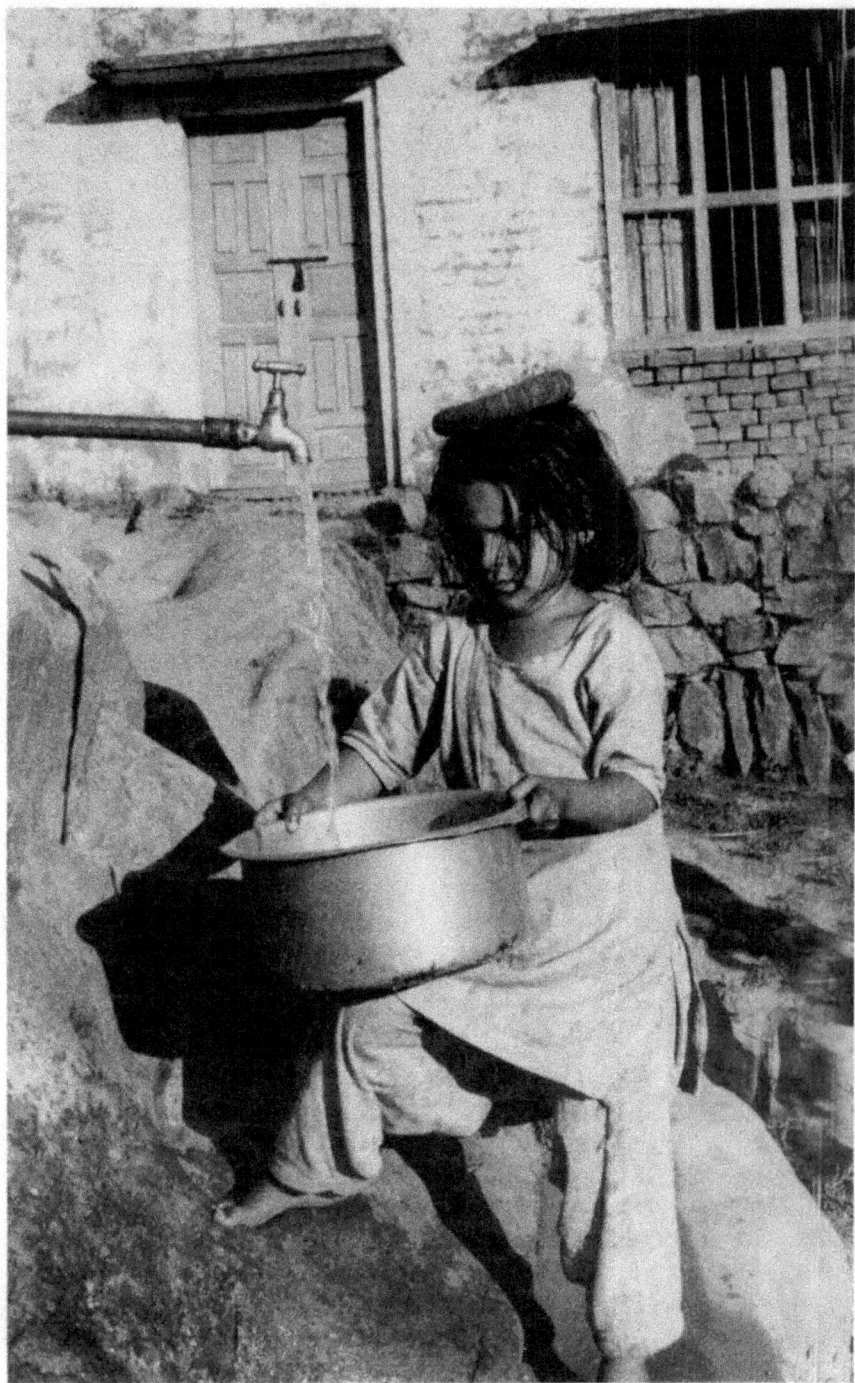

A single tap for health and hygiene in Pakistan (UNICEF/ Rehman)

Village women's meeting

Upon arrival in the village, the project team called all the village women together, through the ten cell-leaders. Approximately 100 women turned up, and we told them about the project in general and our plans for putting it into practice. The women present were given an opportunity to suggest changes. Generally, they expressed support for the project, and 16 women were chosen as village health promoters during discussions with the other women, so the training was carried out with everyone sitting in a circle.

The topics under discussion were not new to the women. They made suggestions, comments, asked for clarifications, different views were aired and deliberated upon. They did not agree all the time, and sometimes the discussions were lively. Most of the women were very vocal and knowledgeable.

Had the women health promoters been chosen by the project staff, they would most likely all have been literate. Table 1 shows that no single variable stands out when characterizing the women selected by their peers.

Eighty-two per cent of the women were married, and their average age was 30 years. Almost 40 per cent did not have any children, and 50 per cent were illiterate. Only one woman held any formal position in the village, while four were married with husbands holding some influential position in the village. The amounts of land they cultivated were average for the area.

We believe that these women were chosen because they were known to be outspoken on issues of village concern. All of them were known to take

Table 1: Description of village health promoters

Sample No	Age	Marital status	No of children	Educational background	Position of husband	Acres of shamba
1	34	Married	10	none	none	4.5
2	22	Married	0	Std.7	none	7
3	24	Married	4	Std.2	balozi	3.5
4	35	Married	3	none	literacy teacher	3
5	22	Married	1	Std.7	vill. govn.	2
6	23	Single	2	Std.7	-	2.5
7	40	Married	0	none	none	0
8	19	Married	1	Std.7	none	2
9	50	Divorced	0	none	-	1
10	36	Widow	0	Std.4	-	7
11	30	Married	6	Ad. class	none	4
12	30	Married	0	none	medicine man	6
13	25	Married	2	Ad. class	none	10
14	25	Married	3	none	none	0
15	47	Married	1	none	balozi	2
16	29	Married	0	none	none	3

good care of their families and to keep their houses clean. The fact that 40 per cent of the women did not have children may also have given these women more time to spend on project activities.

The project team would not have been able to choose the same women based on any formal criteria because we could not quantify the variables which village women felt would assist the project. The cleanest house in the village was kept by a 40-year-old illiterate health promoter.

Discussion groups

After the training of the 16 health promoters, groups of women were formed among the neighbours of each health promoter. To cover the whole village, nine groups were formed with two trained women health promoters in most of the groups, one of whom was literate. They were to act as discussion leaders. For a majority of them, this was to be their first experience of addressing an audience in public, and we thought that two women together would give each other moral support.

The primary role of these village health promoters was to lead and guide the discussions, and also to encourage each woman to participate and contribute ideas to help solve the problems being discussed. An indication of the success of any project is found in the number of people attending during the project period. From Table 2, we see that almost 40 per cent of all the village women (346) attended the meetings.

Table 2: Attendance of health education sessions

Group	No of members	1st meeting	Attendance 2nd meeting	3rd meeting	Mean
A	36	12 (33%)	19 (53%)	20 (55%)	47%
B	51	22 (43%)	32 (62%)	31 (61%)	55%
C	31	18 (58%)	13 (42%)	13 (42%)	47%
D	59	13 (22%)	25 (42%)	24 (40%)	35%
E	29	20 (69%)	15 (52%)	15 (52%)	57%
F	30	none	15 (50%)	13 (43%)	31%
G	41	21 (51%)	14 (34%)	21 (51%)	45%
H	44	32 (73%)	25 (57%)	14 (31%)	53%
I	25	16 (64%)	18 (72%)	13 (52%)	62%
TOTAL	**346**	**154 (44%)**	**176 (51%)**	**164 (47%)**	**47%**

The relatively high attendance was attributed to the following factors:

O The participants never had to walk far, since they were selected from among the neighbours of the particular village health promoter.

O The participants themselves choose the meeting times from days given to them by the project.

O All group meetings were supported by the project team who were able to supervise all meetings at least for some time.

O The *balozis* concerned informed participants of the locations and times of the first meeting and reminded them of subsequent meetings.

O Each meeting was planned in such a way that whatever topic was raised within the theme of water, health and sanitation, the village health promoter would know how to prompt the discussion further by using a list of key words.

O Attendance lists were kept for each group.

Due to the start of the agricultural season, attendance was never complete. In total, each group had three discussion sessions over a period of two weeks. About 50 per cent of the enrolled women participated in each discussion session. Group F had to cancel its first meeting because the members had not been properly informed.

Outcome

The ultimate test of an experimental health education project is, of course, whether the target group took any action to resolve the problems discussed.

One of the participants summed up our whole pilot project when she said that it was unrealistic to educate the people and tell them not to bathe in the river or not to wash in the river when there were no other alternatives. Only with such faciles might some of the problems raised during the discussions be alleviated.

After lengthy discussions, the participants decided in favour of a rectangular-shaped washing slab and sheltered bathing faciles for men and women. After a meeting was held with the Village Water Committee (VWC), which consisted of three men and three women, the village secretary and the village *fundi* (artisan), the following agreement was made:

O Members of the VWC should supervise the construction of an experimental washing slab and shelter for bathing, carried out by the village *fundis*.

O The *fundis* would be provided with enough labour on each of three working days normally used for communal activities.

O The project would supply cement, and other building materials not available locally.

O The village would supply locally available material such as sand, burnt bricks and skilled and unskilled labour.

After the meeting we paid a visit to the dispensary, and decided to build a demonstration washing slab in the compound.

Improvement

Though one cannot expect changes in attitude in the short term from health education in general, a noticeable improvement in the village environment took place during the health education week.

Latrines appeared to be much cleaner, a few villagers without latrines were observed to be digging fresh ones, and among some of those who already had latrines, a few were engaged in renovating them. The houses looked much better than they had during a preliminary visit five months earlier. Floors and walls were being smoothed and cracks filled in. There were also freshly dug rubbish pits. The yards and plots surrounding the houses were in many cases cleared and grass burnt, ready for the rainy season.

Altogether, the project staff spent about 10 weeks in the village from planning to implementation. At the time of finishing the experiment, the 34 households which were part of the baseline study were visited again. Table 3 shows that changes had taken place during the intervention period as far as sanitary and hygiene conditions were concerned.

Table 3: Sanitary conditions among households before and after experimental health education

Characteristics of sanitary facilities	Percentage of households before and after health education	
	Before	After
Without pit latrine	12	3
Dirty pit latrine	18	9
Yard dirty	53	44
No pit for refuse	50	15

Though this study in no way pretends to be scientific, it has nevertheless shown that it is possible to use almost untrained village women as health promoters, even without a honorarium.

It was found that the villagers in most cases were aware of the more important diseases caused by contaminated water, poor sanitation and hygiene. What apparently was required to change the undesired behaviour was prompting. Once a concensus had been reached in the discussion groups about which action to take, the project staff assisted with the required materials. This suggests that availability of appropriate technology plays a decisive role in changing behaviour patterns.

(Waterlines Vol. 4 No. 3, January 1986)

Sanitation training in Nepal

VANESSA TOBIN

In most developing countries, water-supply programmes are developed separately from sanitation programmes with little co-ordination. In Nepal, it was decided to introduce sanitation into the Government rural water-supply programme, since this had already been organized and would require minimum extra assistance, whereas setting up a separate sanitation programme would require additional manpower and resources.

We introduced sanitation into the water-supply programme on an experimental basis for a year before it was officially adopted. We started to train the Nepali technicians already working in the government water-supply programme in 1981.

The programme is run by the government with assistance from UNICEF. In each village:

O Latrines are constructed by technicians at the local school, health post and government buildings. We use the Ventilated Improved Pit type, chosen for its minimal water-use and maintenance requirements. The villagers provide local materials and unskilled labour.

O The government provides all other materials and skilled labour.

O The technicians construct a demonstration household pit latrine made entirely from local materials at the house where they stay during construction. The technicians also supervise any villager who is interested in constructing a latrine at his home. Households provide all the materials and labour for the construction of their own latrine. Health-education materials are given to the local school and health post and distributed in the village by field staff who also assist in explaining the benefits of sanitation.

Introducing sanitation is no economic burden to the programme since the cost per project is only 3-5 per cent of the total cost of the water-supply system. Commitment and belief, though, is required from the project staff in order to convince the villagers of the benefits of sanitation. We found that the best technicians at promoting sanitation were the ones who believed in it, not necessarily the ones who were the best technically. The programme is now being expanded, and new staff have been recruited to work solely in sanitation and health education in each project.

Objectives of sanitation training

The prime objective of training in sanitation for field staff was to increase their awareness of the need for introducing sanitation into the rural areas of Nepal. Only then could they hope to motivate the villagers to construct their own household latrines. The training courses given to the field staff constantly stressed the health impact that combining water and sanitation would have on the community. However, we expect that it could take 3-5 years to motivate the staff properly before we see any significant results in the villages. We aimed to develop a good training programme that concentrated not only on the technical aspects, but also on methods of convincing the field staff to change their own attitudes and present sanitary habits, so that they could change those of the villagers.

Programme field staff

There are four levels of field staff working within the Community Water Supply and Sanitation (CWSS) Programme at present. They are: Engineer, Overseer, Water & Sanitation Technician and Community Sanitation Worker. Sanitation training is given to all levels of staff except Engineers. Their roles within the programme and their sanitation duties are briefly described below.

The Engineer is responsible for the overall supervision of construction of approximately 10 to 12 water-supply projects within his region and will organize their surveying, design and construction. He also has to ensure that latrine construction is implemented according to the policy of the Ministry, and supervise the other field staff. He will co-ordinate and exchange information and progress reports with other regions through the Sanitation Unit of the Ministry.

The Overseer, who is trained to diploma level, is responsible for supervising the construction of between one and three projects, depending on their size and location, and will spend time living in each project village. He will supervise the work of the Technicians closely and ensure that the level of construction is up to standard. He will assist Technicians in promoting sanitation.

The Technician is usually an artisan recruited from local villages and trained for six weeks by the Ministry. One or two Technicians are assigned to each village, where they live during construction. They supervise local skilled and unskilled workers in the construction of the water-supply system and the institutional latrines, while training local village maintenance workers and supervising villagers in building their own latrines.

The post of Community Sanitation Worker (CSW) was only introduced into the programme in August 1983, and, at present they are only working in 10 selected districts on a trial basis. The CSWs are either local artisans or teachers recruited for their communications skills and any previous health education or construction experience. They are interviewed by project staff selected from local villages and interviewed by project staff. The CSWs live and work within a group of two or three project villages each year. They are paid the same salary as the Technicians and have the same level of responsibility. They supervise the construction of household latrines and visit every home in the village to discuss the health benefits of water and sanitation. They assist the Technicians in motivating the community to construct latrines at schools, health posts and government buildings. CSWs also supervise the water quality and drainage aspects of the project. Staff are all male at present.

Training courses

The first sanitation course was given to Water Technicians in Nepal's Eastern Development Region in July 1981. Those who successfully completed the course were upgraded to Water & Sanitation Technicians. This initial training course was used to develop a suitable job specification of the sanitation aspect for the Technicians and also to test new designs for the latrines built at institutions.

The training course was then incorporated into the water-supply upgrading training courses. Sanitation training has been included in all training courses for Technicians throughout the country since 1982. Refresher courses are given each year. The courses consist of a series of lectures, and practical latrine construction sessions are organized by engineers of the Ministry of Panchayat & Local Development with the assistance of health educators and sanitarians of the Ministry of Health.

Sanitation training courses include the following topics:
O Causes and transmission routes of water-related diseases. An explanation of the different paths of infection were given and of how sanitation provides an effective barrier to the spread of excreta-based diseases.
O Specific diseases caused by poor water supplies and sanitation. A brief simple description of the major water-related diseases, their symptoms and control measures.
O Personal and home hygiene. It is important for the Technicians to stress the significance of a clean environment to prevent the spread of disease when they are working in the villages.
O Different technical options. A brief summary of all the different types of latrines, especially those more suitable for hill conditions.
O Communications techniques within the village. The Technicians are trained in different methods of teaching health education and for arousing interest within the village.
O Distribution of and the use of suitable health education materials. The Technician is given a water and sanitation kit consisting of a health education textbook and a set of posters to give the teachers at the local school. He is taught how to use this effectively to support the teachers.
O Construction of latrines. These are constructed in project villages near

the training sites to ensure that the Technicians are proficient in their construction.

Technicians are also trained to use the subject of oral rehydration therapy to make contact with village women and gain their confidence. If a child has diarrhoea, the Technicians will explain that bad sanitation is often a root cause and show the mother how to make home-made oral rehydration solution. This sort of information reinforces the link between sanitation and health in the villagers' minds.

Training courses for new technicians are shorter and are usually of one week duration since they initially require more time to familiarize themselves with the water and sanitation programme as a whole. Other technicians usually receive two weeks training.

Overseers are given four-day training courses to brief them about their responsibilities for sanitation. They cover technical options; water-related diseases; procedures for sanitation and communication techniques in order to persuade the villagers of the benefits. Doctors of the Ministy of Health and a sanitary engineer from India assist in the courses.

New Community Sanitation Workers are given a six-week training course in one of the more remote regions of Nepal. It has to be far more extensive than the training the Technicians received since the CSWs need far more training in health education. They are trained in the diagnosis of simple common illnesses, and taught some basic medicine.

The CSWs also need more basic training in construction since their previous experience is limited. Their training is interspersed with field visits to the CWSS projects for practical construction sessions and to familiarize them with the role they would play. It is very important that they develop their technical skills so that they can demonstrate practical ways of improving environmental conditions. CSWs are also trained in chlorinating a new water-supply system; constructing a simple soakpit; making simple clay-pot water filters and providing adequate drainage at tapstands.

The training courses were used for testing new latrine designs, and, from these, standard designs were developed for the programme. Ideas from other countries were assessed for their suitability in Nepal. Field staff are encouraged to assist in developing new designs. It is very important that all designs are thoroughly tested prior to their introduction to project villages and that field staff are proficient in their construction.

Evaluation

The work of the field staff has been closely monitored for the past two years to assess how effective their training courses have been. In the Mid-Western Region, which is classified as 'remote', at least 80 per cent of the villagers had constructed their own latrine in 8 out of 10 of the projects. One of the Technicians in this area who had worked closely with four villages for two years had succeeded in motivating 85 per cent of the people to construct their own latrine. His major complaint was, though, that he had had insufficient time to supervise the construction, and, therefore, the standard was not as high as it should have been. Most of the Technicians felt that they needed more time to motivate the villagers effectively and that the programme did not allow for this.

The most successful areas were where the Technicians were given constant encouragement and support by their Overseers and Engineers. In some areas, however, there were greater pressures, caused by the need to satisfy government targets for the construction of water-supply systems. Therefore, sanitation was given less attention. In general, it was considered that the training courses had succeeded in starting to motivate staff, but that they needed to be expanded.

Initially both the Overseers and Technicans had not been enthusiastic about receiving sanitation training. They were more interested in the health education component, because they were keen to learn more about how they could improve their own health and that of their families.

Survey of Technicians

During training a survey was performed in which the Technicians were questioned about their own health. In one survey held in the more developed Eastern Region, all 50 Technicans had suffered each construction season from some excreta-based disease. The most common illnesses were dysentery, round-worm and hookworm. Only 30 per cent of the Technicians, though, had any sanitary facilities in their homes. It was therefore vey difficult for them to be effective in promoting sanitation in project villages, when they felt no strong need for sanitation themselves. Appealing to their interest in improving their own health gradually persuaded them to take a much greater interest in sanitation.

Conclusions

The field staff of the Community Water Supply & Sanitation Programme have gradually started to include sanitation in their own work. This has been mainly due to the training courses effectively encouraging staff to accept sanitation as an integral component of their jobs within the programme rather than an extra work burden. It is very important not to put pressure on field staff to perform their duties, but that they should feel motivated enough to want to do the work. The Technicians and Overseers live within rural villages and are aware of the health problems. As they become more motivated, they will play a significant role in improving environmental conditions.

In Nepal, sanitation has always appeared a formidable problem. Progress is now being made, slowly. The continuing success of the CWSS programme depends upon providing the necessary support to field staff through training courses and feedback sessions in order to find out their problems and ensure that they are aware of the importance of their role in improving conditions in their country.

(*Waterlines* Vol. 4 No 2, October 1985)

A demonstration sanitation project in the Gambia

D. M. B. JAGNE

The Gambia College School of Public Health set up a sanitation project at Kerr Seringe to create an awareness of the dangers of inadequate water supply and waste disposal, and to provide the School of Public Health with a demonstration area equipped with well-constructed wells and latrines.

The project was supervised by the school and was financed by the International Development Research Centre, Canada. The building of wells and latrines was supported by health education programmes given by the students and staff of the School. The aim was to find out how acceptable these structures would be to the residents. Furthermore, through the provision of the health facilities, it was hoped that the sanitary environment of the village would be noticeably improved, leading to improved health in the village.

Assessment of needs

In order to determine the appropriateness of the project, the needs of the village had to be assessed. Over 95 per cent of all those questioned declared without reservation their need for good sanitary wells and public latrines. A comprehensive sociological survey was made to identify the tribal groupings, customs, cultures, habits and taboos. This was followed up by a demographic survey and geographical reconnaissance. In developing the concepts and strategies of health education, these factors had to be borne in mind:
O The narrow educational background of the village health educators chosen by the people. They needed instruction in the scientific theories of the causes of diseases. They were therefore taken from the village to the School of Public Health where they underwent three month courses on various aspects of health education with emphasis on prevention of water pollution, waste disposal and food hygiene.
O The literacy rate in the village is extremely low. Only 13 per cent of the

population have had any formal education. Of these, only 3.9 per cent
had reached secondary school level. The standard of education among
females is much lower than among males, probably due to a cultural
restriction on female education.
O There are two main tribal groupings in the village, each group being
sensitive to what the other is doing. We took advantage of this division
by generating competitive programmes based on issues directed towards
behavioural change in accepting the new technologies.
O The students of the School, although keen and enthusiastic, lacked the
experience of dealing with rural dwellers. The concept of developing
receiver-oriented programmes rather than source-oriented ones had to be
established with all groups of students. The students' feeling that their
ideas had to be accepted by the villagers had to be abandoned.

The Village Health Educators regularly hold talks with the people in the
village. Experience taught them to encourage small groups rather than large
crowds. They develop different routines for different days. On Monday
evenings, they visit the spot in the village called *bantaba*, where the issues
of the day are sometimes discussed. On Wednesday evenings they make
home visits and concentrate on teaching nursing mothers and households
about sanitation. On Thursday mornings, they make several calls at the old
well on the outskirts of the village where womenfolk congregate to do their
laundry and talk. On Saturday evenings, they usually go to the open field
south of the village where boys meet to play and watch games.

Each of the three classes at the School of Public Health pays regular
visits to the village, and students work with project officials on various
health education aspects and data collection. In order to satisfy the needs of
all those involved in the project, villagers, students and the investigating
team had to be involved in the health education concepts. Two of the
villagers were trained as Health Educators to work with their own people.
This gave more confidence to the others, who realized that if their own kith
and kin could be trained to discuss such matters with them, they were then
capable also of understanding and putting the new ideas into practice. This
was found to to be a very effective technique.

The needs of the students also had to be satisfied by taking them to the
village regularly to see methods used in construction, highlighting what
should be avoided and what should be incorporated, giving them practical
lessons in the health education theories covered in class and exposing them
to some of the conditions they would face in the rural areas when they grad-
uated.

The third group involved is the Investigating Team at the School. Its
members have supervised the construction team at the village, the Village
Health Educators, and the students during visits. Since the team co-ordi-
nates the efforts from all sectors towards the success of the project, it is the
motivating force.

Implementation phase

After establishing that provision of public wells and latrines were the priority of the villagers, the implementation phase was started by forming the main village committees and assigning tasks to the various groups.

The village community was to provide labour for digging wells and latrines, moulding blocks for the walls, and providing sand and fetching water for the workers. IDRC agreed to provide the other construction materials, a vehicle, and fuel. The staff and students of the School of Public Health had the responsibility of supervising all aspects of the project, including collection of data and interpretation of results.

Well digging and rehabilitation

Wells are the main source of water. Before the project started, there were only 10 household wells and three public wells serving the village. There were 38 households without wells. None of the 10 private wells was lined with concrete, and most of them were known to dry out during the dry season. From a survey made to determine the amount of water used in the village each day, it was found that an average of 300 gallons (1,350 litres) could be drawn from the three public hand-dug wells using ropes and buckets each day. The 10 private wells were therefore estimated to give 3,000 gallons (13,500 litres). For a population of about 250 people, this was found to be quite inadequate. The project dug seven new wells and rehabilitated two of the public wells. The public wells were lined with bricks and will be sealed with cement slabs fitted with suction model handpumps.

The quality of the water appears to be greatly improved due to the construction of the new wells, better methods of retrieving the water and the changes in the attitude of the people towards the way they now use the wells. This has come about mainly as a result of their participation in health education.

Sanitation improvements

There were no public latrines in the village. Of the 48 households, 26 had latrines. The rest used the bush. The household latrines were found to be generally poorly constructed. Eighty-five per cent were made of straw and palm leaves that only last for short periods. The other latrines were made from mud bricks that could not withstand heavy and prolonged rain. Virtually all the latrines had no roofs, were not fly-proof and gave little privacy. The project built seven sets of public latrines based on the Ventilated Improved Pit (VIP) model in different parts of the village. Each latrine had a pit 3m deep, 1m wide and 2m long, with reinforced concrete slabs supported by seasoned hardwood sticks laid across the trench. The walls were built from cement blocks, and the roof from corrugated iron sheets. The vent pipes face the path of the sun. Investigations revealed that after the commissioning of the public latrines, all members of the 22 households now use them.

Health Education concepts, spread through the village health workers and the school, will continue to provide motivation and reinforcement, which has thus been incorporated into the village's internal structure.

Ebb and flow of enthusiasm

The enthusiasm of the community at the planning and implementing stages of the project was overwhelming. But as things progressed, this enthusiasm evaporated to the extent that people had to be literally dragged out of their houses to give their expected quota of labour. The lethargic and nonchalant attitude became quite obvious when rumours started going round the village that all the workers were going to be paid. Willingness to volunteer therefore quickly disappeared.

A series of meetings with the committee and other groups had to be arranged to acquaint all those concerned with the contents of the project document. Community participation returned to a high level after all the misconceptions were ironed out. Enthusiasm gathered again when most of the superstructures were taking shape and people began to see the fruits of their efforts. Towards the end of the construction work, all those who had disappeared earlier started to re-emerge, wanting to be identified with the project. The village's pride in the project and the envy of the other villages was highlighted by the fact that in two years the Area Council, the local government of the area, was hotly debating which village should have the one well which it could provide.

The students' perspective

Most of the students had not been exposed to the customs of people living in the rural areas before, and saw the project as an opportunity to acquaint themselves with this way of life. Students who did have a rural background saw themselves in a different context in the project. They felt that they were going back to their own people to convince them to adopt technologies which have proved beyond doubt to foster good health. The students' general feeling was that the project afforded them the opportunity to see in reality in the field what they have learnt in class. They expressed the view that people in rural areas (if those in the project area could be taken as an example) seem to be slower to adopt new ideas than those in urban areas.

The students' participation in the project has helped them to clarify many misconceptions they had about theories, methods and techniques in health education programmes. They will now go out into the field equipped with ideas and techniques that have been tested. They will also be competent to supervise the villagers in the construction of sanitary wells and VIP latrines, using locally available materials. The collection and interpretation of data, planning and performing social surveys are also useful concepts which they have learnt from the project and these will be invaluable in their careers.

Opportunities for replication

One of the main objectives of the project is to introduce suitable sanitary structures which could be replicated in other areas using local expertise and materials. We believe that with the experience, knowledge and resources available to us, the project could be replicated in other areas with some changes and amendments. The provision and protection of water supplies, sanitary ventilated pit latrines and refuse incinerators should still be the main priorities.

Amendments to the project should include the following, if it is to be replicated in other areas:

•A limited number of public latrines to be erected on demonstration basis so that heads of households can see how locally produced materials can be used to build such structures. Each household should then be assisted with the siting and construction of the structures. Before any household can qualify for such help, they should fulfill certain conditions such as digging the pits and moulding the required number of bricks, while also undertaking to provide the necessary labour during construction work.

•Public wells protected and furnished with handpumps will provide safer water in larger quantities than the many shallow and unprotected private wells which exist in the area at present.

•It is a good idea to work through the Primary Health Care Village Committees, where they exist. They should select village health workers and supervise the construction of latrines according to well-set-out specifications and dimensions

Acknowledgement

The school would like to thank Dr Karl Smith from IDRC for his assistance.

Helping women to help themselves

CHRISTINE VAN WIJK-SIJBESMA

There are various ways to stimulate women to make improvements in water supply and sanitation: for instance, through separate women's programmes which are part of community development services, through appropriate technology programmes and through co-operation between national and international women's organizations and local women's groups.

In the 1970s, many rural development projects and services introduced separate women's programmes. Unfortunately, these programmes have frequently been limited to hygiene, nutrition, and home improvements, without atttention to other important tasks of women, such as agriculture, food processing and water collection. In some cases, integrated programmes have been re-adjusted to focus on domestic aspects only. Increased awareness resulting from women's studies and more participatory approaches are gradually changing this situation.

In Cameroon, the Community Development Department has a separate women's programme, which includes nutrition and child care, home management and improvement, handicrafts, and agriculture. In addition, the programme has introduced appropriate technology to reduce the time and effort required in food processing, for example palm-oil presses and cassava graters. Training has also included appropriate technology for drinking-water. The 50 promoters have received mobylettes (a light motorcycle) from UNICEF and some cement. They have organized cleaning and repair work of spring catchments, construction of rainwater-collection tanks and laundry facilities.

The technical activites originally started with a revolving fund to provide village women with grain mills. To pay back the loans, the women have formed milling societies to which members pay a small monthly fee. In total, 200 societies with about 18,000 members were formed, which also became active in other self-reliant development activities.

A constraint to the implementation of village technology projects reported in the literature is the lack of cooperation and coordination with engineering agencies. In Cameroon, men and women community development workers work on separate programmes. While the women work on self-improvement for the community, the extension work relating to piped water supplies is carried out by men promoters only, and not in cooperation with the women's programme.

Primary health care

In many countries village health workers, many of them women, also play an important role in environmental health improvements. In the People's Republic of China, India, Papua New Guinea, Ethiopia, and the Philippines, they have organized latrine campaigns and water-supply improvements. In Botswana, family welfare educators are trained to construct water carts, water filters and latrines, and to promote them through popular theatre at health centres.

In Kaani, Kenya, a village assembly initiated by a woman health worker decided on a village self-improvement programme, which included the construction of rainwater-collection tanks, spring protection, and latrines. In Thailand, rainwater-collection tanks and water-seal latrines are part of the national primary health care programme for safe drinking-water and sanitation. Health workers provide master moulds and train villagers selected by the community to make concrete slabs for water-seal latrines. Both men and women are trained, including village headmen and teachers. Health workers have now requested that half of the trainees be women. They will work alongside the men in learning to mix concrete, pour latrine bowls and cast rainwater jars. Workers are paid a reasonable compensation by their community development committees.

Self-improvement in water and sanitation may also be stimulated by the development and diffusion of appropriate technology, such as locally made rainwater-collection tanks, water transport facilities, and household water filters. Many bibliographies and manuals on appropriate technology, which include self-improvements for water supply, sanitation and hygiene, have been prepared. However, it is not always clear whether they reach women's organizations in rural and urban fringe areas. Village technology centres have been established in Kenya, Swaziland, Ghana and Papua New Guinea, and also in India and Latin America. However, centres in large cities are difficult for rural women to attend or to obtain information and technical assistance from. Evaluation of the Development Technology Centre in Bandung, Indonesia, showed that most of the target groups have never heard of their three field stations for village technology, in spite of intensive promotion in the mass media. Direct contacts were found to be the most effective extension method.

Target groups

Some programmes have made special efforts to reach target groups. In Indonesia, the Ministry for Women's Affairs has published a handbook on appropriate technology for village women. Copies have been distributed to the wives of village headmen, who usually chair the meetings of local women's organizations. In other countries, courses have been organized to train women leaders and women's groups in labour-saving technologies. Several cases of local women's groups starting income-generating projects to improve family living conditions, including water supply and housing have been documented.

A well-known case are the women's groups in central Kenya who have worked as paid labourers in the peak agricultural season. The income generated has been given to each member in turn to purchase a corrugated iron roof, gutters and a rainwater collection tank. In Polynesia and eastern Kenya, women's groups have sought training in masonry work. They have constructed rainwater tanks and built water-seal latrines for their own use and to generate income. They have also trained other women's groups in these construction techniques. In a South Korean community, a women's club initiated by the wife of the assistant headmaster started to sell compost and to raise funds in several other ways. The proceeds were used to make kitchen improvements and to protect local wells. Their example was followed by women in 11 other villages.

Professional intermediaries

In other cases, professional women have acted as intermediaries to mobilize local women to initiate and manage local projects. Women in a Karachi squatter area responded to the efforts of a concerned woman architect-planner to get them to undertake the improvement of their own community. Despite statements from male community workers that only men did that sort of thing, the inspired women harnessed the efforts of their out-of-school adolescent boys to carry rock fill from a nearby hill, and dredge the stagnant canals in the neighbourhood. The women were right there directing the work all the way.

Co-operation is increasing between women's groups and national women's organizations in developing and western countries. The latter often work through international programmes, such as the UNESCO Co-action Programme and the Voluntary Fund for the United Nations Decade for Women, and, of necessity, provide support rather than participate in joint field-work. National women's organizations have more opportunity for co-operation with women's groups in the field in such a way that both parties increase their understanding of the factors which hinder escape from poverty and help to break down these constraints through joint efforts and solidarity.

Two cases of co-operation between development-oriented national women's organizations and local women's groups in water supply and sanitation have been reported in Honduras. In the first, a mass media campaign on environmental sanitation stimulated the Union of Honduras Women to co-operate with a village group in a latrine construction project. Extension of the project to other communities is planned. In the second, the Federation de Associaciones Femeninas de Honduras assists women's groups from poor *barrios* (squatter towns) threatened with eviction from their land. They also provide support for rural water-supply and sanitation improvement in co-operation with the Office for Squatter Settlements of the metropolitan authorities.

Little recognition

So far, programmes for self-improvement have received little official recognition. The only account of a combined effort for total coverage based on national policy decisions identified in the literature concerns a programme in Paraguay.

At the conference on the role of Amercian volunteers in the National Service of Environmental Sanitation (SENASA), held in Paraguay in 1982, it was decided to station Peace Corps volunteers in areas not being served by SENASA. Their tasks are to assist communities to make self-improvements using local materials and craftsmen, and to help them to set up local enterprises to construct latrine slabs, well covers and handpumps. They co-operate with local teachers, who are often women, to organize the community. The names of local craftsmen and community motivators are reported to SENASA so that, when the government programme is expanded to new areas, their skills can be used.

The many women's programmes and organizations, some of which are mentioned briefly here, are rich resources for community self-improvements in water and sanitation. Their efforts deserve to be incorporated and supported in national programmes and by donor agencies, aiming at the establishment and use of water supply and sanitation improvements for all.

(*Waterlines* Vol. 4 No. 4, April 1986)

CHAPTER 9

Community Education and Participation

The title of this chapter and its acronym CEP, is now accepted as a fundamental factor for the success of any project. As stated by Charles Chandler in his article in Chapter 1, 'Community education and participation (CEP) helps to overcome any gap that may exist between people and planners as a result of their different perceptions of community needs. The objective of CEP is to improve communications so that planners can come to understand community problems, and people can participate in decisions regarding how to meet community needs through development projects.'

Arnold Pacey identifies a high literacy rate as the most important factor for improved hygiene. He illustrates his view by reference to Kerala, where people have exploited opportunities for technological development more fully than the rest of India, although it is one of the poorest states. He suggests literacy programmes may be the most effective medium for health education.

Bob Linney and Ken Meharg run poster-making workshops in India for health and community workers and have their own poster studio in the UK. They stress the importance of pre-testing posters about water and sanitation to ensure that they communicate the intended message. They discuss examples from their own experience illustrating how a completely wrong impression may unintentionally be given.

The importance of the evaluation of the media prepared by development workers is also stressed by Sue Laver. Material which is haphazardly compiled and hurriedly put out can be damaging. She describes how she and her colleagues developed visual aids to back up Zimbabwe's vigorous low-cost sanitation programme.

Lesotho's Urban Sanitation Improvement team is committed to teaching safe hygiene practices at primary schools as a way of achieving good health not only for students and teachers, but for the community as a whole. Virginia Dlangamandla outlines the approach adopted.

Many projects are faced with the prospect that they were started before the need for the CEP component was appreciated. The article in Chapter 11 by Joanne Harnmeijr indicates how this omission can be rectified.

Hygiene and literacy

ARNOLD PACEY

As piped water supplies and sewers were built in the industrialized countries during the last century, health improved remarkably. We hope that something similar can be achieved for the Third World during the IDWSSD. However, our hopes may not come to fruition if we do not understand clearly how and why past improvements in health occurred.

David Bradley,[99] Richard Feachem, and their colleagues frequently remind us that, with many diarrhoeal diseases, what matters is not just the technical improvement of the water supply, but how much water people use and for what purposes. In other words, people's behaviour is very important. It is 'changes in hygiene behaviour that bring the greatest benefit', especially to individual families in places where there are no 'wide-spread changes in the community'[100].

In analysing historical improvements in health in Britain, Thomas McKeown[101] sees human behaviour as a major factor, but mainly in the context of child care and birth control. What he says about hygiene and sanitation tends to emphasize the benefits of hardware — taps and water closets — and makes little mention of social changes that might have influenced hygiene behaviour.

The construction of better water supply and drainage systems in British towns during the middle decades of the 19th century is probably sufficient to explain the ending of cholera epidemics — the last one was in 1866. But the decline in other diarrhoeal diseases followed much more slowly. Only after 1900 do we find evidence of a consistent decline in diarrhoea among children, which is reflected in a falling infant mortality rate (Figure 1).

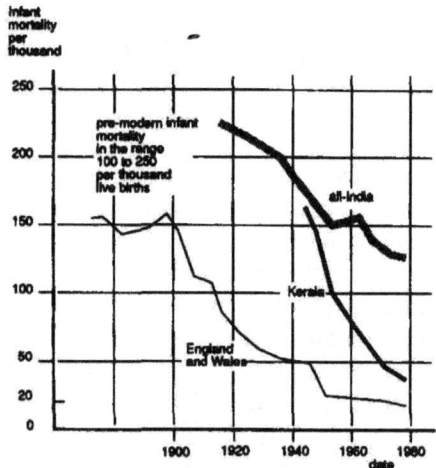

Figure 1. Mortality of infants during the first year of life in India and Britain, per thousand live births

Data for England and Wales are discussed by McKeown and Lowe (see reference 101). The much more approximate estimates for India are assessed by Cassen, Dyson, and other commentators (see reference 105). For early Kerala data refer to Travancore-Cochin only.

Social and technological changes

Technological changes which could have contributed to this include the slow spread of the hygienic bottling of milk, and the installation of bathrooms in urban housing. But at the same time there were social changes which may have had an influence: universal primary education was introduced in Britain in the 1870s, and, by 1900, included many classes for girls in cooking, laundry and hygiene.[102] Health education aimed at expectant mothers became fairly widespread between 1900 and 1914.

Thus only in 1900, and not before, could one say that most babies were born to tolerably well-educated mothers. And that was just the time when the turning point in infant mortality occurred.

The possible influence of education is always difficult to assess, but there is evidence from many parts of the world that it can have a marked impact on hygiene behaviour. In the 1930s, missionaries working among Miao hill tribes in western China noted that as people learned to read, they also became more concerned about personal cleanliness. More recently, sociologists working in South America and India found a close correlation between functional literacy and innovations in the home such as the installation of latrines and medicine cupboards. In all these instances, it seems to be literacy that is the key, not just health education. Literacy, it is said, is 'the basic personal skill that underlies the whole modernizing sequence'.[103]

High literacy rate

Some of the best evidence for this comes from the south Indian state of Kerala where, in 1981, some 69 per cent of the adult population were literate, as compared with an average literacy rate throughout the whole of India of 36 per cent.[104]

Table 1 (page 244) quotes a miscellany of statistics from Kerala which indicate that mortality rates are remarkably low by Third World standards, so that life expectancy at birth is about 66 years. This is about 11 years longer than for India as a whole.[105] In the last two decades, Kerala's health statistics have come to resemble those of the developed countries more closely than they resemble data from most of the rest of India (Figure 1).

Contribution of technology

What contribution has been made to Kerala's achievement by improved water supplies and sanitation? In 1965, a social survey in a rural area reported that latrines were almost totally lacking — people used the bush instead. Drinking-water came from badly protected wells which were muddy in summer. Some 32 out of 72 deaths in the area just prior to the report were attributed to typhoid and dysentery.[106]

Since then, there have been reports of latrine building in rural areas and of the high efficiency of night-soil collection in towns. In two places, Quilon and Trichur, experiments are in progress in which biogas digesters process the night-soil from substantial urban populations, and at the village of Mynoor, one agency is installing a night-soil biogas plant to serve between 30 and 40 families.[107]

Such reports imply a highly significant technological contribution to improvements in health. But one of the paradoxes of Kerala is that in terms of per capita income, it is one of the poorer states of India (Table 1), and spending on public health during the 1970s was substantially less than average for the subcontinent.[108]

Admittedly, Kerala has a moist climate, and improved water supplies can often be installed at a lower cost here than elsewhere. But even allowing for this, material development in water and sanitation is not so much in advance of the rest of India as the health statistics would lead one to

Table 1. Some indicators of health and economic conditions in Kerala and for the whole of India during the 1970s

Health indicators*	Year	Average for Kerala	Average for all India
Crude death rate per 1,000 population	1975-76	8.3	15.4
Crude birth rate per 1,000 population	1975-76	27.9	34.8
Infant mortality per 1,00 live births	1961-70	61	156
(compare Figure 1)	1978	40	130
Percentage of married couples using family planning	1981	29	22
Average annual rate of population increase	1971-81	1.74	2.21
Economic indicators**			
Income per capita (Rupees)	1972-73	579	698
Average food intake per person per day (Calories)	1972-73	1840	1985
Electricity consumption per capita (kWh per year)	1972-73	81	97

* Sources: Tim Dyson, 'Preliminary demography of 1981 census', Economic and Political Weekly (Bombay), 16, No. 33 (August 15, 1981), pages 1349-54; and P.M. Blaikie, Family planning in India, London, Edward Arnold, 1975; see also reference105.
** Sources: B.L.C. Johnson, India, Resources and Development, London, Heinemann, 1979; and P.D. Henderson, India: the energy sector, Delhi, Oxford University Press, 1975.

suppose. Technological developments have created opportunities for better hygiene, but the significant point seems to be that, in Kerala, people have exploited these opportunities more fully than elsewhere.

In trying to explain why, we are brought back again to the question of literacy. In Kerala, it is said, 'sanitation is good because the people are educated', and that means they take care over refuse disposal, defecation, washing, and night soil collection. One account of a rural latrine-building programme traced its origins to a women's literacy class which had stimulated thought about how conditions in the village might be improved.[109]

Breaking the vicious circle

Conventional explanations of Kerala's good health also place considerable stress on the good quality of primary health clinics in Kerala[110] and the high take-up of family planning.[111] Because many women are literate, the argument goes, they make better use of the available health-care facilities than in other places.

Rapidly falling infant mortality (Figure 1) implies better feeding of children and a much reduced incidence of diarrhoea due to better hygiene. But this is hygiene in the context of child-care, not general hygiene, that is the outcome of technological improvements. Thus the question of the mothers' education definitely seems to be important.

Many experts 'view literacy instruction as the best possible means ... to break the vicious circle of low incomes, high birth rates, and slow development'.[112] Kerala's experience seems to confirm this, but how it happens is infuriatingly hard to explain to anyone more used to dealing with the engineering aspects of public health.

Some of the practical advantages of being able to read are obvious. A mother can 'store' information about child care and health without having to rely on memory; she can read instructions on food packets and medicine bottles. More important, though, reading gives the individual the ability to control the rate of 'information input' and think about it, and this may unlock unused mental abilities. It sometimes seems to make people more self-aware, and this alone may be a stimulus to more care in personal cleanliness. Some accounts imply a connection between greater self-awareness, changed standards of decency in dress, and a greater demand for privacy during ablutions. In one area, it was reported that as women began to wear blouses and fewer 'nude busts' were seen, lack of privacy was more keenly felt, and people became more concerned to build and use latrines.[113]

Evidence to back up many of these points is scarce, and interpretations are speculative. However, social research currently underway in Kerala should soon shed more light on the mechanisms involved here.[114]

Important questions

Meanwhile, we ought to be provoked into asking a number of questions. In the industrialized countries, how much did technology contribute to improved hygiene and how much was due to the spread of literacy? In planning health education in conjunction with the Water Decade, what impact can we expect where literacy rates are low?

We are told that many 'thousands of health educators all over the world continue the search for an effective visual language' for communication with 'pre-literate' people.[115] Visual aids and readily understood symbols of all kinds are under investigation. But much of this work presupposes that there will be little improvement in the present low level of literacy, which is regarded as outside the health educator's control. That will certainly very often be true.

But might there not also be instances where literacy programmes will be the most effective medium for health education? Or where literacy is a necessary pre-condition to full use of the water and sanitation hardware introduced as part of the Decade campaign?

Acknowledgement

I am indebted to Tim Dyson, Lecturer in Population Studies at the London School of Economics, for allowing me to see two unpublished papers in which he discusses the significance of regional variations in health and demographic statistics for India.

(Waterlines July 1982)

Pre-testing posters for communicating about water and sanitation

BOB LINNEY

If you happened to live in a village in the southern part of the Indian Punjab, the chances are that your teeth would be yellow. You might also suffer from back-ache, pains in your joints and stones in your bladder. Why? Simply because the only drinking-water available — that from the village well — contained excessively high concentrations of mineral salts.

At a poster workshop conducted by myself and Ken Meharg in Chandigarh, one of the participants designed a poster on this problem of salty subsoil water. In it, he drew what he meant to be a typical male villager from the southern Punjab. The man's teeth are bright yellow, and, to associate this with the water he has been drinking, a well is shown. When we field-tested the design, by interviewing village people in order to see what message they were receiving from the poster, one person gave the following explanation - 'The man is smiling. He is happy because there are clouds in the sky. It will soon rain and fill his well, so he will have plenty of water for drinking and for growing his crops.' This is a perfectly reasonable and logical story, but it is not the one that the designer intended. It illustrates one of the many ways in which a poster can fail to communicate its intended message. In this particular example, failure results from the inclusion of irrelevant background detail, in the form of clouds.

Misinterpreted messages

Looking at the more general situation, it is likely that the *majority* of posters for health and development education don't work, in that they do not get their intended messages across to their intended audiences. A poster I saw in India showed a pregnant woman, her hands resting on her stomach. Beneath her were shown the fruits and vegetables that pregnant women are advised to eat in order to avoid anaemia. Many village women to whom we spoke thought that the pregnant woman had been poisoned by eating the foodstuffs shown, and that such foods should, therefore, not be consumed during pregnancy.

A poster used in Pakistan to encourage people to use iodized salt to prevent goitre, showed an attractive, unveiled young woman. When it was displayed in rural areas, it was torn down by members of conservative Muslim communities to whom the picture was offensive: the woman was thought to be scantily clad because she was not wearing a veil.

A third poster was designed to encourage people to cover food to protect it from flies. When it was displayed in one African village, the inhabitants fled into the bush, afraid that a plague of enormous flies was about to descend on their settlement. And so on. Massive amounts of money, time and energy (not to mention trees) have been wasted in producing posters that don't work.

There are many reasons why posters can fail. Yet there is a straightforward means by which failure can be avoided. That is by pre-testing designs before they are mass-produced. Pre-testing means that you produce an initial, draft design and simply ask a sample of the audience to suggest how the draft design could be improved so that it gets its message across more effectively. On the basis of their suggestion, you can change the initial draft and make a second draft which can, in turn, be pre-tested. This procedure is repeated until you end up with a design which is clearly communicating its intended message to a large proportion of the audience. All this testing is carried out before the final poster is mass-produced.

The workshop approach

To help people improve the effectiveness of health education posters, Ken Meharg and I have developed a practical workshop approach. Workshop participants are all health and/or development workers, usually with no previous artistic training. We emphasize that you do not have to be an artist in order to produce effective educational posters. Indeed village level workers, some of whom had rarely even drawn a picture before attending the workshops, invariably managed to print their own designs. In such cases, posters were being made for particular communities by people who were themselves integral members of those communities, with all the advantages that come from the designer having an intimate knowledge of the local customs, beliefs, superstitions and styles (of housing, dress and even hair) of the people at whom the poster is directed.

Each workshop consists of two parts. In the first stage, participants specify their intended audience and then design and print 20 or so copies of their poster. We use a simple low-cost silk-screen technique in which stencils are made by hand-painting water-based glue directly on to the silk-screen. In the second stage of the workshop, we go out for pre-testing. This is done by interviewing members of the audience using a questionnaire that we have developed. Questions are designed to determine how well the poster's message is understood, as well as to provide information on whether or not the respondents find the design clear, attractive, acceptable and relevant to themselves.

One of the posters made at a workshop in Calcutta was meant to encourage people to boil water before drinking it (Illustration 1). The four pictures were meant to be 'read' in sequence from left to right — boil the water, pour it into a jug, let it cool, and then drink it. During pre-testing it became

Illustration 1 : 'Boil water before drinking it' (Calcutta)

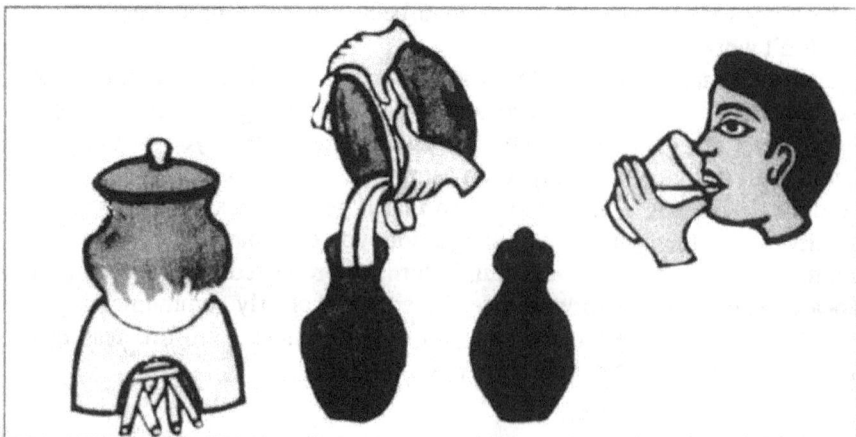

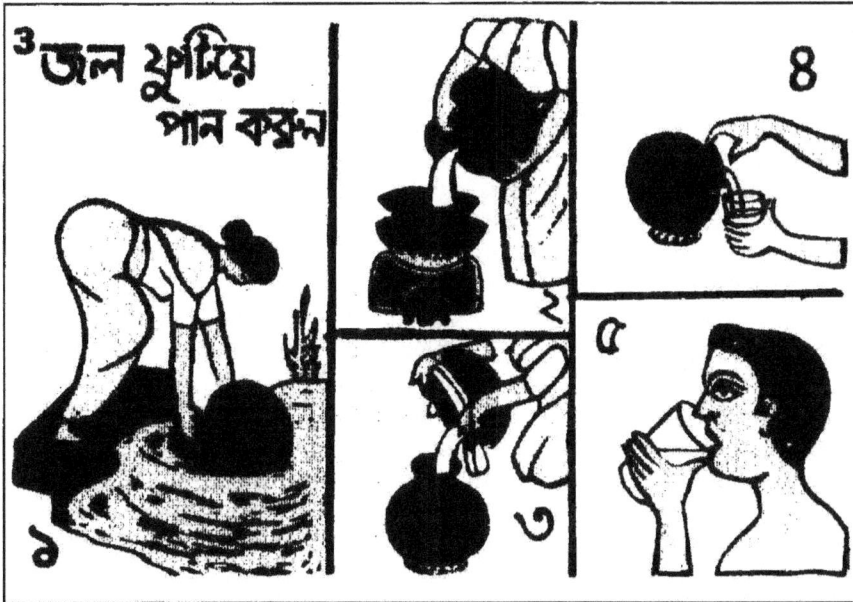

Illustration 2: Improved version of 'boil water before drinking it'

clear that this design was not being understood well. Some people thought it was about drinking milk, because of the white colour of the 'water', others thought it was about boiling rice; and some thought it was about making a cup of tea. The majority of respondants didn't understand that the four events were meant to occur in temporal sequence from left to right. Many saw the four pictures as happening simultaneously and were confused about the message. Further confusion arose from the isolated head and hand which were not always perceived as being connected to a complete body.

A revised version of this design, based on the results of pre-testing, was made (Illustration 2). A full figure has been drawn in the first frame, to reduce the problem of isolating parts of the body. The frames themselves have been separated, one from another, by thick black lines, while the intended reading sequence has been clarified by the inclusion of the Bengali numerals 1-5. The designer has also used words, in spite of the fact that the majority of the poster's audience was not literate and could not read them.

Another poster from the workshop was intended to convey the message 'Avoid drinking contaminated water'. In spite of evidence suggesting that among poor people in developing countries most of the spread of organisms which cause diarrhoea is by faecal-oral routes that do not involve drinking contaminated water, the topic of this poster is an important one. The poster, however, was not a success. Again, the intended sequence in which the four frames are meant to be read is unclear.

Difficulties with visual conventions

Another factor contributing to the failure of this poster concerns the proportions in which some of its visual elements are depicted. The water container that the woman is carrying is smaller in relation to the figure than it would appear in reality. More extreme still is the size of the barely discernible glass from which the man is drinking in the bottom-left frame. As a general rule, it is best to show figures and objects on a poster as close as possible to the same relative proportions as they appear in everyday experience.

A poster on the theme of oral rehydration therapy (ORT) showed an ill, malnourished baby drawn by the village health worker in a simple two-dimensional representational style. Beneath the child are shown some sugar, salt, a slice of lime and a glass of water coloured blue. Again this poster was not successful in communicating its message — that ORT is an effective treatment for diarrhoea.

It does, on the other hand, raise one or two interesting points. What can one learn, for example, from the fact that one non-literate respondent thought that words written along the bottom of the design were meant to represent stools? And what colour is water? Sometimes blue, sometimes brown and sometimes more or less colourless or transparent. Another poster from the Calcutta workshop was on the subject of fish-culture in the village ponds of West Bengal. A number of people, on seeing the 'realistic' brown-green that the designer had used for the colour of the pond, said that the water should have been shown in blue. This came as a surprise to all of us, since by no stretch of the imagination could one see the water in the pond as being blue. I have already mentioned the white colour of water in the 'Boil drinking water' design and how it led people to think of milk or rice. It is, indeed, quite difficult to know what colour to use for water in a design intended to be for people who are not exposed to pictures very often.

There are other problems with water. Lines used to depict ripples on the surface of a pond may be confusing to people who do not know that such lines are meant to represent moving, spreading ripples. Health posters sometimes use dots or small lines to represent the spray of water particles that come from a person's mouth during coughing or sneezing. This, too, can be easily mis-interpreted by someone unfamiliar with such convention.

Another visual convention which causes trouble is that of symbolism. The rather obvious point to remember is that the symbol must mean the same to the members of the audience as it does to the designer. A variety of symbolic conventions are used in the West when we try to represent water in a picture. Most of these, along with the other visual conventions that we take for granted (such as our acceptance of the convention in which we imagine a third dimension in a picture were it does not physically exist) have not been learnt by many people, particularly by those living in the rural areas of poor countries. In the same way that we do not all share the same verbal language, neither do people from different societies necessarily share the same visual language.

The Xerophthalmia campaign

Having mentioned some of the pit-falls which await the designer of educational posters, I will briefly describe one of my recent attempts to put some of these ideas into practice. I have been helping a small group of medical and social workers to develop a poster for use in Dharavi, Bombay. Dharavi is, in population terms, the largest slum in the whole of south-east Asia, with 600,000 people living in one square mile. Water supply and sanitation are, to say the least, poor, with one tap per 400 residents and a network of open gulleys into which waste is poured. One of the many health problems suffered by the residents of the slum is that of xerophthalmia, a disease which causes about 40,000 Indian children to become blind every year. Xerophthalmia results from a dietary deficiency of Vitamin A and, hence, residents of Dharavi are being encouraged to eat cheap foods containing Vitamin A. As part of this campaign we are producing a poster whose message is 'For healthy eyes eat dark green leafy vegetables'.

In the initial draft design, I drew what I meant to be a healthy young boy carrying a basketful of recognizable, locally available, vegetables rich in Vitamin A. We tested the design by interviewing 36 young mothers from the slum. Almost without exception, they said things like 'The boy is unhealthy because he has not eaten these vegetables' or 'Make him look chubbier so that he does not look sick'. Other suggestions included 'Make skin lighter', 'Make pupils darker', 'Remove highlights from hair' and so on. A revised version of the design is currently being tested. Eventually I am hoping to learn from the audience how to draw a boy who, to them, looks healthy. When this happens, we will mass-produce leaflets and posters for distribution at Dharavi.

Supply scheme

Lastly, it may be useful for readers to know about a scheme I am initiating to help projects which do not have enough money to produce their own posters. In outline, this 'supply scheme' involves somebody from the project producing an initial design, pre-testing, revising and testing it again until a design is made which communicates its message to a large proportion of the audience. At that stage, we will print posters and send them back to the project for use. We can provide this service free of charge, though, obviously, we need to be fairly selective. Interested readers should contact me.

Although not of such fundamental importance as water-supply, I think that poster-supply may be useful to many people working on health and development education.

Further reading

1. George McBean, Norbert Kaggwa, John Bugembe, *Illustrations for development*, Afrolit Society, PO Box 72511, Nairobi, Kenya, 1980.
2. *Communicating with pictures in Nepal*, Report of a study by NDS and UNICEF, Kathmandu 1976.
3. Marina Maspero and Elinor Kennedy, *I see*, Report of FAO study, Rome, 1978.
4. Bob Linney and Ken Meharg, *Posters for health in India*, Workshop Report, 1985 (photocopied).

(Waterlines Vol. 4 No. 2, October 1985)

Communications for low-cost sanitation in Zimbabwe

SUE LAVER

The impact of practical research on the development of low-cost technologies for water and sanitation in rural Zimbabwe is significant, and progress in this field is widely recognized both within our borders and outside the country. Simple low-cost devices for raising water in villages have evolved through vigorous field testing. Other new technologies for drilling shallow tubewells have also been developed. Low-cost sanitation is becoming a reality for more and more families, and home-built Blair Ventilated Improved Pit (VIP) latrines are viewed with pride by their owners.

These developments are the result of a team effort which involves not only the village-based extension workers, but the people themselves. The Minsitry of Health has official responsibility for developing low-cost water and sanitation, but other ministries and non-governmental organizations have contributed significantly to projects. Projects are co-ordinated locally through village development committees (VIDCOs) and Ward Development Committees (WARDCOs).

Communicating with the community

Development workers have adopted the philosophy that technical progress in rural Zimbabwe should not be dependent on machinery alone and that development should be approached through the people. The essential components of this concept are good management and a well-informed community — which depend on effective communication.

Communication at project level can take place either by personal contact through extension workers, by media such as instruction leaflets, posters and other visual aids, or by a combination of these strategies. However, with a growing demand for low-cost technologies from villagers, the one-to-one approach to sharing information is limited by lack of time and manpower. Under these circumstances, we think that visual media will have to play a greater part in assisting the transfer of technical information at community level. They should also play an important role in promoting the programmes, by stimulating changes and creating a better understanding of the reasons for technical intervention in rural Zimbabwe.

We needed to develop visual aids both to teach people and to promote the programme at the planning, mobilization, implementation and maintenance phases. We could not use video or film, but we did use drama to enhance people's understanding of key issues. We therefore developed a Communications Support Guide to help project workers select the best combination of media to use, and it appears as Table 1 on page 254.

A background survey[116] provided a lot of useful information about how well people understood the latrine technology, their grasp of how to measure the latrines during construction and their concept of management. Important questions were where to site the latrine, how to divide up labour and what the community should contribute to the project. Our study was closely linked to an earlier survey by Boydell[117].

Using survey results

When compared and combined, the results of both surveys confirmed that local builders were unclear about many basic questions to do with construction. For example, untrained local builders varied in their conception of how high the vent-pipe or how thick the slab should be. This was consistent with the findings of Boydell's study.

Our findings reinforced the need for standardized instruction for project workers, so we developed a Builders' Instructional Manual, covered in plastic, with simple step-by-step information for building a latrine.

Posters were also designed to promote a community-based approach to latrine projects, and the caption 'The people of Zimbabwe are building latrines — join them' has been widely accepted by project workers and has even been quoted by community leaders.

To put across the message 'Care for your latrine', we developed a plastic-covered leaflet and, slightly less orthodox, local potters designed a series of hand-painted ceramic tiles illustrating maintenance and hygiene procedures. The tiles have proved to be an eye-catching way of reinforcing the informa-

Table 1: Communications Support Guide: which media to use

Project phase	Key issues	Method of communication support
Planning phase	Establish contact with key leaders	Face to face contact with key leaders
Community needs survey	Community needs survey eg. assess problems, needs and priorities	Small group discussions
	Discuss technology options/project benefits	Visits to other projects
	Explain about support organizations and structures	Psycho-social methods for problem solving eg. picture codes
Mobilization phase	Facilitate decision-making through groups	Group/public meetings/ promotional media
	Discuss community objectives/contributions	*Poster 'The People of Zimbabwe are Building Latrines — Join Them!.
	Facilitate community organization through local management structures	*Leaflets, ie. summary leaflets 'Build a Latrine'
	Choose project site with the people/leaders and community-based workers	Visits to other successful projects
Implementation phase	Provide information support	
	Facilitate delivery support materials i.e. cement etc	*Instructional support ie. Builders Instructional Manual
	Encourage maximum community support for project	*Information leaflets ie. summary leaflets 'Build a Latrine'
	Encourage completion of project	On-site assistance where necessary
	Facilitate visits by key leaders/local authorities	
Maintenance phase	Encourage placement of high value on facility	Maintenance training eg. personal approach
	Facilitate selection/training of maintenance personnel through local management structures	*Maintenance reminders ie. encapsulated leaflets 'Care for your Latrine'
	Establish support/referral system for maintenance through local management structures	*Ceramic tiles for plastering into completed structures
		Other hygiene interventions (handwashing etc.)

*Asterisk indicates promotional and instructional support media developed for Zimbabwe project

tion communicated more conventionally through the leaflets and the Builders' Instructional Manual at demonstration latrines at schools and clinics.

The visual aids were developed by continuous liaison between long-suffering illustrators, technical experts, project workers and the author and her co-workers.

Evaluation is a must

Evaluating the media they have developed almost seems the last straw to many development workers, for it always involves a mammoth effort and readily reveals inadequacies. So it is often neglected, but material which is haphazardly compiled and hurriedly put out can be damaging.

We consider that evaluation is a 'must', not an 'option', as shown by the results of the Zimbabwe study. We invited interested health workers, experts and development workers throughout Zimbabwe to assess our visual media for communicating about sanitation in an objective way. Groups and individuals reviewed the content, illustrations and appropriateness of the media for us.

We gave copies of the Builders' Instructional Manual to groups engaged in building, and asked them to construct a latrine from the information given. Each stage in the process was observed, problems were noted and the completed latrines were measured to find out how closely they lined up with the instructions. This was very valuable, and exposed many errors. If we had neglected the evaluation, many technical inconsistencies would have been perpetuated through inaccurate illustrations and omissions in the text. We are now confident that the end result is nearer to what the people want — and need — to support the development of sanitation in Zimbabwe. The procedure will help us move on to develop a wide range of communications media to support low-cost water development projects.

Acknowledgements

The German Agency for Technical Co-operation (GTZ), in collaboration with the World Bank's Technology Advisory Group, generously funded the Media Development Project described in this article. Assistance was also given by the Research Board, University of Zimbabwe. Thanks is also due to the illustrators, in particular Kors de Waard and Colleen Cousins.

(*Waterlines* Vol. 4 No. 4, April 1986)

Hygiene and health education in primary schools in Lesotho

VIRGINIA DLANGAMANDLA

The provision of improved sanitation in Lesotho's schools is a means of improving the health of all students as well as promoting good hygiene practices among both the students and the broader community as a whole.

As a general rule, hygiene is incorporated into the school syllabus in Lesotho. The Ministry of Interior's Urban Sanitation Improvement Team (USIT), through its community section, commits much of its time to teaching hygiene at those schools provided with adequate improved sanitation facilities, such as the multiple Ventilated Improved Pit (VIP) latrine.

The community section becomes involved when the latrines have been completed, just before they begin to be used. They provide user and health education to teachers, who in turn arrange for students to have lessons. The role of the teacher in emphasizing good hygiene and sanitation practices is an important area of discussion. Possible ways in which to integrate health education into day-to-day subjects such as nutrition, language, biology and science are also considered.

Using latrine-cleaning as a form of punishment is discouraged, as it tends to lower the status of VIPs; schoolchildren need more positive incentives. Teachers are encouraged to produce their own teaching aids, which they feel will be easily understood by their pupils; these are then printed by USIT. So far, only posters have been produced in this way.

The time spent by USIT members in each school varies between three to seven days depending on the number of pupils, distance, and availability of USIT members giving the health and user education lecture. Since health education on sanitation cannot be taught in isolation, all factors related to water-borne, water-washed and water-based diseases are covered; personal hygiene is also taught.

Programmes and methods

USIT has prepared different tape-slide programmes for audio-visual aids, including one for school managers and teachers entitled *Hygiene and health in our schools*, and another for students called *A new start for health*. A generator is used to run the tape and slide equipment in rural areas.

The programmes discuss in detail how faecal-related diseases are spread. They show how such disease can be prevented by building and using VIP latrines, as well as emphasizing the importance of hygiene and proper maintenance. The tape-slide programme for pupils includes a 10-point programme, a reminder of the health education programme, which is also made into a wall chart for display in each classroom. Booklets are provided for pupils, which summarize the information in the tape-slide programmes. In addition, self-adhesive posters are put up in each latrine; these stress simple practices that are easily forgotten, such as washing hands and closing seat covers.

USIT has prepared two poems on VIPs, which are aimed at reminding students of their responsibilities towards their own health, as well as the care and maintenance of latrines. A song has been composed, too, which is suitable for both teachers and students: this is sometimes used by the Ministry of Health in its health education programmes on national radio, especially when faecal-related diseases are being discussed. The radio is frequently used to communicate information on health education to both pupils and the general public, as are newspapers.

Since teachers are key people in communities, they are encouraged to disseminate information on the need for improved sanitation in their own communities. This is emphasized during training lectures provided by USIT at the National Teachers' Training College. Teachers have close contact with parents, so it makes sense for USIT to use them as a mouthpiece. Teachers in the field are often called together in workshops to discuss health hazards they have to face in their schools; they advise each other on how to overcome these problems. As soon as target health standards have been achieved, USIT becomes involved in technical problems. Every three months schools are visited for an inspection of the latrines.

Co-ordination with the ministries

The Health Education Unit and Rural Sanitation Programme of the Minsitry of Health work hand in hand with USIT to promote health education in schools and to cope with any problems that may arise. The Health Education Unit provides some of the display and teaching materials for teachers and pupils, while USIT provides lectures on sanitation to health assistants, nurses and village health workers, whenever necessary. There is therefore continual co-ordination between USIT and the Ministry of Health.

The Ministry of Education, through its National Curriculum Development Committee, also works closely with USIT. The design and modification of the health education syllabus for primary schools involves USIT, health education personnel, nutrition departments and other organizations concerned with health promotion. Training teachers on how to tackle the syllabus is also an important joint venture of these departments.

Constructing latrines in schools is part of a co-ordinated effort with the Ministry's Training for Self-Reliance programme, including constructing VIPs in schools in Lesotho, a project which could not proceed without consultation with USIT. Plans have to be designed by USIT's Community Section. No latrine is supposed to be constructed by any builder in any school without USIT's approval.

As far as schools are concerned, USIT helps all individual schools that need help both within project areas and outside. However, health education by USIT alone would not solve all the problems that are experienced in Lesotho, hence the integrated effort of all the departments. Working together in the promotion of health also avoids duplication of jobs, a common problem in many places.

Education for all

Health education is a key component of all water-supply and sanitation programmes. It involves various important elements including motivation, counselling (door-to-door or person-to-person), advertising and basic hygiene education.

Sanitation in schools is beneficial to the children who learn good health and hygiene practices and pass their knowledge on to their older relatives at home. However, if the latrines at school are not properly used and maintained and become a health hazard, this could have a negative impact on the community, and on the sanitation cause as a whole. USIT's experience is that it is important for the recipients of sanitation improvements to be committed to the proper use, care and maintenance of hygienic sanitation facilities. Success willl encourage other schools to seek similar improvements.

(*Waterlines* Vol. 6 No. 4, April 1988)

CHAPTER 10

Programme Planning

Following on from the last chapter, John Hubley describes why both communication and health education are vital components for sanitation programmes. He briefly describes the role played by communication at different stages of a programme and key factors to be taken into account in the design of effective programmes. As he says, many problems can be avoided by involving the community in the planning and implementation process.

WASH has been working with USAID in Belize on the development of low-cost data-gathering techniques. Dan Campbell describes studies using village profiles and household surveys. These have produced some interesting ideas which have been incorporated into the design of village water and sanitation programmes. Communication was through village councils and the vehicle for implementation of the community projects was through the village water and sanitation committee. Goals and indicators have been formulated to monitor and evaluate the project's progress.

Zimbabwe has embarked on an ambitious national programme to bring improved sanitation to every rural family by the turn of the century. As Peter Morgan reports, considerable efforts are being made, and will be required, from the government, donors and rural families alike. Over 100,000 Blair latrines have been constructed since independence in 1980.

A long-term approach to the provision of low-cost sanitation in rural Lesotho is discussed by Phil Evans. He emphasizes the need to establish a foundation based on long-term planning, community self-help, and social and cultural appropriateness in project design, supported by good monitoring and evaluation plus an integrated approach to replication. In a separate article (*Waterlines*, January 1988) not published here, Isabel Blacket of USIT (the Urban Sanitation Improvement Unit) stressed the benefits from co-ordinating a national sanitation programme, both urban and rural, for maximum efficiency, as is being done in Lesotho.

An experimental project in community mobilization has been initiated by Akhter Hameed Khan in a squatter town of Karachi. Sami Mustafa, a consultant for research and evaluation, sets out the problems and achievements. The aim is to organize the people and teach them how to build a sewerage system for their houses themselves. The effect of the self-help programme has been significant, but many problems still have to be overcome. Community involvement and leadership abilities in conjunction with a breakthrough in the technology of low-cost sanitation are vital for this self-help and self-financing programme.

Communication and health education planning for sanitation programmes

JOHN HUBLEY

Communication and health education are essential components for the success of any sanitation programme to promote health. Each stage of a programme must be considered carefully in order to assess where uptake and effectiveness can be improved through a well-chosen communication strategy. This article briefly describes the role played by communication at different stages of a programme, in particular when promoting an improved sanitation technology such as the Ventilated Improved Pit (VIP) latrine. Key factors to take into account in the design of effective communication and health education programmes will also be considered.

Motivation

When the normal practice of a community has been to defecate in the open, one of the most important tasks will be to motivate the people to use latrines. Common objections to latrines often include an unwillingness to share them with others, fear of contact with faeces, smells and flies. Another drawback may be cost, either in materials or time taken for building. It is important to consider separately the various sub-groups, which will require quite different treatment in a communication programme. One sub-group will be those living in their own homes, another will be those people living in rented accommodation, or even landlords, in urban areas.

If the community is already using some form of latrine, such as an ordinary pit or bucket latrine, the emphasis of the communication programme will be on the advantages of the improved latrines, such as the VIPs or the Pour Flush latrine, so that they are apparent.

Construction

Once people have been motivated to build or improve their sanitation equipment, they will need to find out how to build the latrines. The advantages and disadvantages of various latrine types will have to be explained to help them decide on the design and materials most suited to their needs. This communication should be directed at householders, community leaders, local officials and people responsible for institutions where latrine provision is desirable, for example, schools, health centres, markets and other public places.

Only a basic level of advice and support will be necessary to enable the householder to construct the simple latrine types made out of local mud or using thatch. More detailed advice and technical support will be required for solid and permanent latrines, such as the alternating twin-pit VIP latrines with a stone or cement-block superstructure and reinforced concrete slabs. The communication approach most appropriate would probably be a latrine construction workshop, where all the necessary practical information and skills are provided for latrine construction. This would include detailed information on materials, construction techniques, how to follow blueprints and choose sites, and, where necessary, a list of builders familiar with latrine construction.

Correct use

Communication programmes must stress the importance of the whole community using the latrines. This need should be explained to older people, and a special effort will be needed to ensure that they are properly used by children. They may be afraid of falling into the pit, or may have difficulty climbing on to the seat. Another problem may be parents locking the latrine for security, to prevent unsupervised children getting in. Some parents may regard children's faeces as harmless, but even the faeces of very young infants should be disposed of in the latrine.

There may be special requirements according to the latrine type: if, for instance, the VIP latrine has a door, advice will be required on how to close it to keep the interior shaded. Information about cleaning the latrine, seat and door handles will also be needed. If disinfectant is to be used, it is important to stress that this should not be poured into the pit, as it would prevent bacteriological action. Using the pit as a refuse dump should also be discouraged.

Maintenance

A latrine that is not working properly is more of a danger to health than no latrine at all! It can undo all efforts to convince the community of the value of latrines, providing substance for beliefs that latrines are smelly, dirty and filled with flies. Maintenance requirements for the VIP latrines include checking the fly-screen for tears, ensuring that the pit is completely sealed at the base and checking for broken slabs. The need for regular inspection and maintenance must be discussed with the community.

It will be particularly important to explain the need to set aside funds for maintaining the latrines in schools, health centres, public places, and other institutions where they will be subject to much use. Lack of maintenance and repairs is one of the most serious problems in the institutional and public provision of sanitation.

Hygiene and health

On their own, the provision of protected water supplies and the use of latrines will not lead to improvements in health. It is dangerous to promise the community that all their health problems will disappear once they begin to use latrines. One of the main routes for infection lies in direct contact with faecal matter, and improved sanitation will only lead to better health if it is accompanied by a package of hygiene measures.[118,119] These include:

O Washing hands after using the latrine, handling infants' nappies, after defecation and before preparing or eating food.

O Covering food (especially if there is a time interval between preparation and eating), and clean storage of cooking utensils.

O Clean storage of drinking-water, using clean cups to remove water for drinking and avoiding contamination of drinking-water by dirty hands.

O Cleaning surroundings, disposing of children's faeces, disposing of waste water (sullage) into soak-aways.

O Personal cleanliness, especially washing infants, soiled nappies and disposing of the water used to wash them.

There are a range of general health measures which must be carried out by those looking after young children. These might not be considered part of a traditional sanitation programme, but they are essential if sanitation improvements are to lead to health benefits. Such child health measures are concerned with the prevention and control of diarrhoea and include the promotion of breast-feeding, discouragement of bottle-feeding, early recognition of the signs of diarrhoea and how to administer oral rehydration therapy. But other child health measures are also important, such as immunization against childhood diseases, especially measles, which interacts with diarrhoea to make it so serious that it can sometimes be fatal to the child.

Communication guidelines

The following guidelines show how to incorporate effective communication and health education into sanitation programmes.

The emphasis should shift from latrine construction to the promotion of health. Pressure is often placed on field projects to generate quick results in terms of completed latrines, rather than more meaningful objectives such as the actual use of the latrines or health improvements. This involves incorporating into the programme the objectives described above which relate to use, maintenance, hygiene practices and general health measures. The importance of communication support and health education should be recognized at the outset and built into the planning process. The function of communication support should not be seen merely as a device to make the community accept and use the sanitation technology provided. A communication programme cannot persuade people to carry out actions which conflict with their cultural beliefs. An appropriate latrine design should be compatible with the culture of the community, technically feasible using locally available skills and materials, require the minimum of user maintenance and be simple to use. Carrying out a social and cultural survey[120, 121] of the community combined with a community participation approach will provide the guidelines for technical personnel on appropriate latrine designs. It must be remembered that a communication programme will only influence people's actions if they have the resources to do what is asked of them. The programme should ensure that:

O Adequate provisions are made for designs using low-cost, locally available materials.

O Builders have been trained.

O Materials such as fly-screens are available.

O The method of payment to individuals, the community or schools has been properly considered and suitable arrangements made, such as credit schemes.

Sanitation programmes should be accompanied by other programmes, especially water supply, housing, women's programmes and primary health care. This is often preached but less often practised. People cannot be expected to practise hygiene if they do not have enough water or live in poor housing. Another important resource is time, especially for women who carry out a double role in agriculture and the home, and are expected to shoulder the considerable burden of improving home hygiene. Achieving improvements in hygiene and child health practices is a massive task to be shared with primary health care services, schools, home economists and other services. Health education is particularly vulnerable to lack of co-ordination between services; the community is often exposed to inaccurate and conflicting information from different agencies and can become confused.

Keep the advice to a minimum and make it as easy to follow as possible. There can be a tendency to ask the community to do more than is really necessary. A good example[122] is the frequently delivered — and usually ignored — exhortation to boil drinking-water, an exercise which takes time, uses scarce fuel and does not interrupt the main channels of infection of water-washed diseases. It is important to continually explore simple technologies, such as the disinfection of water using sunlight.

Building on existing practices

One of the most important characteristics of effective health education is to build on concepts, ideas, and practices that the people already have[123,124]. It is not necessary to convince people of the germ theory in order to use latrines and practise measures of hygiene. That is a long-term process which is best done in the schools for future generations. It is possible to find supporting ideas in many traditional beliefs, and an appeal can be made to non-health advantages, such as comfort and privacy.

Building on existing practices applies to communication methods. Traditional media, such as drama and story-telling, offer rich potential and have often been used in sanitation and hygiene programmes.[125] On the other hand, problems arise when unfamiliar media are used, such as drawings or diagrams, which can be ambiguous unless the artist is very careful.

Overall, demonstration is one of the most powerful forms of communication, particularly if it can be seen to produce observable benefits in the short term; installing a demonstration latrine in a well-chosen location is certainly worth trying. Unfortunately, the health benefits from hygiene can take time to materialize, so it is best to emphasize the immediate benefits such as comfort and freedom from flies and stench.

Another valuable method is the use of local people who have already been convinced. Those who have already improved their sanitation or hygiene and are pleased with the results are the best people to spread the message to the rest of the community.

Mass media such as radio can be used for rapidly disseminating information to large numbers of people[126]. Care must be taken to synchronize the availability of latrine components and technical support staff with broadcasts. Problems can arise when people outside the project area hear the programme and want to take part.

Bringing about the fundamental changes that are required to improve sanitation and hygiene requires an intensive programme of face-to-face communication by fieldworkers in the community[127]. If the number of project field staff in sanitation programmes is limited, it will become essential to involve field personnel from as wide a range as possible such as health assistants and health inspectors, nurses, village health workers, teachers, agricultural and rural development staff, rural home-makers, and adult-literacy and adult-education workers. It will become important to brief all local officials in project areas and to provide training in sanitation and hygiene. A substantial amount of practical communication skills should be incorporated into the training programme, and a range of learning materials developed such as flip-charts, leaflets, posters and models. Valuable source-books on media used by various sanitation and hygiene projects in the field have been prepared by UNICEF[128] and WASH[129].

Many problems can be avoided by involving the community in the planning and implementation process[130]. Community participation from the planning stages will eliminate inappropriate designs and unrealistic changes in behaviour. It will ensure that the latrines are used and maintained, and provide a catalyst for the spread of new ideas through ordinary communication channels.

Underneath the rhetoric of community participation are some genuine problems. The needs of a community cannot be determined at a single meeting, but require a process of active dialogue which will involve discussion and feedback. The emphasis should be on participatory learning methods which are open and promote critical consciousness. To achieve effective participation, fieldworkers must spend considerable time in a community, building trust and overcoming divisions and conflicts that may exist. Thus, it is important to brief development workers on the full implications of community participation and to build into the programme a realistic amount of time for the objectives planned, as well as thoroughly trained field staff. Community participation should not be seen as merely another method of coercion; it is a philosophy which should be incorporated throughout all programmes.

A great deal can be learned from communication and health education programmes in other countries. The unique characteristics of each community must be taken into account. What is needed is a flexible approach using a range of methods that are continually modified and monitored in the light of evaluation and experience.

(*Waterlines* Vol. 5 No. 3, January 1987)

Data collection for the design of water and sanitation projects in Belize

DAN CAMPBELL

The collection of data for planning and designing projects can be a difficult and complex process. Problems may include the questionable reliability of the data collected, high costs and the time factor. In response to these problems, the United States Agency for International Development (USAID) has published a report describing gathering techniques for conducting low-cost studies within reasonable time limits.

The Water & Sanitation for Health Project (WASH) has assisted in developing surveys in northern Belize for the village-level water and sanitation project, a three-year programme focusing on 1,600 households in the

Corozal and Orange Walk districts. The water-supply component of the project includes the construction or rehabilitation of 160 tubewells, and the installation of 160 India Mark II handpumps. Specifying a standard hand-pump has simplified the stocking of spare parts and repairs of broken pumps. Meanwhile, the sanitation side of the project plans to construct or rehabilitate 1,600 latrines. A strong emphasis has been placed on health education for all age groups and will include both formal school-based programmes and informal community-based education.

Survey and profile activities

As well as developing a household baseline survey, the WASH consultant helped to develop water and sanitation profiles on all the villages to be used for selecting and ranking villages to participate in the programme. The consultant also trained project staff in survey design, enumeration, and analysis. Villagers were involved in all phases of the survey and profile activities, including survey design, counting the responses, and the use of the survey results for designing a local water-supply and sanitation programme.

The village-level surveys were designed to collect information in three areas. First on environmental health knowledge, to assess local awareness of the connection between clean water, excreta disposal and good health. Secondly, to find out villagers' attitudes to water use and sanitation: what water is valued for, what cultural beliefs related to excreta disposal or personal hygiene exist and the causes of ill health, especially in children? The third area was an assessment of water usage and sanitation practices, to find the answer to the questions: What are the current water sources? What is water used for and in what quantities? How is excreta disposed of? What are the problems faced when trying to meet household water and sanitation needs?

Summaries of some of the findings in the village-level surveys showed that:

O Villagers have a good understanding of the necessity and importance of latrines. Latrines are used by both adults and children.
O Hand-washing after using latrines could not be observed, as latrines are located at least 100ft (30m) from pumps and household water buckets.
O Although villagers wash their hands before eating, they usually share a common basin with other household members.
O Because water is transported and stored in buckets, villagers need to be taught the importance of covering the buckets at all times and cleaning them regularly.
O Traditional water sources, particularly rain-water and dug wells, were used when potable water was supplied from handpumps located more than 150ft (45m) from the house. To ensure an adequate quality of

drinking-water, health education efforts should include information and instructions on how to improve traditional sources.

Data collection and information exchange between villagers and project staff was carried out in each of the following activities:
O Implementing a village water and sanitation profile for all villages in the Corozal and Orange Walk districts.
O Using the profile to select project villages.
O Holding village meetings to explain the purpose of the project and to discuss the contribution expected from the villagers.
O Implementing a baseline household survey of water and sanitation conditions for design, monitoring and evaluation purposes.

Water and sanitation profile

The water and sanitation profile was completed in all 58 villages of the Corozal and Orange Walk districts. It was accomplished through visits to each village and by collecting data from a variety of sources outside the village.

A typical site visit lasted three or four hours and included meetings with the village council members and teachers. Project staff discussed the technical feasibility of working in the villages with well-drilling teams, handpump maintenance crews and the Ministry of Health. These discussions covered issues such as road access, the existence of shallow bedrock and wells with a history of unsuitable drinking-water.

Selection of villages

Using the village water and sanitation profiles, 16 villages were selected to participate in the project. Selection criteria were agreed on, and a ranking of villages established. The rankings were determined by comments from the Ministry of Health. Considerable discussion took place between CARE, the Ministry of Health and USAID before determining the following criteria for the selection of the villages:
O Population must be between 100 and 150 families.
O Roads accessible in all weather.
O Existence of community infrastructure or past involvement in community-based projects.
O Present water supply located a long distance away.
O History of repeated and/or frequent incidence of water- or excreta-related diseases.
O An existing water-supply system which is functioning poorly.

During the past 18 months, the village water and sanitation profile has been modified. Information is now included on why a certain community has not been selected to participate in the project, and recent project evaluation recommends that the village profile should include more information on indicators of community organization. These would be used to assess the level of readiness of a community by identifying eight or 10 characteristics which indicate a dynamic community. Communities would be ranked on a scale of one to five, with one being disorganized and unmotivated, and five highly organized and well motivated. Separate strategies could then be developed for working with communities at each level.

Communities involved in the project vary considerably in the degree to which they are organized and ready for a project. Some, such as San Antonio and Chunox, are progressive, relatively affluent, and have had experience in community improvement projects. Others, such as Chan Pine Ridge have worse economic problems and have no experience with community action.

Village meetings

When the villages had been selected, meetings were held with each village council — including the general public, school officials, and other local organizations — to explain the project. These meetings covered the purpose of the project and activities to follow; confirmation of the village's interest in seeing through the project; the formation of a village water and sanitation committee; the identification of local enumerators for survey work; and a question-and-answer period.

The vehicle for the implementation of the project in the community is the village water and sanitation committee. Membership is largely voluntary: anyone expressing an interest can join the committee. The committees were organized in an attempt to side-step the political infighting that can arise in village councils. The responsibilities of the village water and sanitation committees include:

O Organizing the distribution of moulds for latrine construction, cement and other materials.
O Carrying out the health education programme.
O Maintaining the system once installed.
O Supervising the construction of latrines.
O Motivating the villagers to participate in the project,
O Resolving the problems and conflicts related to the project.

Each committee has seven to 10 members. Despite the fact that women are the main users of water, few belong to village water and sanitation committees. Following project evaluation it has been recommended that special efforts be made to include women in responsible roles.

The baseline household survey had three purposes. First, to document water-supply and sanitation conditions in each village household. Second, to increase the familiarity of village residents with the goals, objectives, and procedures of the project, and third, to introduce project staff to residents.

Monitoring and evaluation

It was recommended that information collected in the baseline household survey should also be used to monitor and evaluate the project. Goals and indicators have been formulated to assess the project's progress (Table 1).

Table 1. Goals and indicators used to assess project progress

Goal: Provision of adequate water supply	Indicator: Installation or rehabilitation of wells, water systems or springs with a capacity of 30 lcd for 1,600 families by June 1988.
Goal: Provision of an acceptable excreta disposal system.	Indicator: 70 per cent of latrines in the village to be clean and clearly in use by June 1988.
Goal: Increase the health education capacity of the Government of Belize.	Indicator: All schools in the two districts have received both materials and training in health education as relevant to water and sanitation.

Several interesting issues have emerged from the data collected so far. First, sanitary conditions in almost all the villages were quite poor, whereas water supply varied widely, with no uniformity in terms of the type or degree of water problems or their solutions.

A second issue that arose was that many villages did not regard hand-pumps as the most effective solution to their water-supply problems; this conflicted with the emphasis on handpumps in the original project design. The project design was made more flexible to include springs, wells and other village water-supply systems.

The third issue was that villagers were often either unavailable or not interested in participating in self-help projects during the cane-cutting season: this influenced the scheduling of projects. In addition, the involvement of more women in the project allowed some activities — such as health education and information collection — to continue during these times.

Lastly, the development of a village water and sanitation committee in each community has been an effective method of avoiding the political conflicts which often hinder efforts to organize at the community level. In some communities, these committees have provided unique opportunities for villagers to work together to solve their problems. The skills that committee members have learned will undoubtedly be used in other activities, especially in the area of health.

(*Waterlines* Vol. 6 No. 3, January 1988)

Village-level sanitation programmes in Zimbabwe

PETER MORGAN

The Government of Zimbabwe places considerable emphasis on rural development, and the provision of improved sanitation has been adopted as one of the priority areas. The Ministry of Health is responsible for planning and executing rural sanitation projects throughout the country as part of its Primary Health Care Programme, which also includes improving water supplies. Many of these projects are assisted by loans and grants from a large number of donor agenices.

All rural sanitation programmes in Zimbabwe are based on the Ventilated Improved Pit Latrine, known locally as the Blair latrine. The Blair latrine is basically a well-built pit latrine equipped with a roof, and a screened ventilation pipe that acts as a fly-trap and exhaust-pipe (as described in Chapter 6).

Since it was developed by the Ministry of Health 12 years ago, this technique has been strongly backed by the government. More recently, it was chosen as the sanitation technology for rural development in the National Water and Sanitation Master Plan. The Plan also endorsed the method of giving each family a subsidy, in the form of materials, to assist in the construction of their own latrine. The aim is to provide access to improved sanitation for every family living in the rural areas. By the turn of the century, 750,000 Blair latrines should have been built.

Community participation

The concept of the Blair latrine is well established in Zimbabwe. It appears in school curricula, is publicized by mobile cinema units, and is actively promoted in the press and by village health workers and other staff operating at all levels throughout the country. Literature on construction techniques is also available. The Blair latrine is well known, and has been accepted by the user community as a valuable and practical means of improving their living conditions. In most communities, there is actually a demand for units to be built.

Before embarking on a programme of construction, Ministry of Health workers carry out educational and awareness campaigns to motivate the people in a particular village, ward or district. Demonstration structures are made and local builders are trained in the best construction techniques. This takes time, but is vital to the future success of the programme. Community participation is another essential component if any scheme is to be long-lasting, and is made easier as all rural sanitation programmes are based on one latrine per family.

Case study in Chiota

The ward of Chiota West, in the province of Mashonaland East, lies south of Harare and is occupied by 1,300 families. The Chiota Rural Council and the MOH approached a donor, in this case the UK's Save the Children Fund (SCF), for technical and financial assistance to begin a sanitation project. When an agreement had been reached, MOH and SCF field officers began an awareness campaign, operating through village committees, and also trained 30 local builders in theory and practical techniques. Each course lasted one month, and each builder was expected to build two complete latrines to the satisfaction of the trainers. On completion of the course, each builder was given a set of tools.

The programme began in January 1986 and ended five months later; during this time, 622 family structures and eight multi-compartment school structures had been built. In each case, the family was provided with seven bags of cement, 24m of 3mm reinforcing wire, 2m, of 50mm chicken-wire (6ft width) and a fly-screen, a total value of Z$40 (US$25). Each family provided 1,200 burnt bricks, suitable quantities of pit and river sand, and stone. In addition, the family dug the pit to the required depth and paid a builder a negotiated fee of Z$25 (US$15) to construct the latrine. The contribution amounted to Z$70 (US$43), nearly double the donated subsidy, and demonstrates the willingness of rural people to participate in and contribute to schemes of this type. The square spiral structure was chosen, as it was considered larger than the alternative round spiral and more suitable as a wash-room. Woodland is sparse in Chiota, and there is a demand for the construction of facilities in which defecation and bathing can be undertaken in privacy. One of the advantages of the Blair latrine over other models is that it serves as a wash-room as well as a toilet, a feature which has greatly assisted the promotional campaign.

The Chiota Sanitation Programme is one of a number of successful projects which have been undertaken in Zimbabwe. Over 100,000 Blair latrines have been constructed since Independence in 1980. However, the overall programme is not without its problems. While simple in concept, the Blair latrine only functions correctly when built according to the specified designs. The standards of construction are very high in Chiota, and in many cases exceed the standards of construction of the house itself.

Construction standards

While standards are improving nationwide, many examples could be cited of so-called Blair latrines which are poorly built and which offer none of the advantages of an improved pit latrine.

Vent-pipe

In some programmes, the brick vent-pipe is built too small to be efficient at drawing air. This means that, when the wind blows in certain directions, an odour can be noticed inside. The brick vent-pipe is one of the least efficient pipes and must be large to be effective: an internal size of 225mm by 225mm is essential.

The internal walls of a brick pipe are often rough, causing air turbulence and loss of efficiency. Smaller pipes made of PVC, steel or asbestos are more efficient because their internal walls are smooth. However, when built correctly, a brick pipe functions well over a great range of climatic conditions and is certainly adequate for the job.

Fly-screen

If fly control is to be effective a roof must be fitted to the structure and a corrosion-resistant screen fixed to the head of the vent-pipe. Screens made of plastic disintegrate within months, and ordinary steel screens last less than a year. In Zimbabwe, PVC-coated glass-fibre screens last for four to five years, and stainless steel is expected to last for decades. It is known that many latrines still have no screens. Right now, no suitable screen is made in Zimbabwe, but must be imported. Currently, as many as 40,000 stainless-steel screens are being imported every year for the sanitation programme.

Base slab

The construction of the base slab also requires care. It should be made from concrete, 75mm thick, with a mixture of stone (four parts), river sand (two parts) and cement (one part), and suitably reinforced with 3mm-wire at

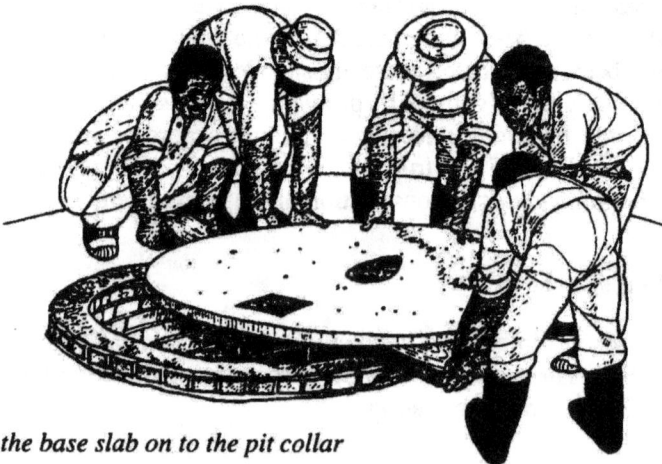

Lifting the base slab on to the pit collar

150mm spaces in a grid pattern. The slab is sometimes made by plastering a layer of cement mortar over wooden poles laid over the pit, which makes the life of the slab dependent not on the life of the concrete, but on the life of the poles. This is clearly undesirable.

Latrine floor

One of the best features of the Blair latrine is that it is odour-free inside. This feature is very popular, and results from the passage of fresh air down through the squat hole and up through the pipe. To keep the latrine odour-free, it is essential for the latrine floor to be kept clean and scrubbed. Not infrequently Blair latrines are made without the essential sloping floor; instead the flat cement slab acts as a floor. This can harbour pools of urine and is difficult to wash down, with the end result that an odour will develop despite the pipe. The floor should be sloped towards the squat hole and made of hard cement, with a mixture of three parts sand to one of cement.

Foundations and pits

A latrine is as good as the time it remains standing. Experience has shown that a good foundation is crucial for any structure, and this is true for the Blair latrine as well. The walls of the latrine should be built on proper brick foundations, which are offset from the pit itself. Occasionally, latrines have

Laying the first course of bricks for the superstructure. Note how the structure is partly offset from the pit, which reduces the chances of collapse.

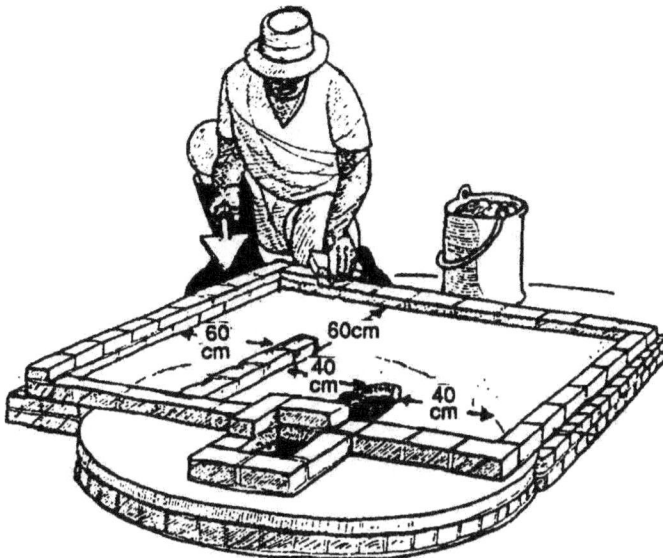

been built on loose soils with the entire weight of the structure taken by the pit collar — a dangerous technique which should be avoided.

With the advent of the double and multi-compartment latrines, it is essential that the pit itself should also be subdivided so that the air-circulation in each unit operates independently. If a single undivided pit is used in combination with several structures, the air pull from one pipe cannot act on a single squat-hole, with the result that air moves about freely from one hole to the next, carrying odours.

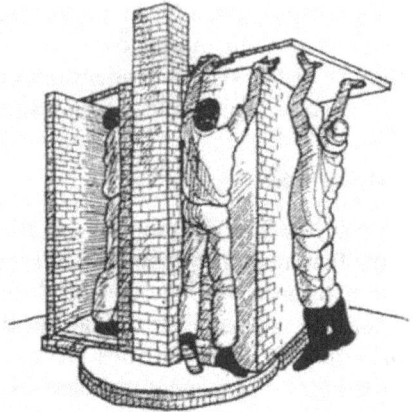

Lifting the roof slabs (made with sand, cement and chicken-wire) into position.

Achieving success

It has been realized for some time that the construction problems outlined above are caused by a lack of understanding of the special properties of ventilated pit latrines. In Zimbabwe, considerable effort is being placed in providing an adequate supply of suitable educational literature, which explains why the latrine works, how to build it properly and how to maintain it. This campaign will help, but it will never completely replace direct, hands-on training. A mobile training unit is now active and tours the country providing the best training in latrine construction techniques.

Zimbabwe's ambitious national programme of latrine construction hopes to provide all rural families with an improved ventilated pit latrine. The programme is being carried out with considerable financial support from a large number of donor agencies. The emphasis is on village-scale projects in which householders are given a subsidy to assist them in the construction of their own family latrine. Clearly this technique is working well, but requires considerable effort not only from the donor but also from the Zimbabwe Government (which provides technical expertise and transport), and from the family itself. The fact that families are prepared to commit their time, effort and money to the programme gives grounds for hope that it can be sustained in future years, albeit at a slower pace, should the flow of donor funding diminish. For the time being, however, every effort is being made by government, donors and individual families to make the national rural sanitation programme in Zimbabwe one of the most successful in Africa.

Acknowledgements

I wish to acknowledge the kind assistance of the Save the Children Fund, UK, for access to their records, and the Provincial Health Inspector, Mashonaland East, for valuable discussion. I also wish to thank the Director, Blair Research Laboratory, and the Permanent Secretary for Health, for permission to publish this article.

(Waterlines Vol. 6 No. 3, January 1988)

Planning self-sustaining programmes for sanitation: the Lesotho experience

PHIL EVANS

If ever anyone thought that improving sanitation in developing countries, particularly in rural communities, was easy, experience gained during the IDWSSD quickly shattered illusions. Many important technical problems have been solved, and adequate technologies now exist for the safe disposal of human waste at a reasonable cost. Nevertheless, rates of installation, adoption and use have been disappointingly low, and far below the pace demanded by the targets set for the Decade.

In seeking solutions to these problems, the idea that a decade is ample time to bring about significant and lasting change must simply be rejected. Instead, serious moves must be made to create the solid foundations on which lasting, self-sustaining programmes can be built.

Long-term planning

The introduction of a new sanitation technology brings with it a whole package of demands, which challenge prevailing patterns of behaviour and urge revisions in long-held views regarding personal and domestic hygiene practices and beliefs about sickness and health. These implications are now widely recognized: simple technical fixes alone are inadequate in bringing about the improvements in environmental sanitation and general hygiene which are likely to lead to wider improvements in health.

The immediate consequences of this recognition are twofold. First, sanitation programmes must be planned in such a way that they include adequate provision for tackling behavioural issues and, where possible, harmonize with existing education and training campaigns. Second, planning must aim for long-term improvements. Short-term gains through, for example, the running of brief, intensive demonstration projects (often heavily subsidized) are easily achieved, but often lead to long-term failure and stagnation when high levels of subsidy cannot be sustained. Changes in behaviour cannot be achieved overnight, but occur gradually as new ideas are considered and tested.

Recent experience in Lesotho, in southern Africa, has shown that long-term planning, with the emphasis on self-reliance and the cultural absorption of new technologies, can yield results which generate optimism in the future development of sanitation programmes in the region. Lessons learned in Lesotho may also be applicable to programme planning elsewhere.

In October 1983, the Government of Lesotho, with financial aid from the United Nations Development Programme, the United Nations Children's Fund and the United States Agency for International Development, and with management support from the Technology Advisory Group of the World Bank, launched a three-year pilot Rural Sanitation Project, with a view to developing and testing a plan of implementation for a proposed National Rural Sanitation Programme. The project was to be based on the principles of community self-help and minimum long-term cost to the government.

Choosing a technology

Choosing the technology was not a major problem. The Ventilated Improved Pit (VIP) latrine had already been introduced fairly successfully in low-income housing areas of the capital, and the construction of improved latrines was already in place. VIP latrine owners in cities were generally satisfied with the technology, and thus the groundwork of acceptability had already been laid for the rural project.

Drawing on this previous experience, prototype rural VIP latrines were designed and built at a test site in the capital of the district selected for pilot activities. Afterwards, consultations were held at a number of short workshops, with groups of people from proposed pilot sites and with representatives of relevant government ministries and donor agencies.

Acceptable designs were identified and an outline implementation strategy was devised, based as far as possible on the views expressed by the workshop participants. Involving the rural population in discussions at this early stage reflected an important element of the project's philosophy and was seen as essential to enhancing prospects for long-term success.

Self-help philosophy

Early in the project, the policy was established that the full cost of latrine construction would be met by the beneficiaries, and that latrine builders would be recruited from, and paid by, the local population. In the short term, this self-help philosophy had implications for the likely rate of construction, but it was felt that such an approach was more conducive to long-term success. In the event, the project's three-year construction target of 400 VIP latrines was exceeded by 50 per cent, with slightly more than 600 completed. Of these, however, roughly 350 were built in the final year, indicating a relatively lengthy lead-up time.

A primary objective of the strategy is to create a situation in which VIP latrine-building becomes absorbed into the local culture. Many of the artisans trained as latrine builders were drawn from existing cadres of skilled local house-builders and general handymen. By attending project training courses, held at village sites, they are able to add the VIP latrine to their repertoire. Ultimately, it is hoped that they will pass on these skills to others, through traditional apprenticeships, and thus reduce the long-term training burden on government.

At the same time as building up local self-reliance in the construction of improved latrines, this approach has also had an important impact on private sector enterprise in the rural areas, creating income-generating opportunities for local artisans and stimulating cash flows within communities. This emphasis on cultural absorption has also been strongly reflected in the promotional and educational aspects of project work.

Primary health care

In Lesotho, a commitment to a primary health care approach, with education campaigns playing a central role, has been government policy for some time. An existing structure thus was in place within which the project could operate.

To boost the effectiveness of these campaigns, the project made studies of prevailing attitudes and levels of knowledge within the rural population, with particular emphasis on sanitation-related disease. These studies suggested that a good proportion of rural people held germ-related theories of disease transmission, though knowledge was often fragmentary and not integrated into an overall theory of prevention and cure. Attempts to improve this situation are being made by integrating sanitation-related messages with other aspects of primary health care education already underway, such as campaigns related to improved water supply, nutrition, mother and child health, and so on.

The full impact of these campaigns is unlikely to be felt for some time, but early evaluation at pilot sites, through the project's built-in monitoring and evaluation system, indicates that some progress has been made on a modest scale and prospects are good for a more substantial impact in the longer term.

A crucial factor in developing a campaign of this kind is that it must take as its starting point the prevailing views and levels of knowledge of the targeted population. By paying attention and giving respect to existing views, a dialogue can be encouraged between extension workers and target populations. Once this is the case, a joint commitment to improving health conditions can be developed.

Government role and predicted success

The emphasis on absorption and self-sustainability, critical to the prospects for success in the field, is equally important at the institutional and governmental level. The principle that attempts should be made to fit the project into existing structures, and to make maximum use of available skills and resources, applies at all levels.

Before the launching of the project, responsibility for improved sanitation in the rural areas lay with the Environmental Health Section of the Ministry of Health, with its staff of trained public health inspectors and health assistants. Rather than establish the project separately, it has been located within this section as a central part of it, using its existing staff.

Similarly, technical staff assigned to the project are employed through the long-standing Village Water Supply Section of the Ministry of Interior. This process of institutionalization is by no means complete, but important first steps have been taken. Not the least of these is the inclusion of rural sanitation activities in the government's 1986-90 five-year development plan. This underlines the commitment to continue with project activities, as a full part of the government's development programme, at least until the end of the Decade.

It would be wrong to suggest that the Lesotho Rural Sanitation Project has had a history of effortless success. This would be far from the truth. Many problems have been encountered, and many more remain to be solved. Sufficient progress has been made, however, to justify the expansion of activities to a national scale. This process has already begun with the participation of the British Overseas Development Administration in the extension of project activities to a further three districts. Interest has been expressed by other donors, and a phased expansion has been projected, which will bring all 10 districts into the programme by the end of the Decade.

The Lesotho experience provides an argument for the wider adoption of a particular approach to the implementation of sanitation programmes. This approach takes as its starting point a long-term view, establishing the principle that strategies should aim for a self-sustaining programme which can be maintained for a long period with minimal government and donor expenditure and maximum self-reliance within the community.

Short-term gains, which result in ephemeral high-profile projects, may look good within the context of brief project cycles, but, in the end, do little for the people they are intended to serve. An emphasis on long-term planning, community self-help, social and cultural appropriateness in project design (supported by good monitoring and evaluation), and an integrated approach to implementation may not speed up the attainment of the immediate goals of the Decade, but may well establish a foundation upon which significant and lasting gains may be built in the future.

(Waterlines Vol. 6 No. 2, October 1987)

Low-cost sanitation in a squatter town: mobilizing people

SAMI MUSTAFA

Orangi is a *katchi abadi*, a squatter town inhabited by 800,000 people in an area of about 5,000 acres. In Karachi division alone, there are 362 such *katchi abadis* with a total population of 2 million people.

For a long time the existence of such large numbers of people living in *katchi abadis* was not recognized by the government, as if these people did not exist. The government felt no obligation to their developmental needs, and accordingly no attention was paid to them until a Directorate of Katchi Abadis was created to look into the possibility of providing the *katchi abadis* with basic services, such as water supply and sewerage.

The improvement of *katchi abadis* in terms of providing water supply and sewerage has involved large sums of money: a rough estimate of Rs1,650 million has been made for initial development. The government agencies responsible for this task, first the Karachi Development Authority (KDA) and, since July 1981, the Karachi Metropolitan Corporation (KMC), have faced difficulties with funding these improvement projects. Neither borrowing the money from foreign countries nor recouping the outlay from the residents proved feasible.

Consequently, a solution had to be found without having to depend entirely on external assistance. The conventional approach of development from above had been shown to hold very little promise for solving the problems of Orangi.

The broad outline of the alternative strategy had been envisaged by Dr Akhter Hameed Khan. It had to be development from below, and local residents would be organized and their resources mobilized. By this method, the creation of effective local organization and dissemination of technical skills among local people would be the key to the improvement. And above all, the success of the methodology would depend on a sound low-cost technology, technical competence, and professional approach of its workers which the Orangi Pilot Project (OPP) has now acquired through much time and effort.

Barriers to self-help improvement

There were three barriers preventing the improvement of Orangi on a self-help basis. First, there has been a 'psychological' barrier both at the 'top' and at the 'bottom'. At the 'top', government departments perhaps feel that the problem of *katchi abadis* cannot be solved because they have insufficient resources. At the 'bottom', some people in Orangi still expected the KMC or the KDA to do the work for them. They also feel that the work of sanitation, water supply, drainage, and so on, is beyond their own abilities and resources.

Secondly, the cost of constructing a proper sanitation system through conventional methods involving government departments, vested interests and corruption, was too high for people to afford.

The third barrier was technical. Where residents have been interested in and motivated towards constructing a sewerage system, they have lacked the technical know-how to do it competently and satisfactorily. The result has invariably led, sooner or later, to failure.

Orangi Pilot Project

The Orangi Pilot Project (OPP) has attempted to remove the three barriers. With regard to the sanitation programme, the experiment has been:

O To persuade the residents that if they do not organize themselves to improve their living conditions, nobody will do it for them, and they will face greater hardships.
O To try to reduce the cost of a standard sewerage system.
O To provide the interested residents with a low-cost technology and the technical guidance and assistance for constructing it, and to train them in its maintenance and upkeep.

The people of Orangi know that collective effort is perhaps the only effective solution to their needs. One problem is that of trust. In their experience, all efforts at organizing them has invariably resulted in either incompetence and waste, or in their being cheated out of their money. Accountability has been difficult, and corruption rampant, even among fellow residents.

In order to reduce the problem of mistrust, Dr Khan started with the lane as the unit of organization instead of the larger mohalla, or neighbourhood. There are between 20 and 30 houses in each lane. The heads of these households get together, discuss the problem of sewerage and the need to rectify it. When they all agree that work should be done on sewerage and that they are willing to contribute their share of the cost, they make a formal application to the OPP office. The OPP office sends its technical team, which surveys the lane and gives the design and cost estimate. Then the residents collect and give the money to elected lane managers. The managers then buy the material and organize the work. Full account of expenses is maintained, and a copy is submitted to the OPP office.

Reducing costs

The OPP has reduced the cost of construction by eliminating kickbacks and profiteering. The cost has been brought down to less than a third of usual rates. In some cases, the cost has been reduced to as low as Rs12.60 per foot as compared to the usual rate of Rs45 per foot of drainage line.

This has been done by improving the design of the manholes for inspection and maintenance, and use of septic tanks. By changing the design of the manholes from block construction to casting them in-situ, the need for expensive skilled masons has also been eliminated. Steel shuttering is loaned to the residents, who use it to construct the manholes themselves under OPP supervision.

It is fully realized that the reduction in cost should at no stage compromise the quality of work. By improving the design of the manhole and also by simplifying the system by putting a 'T' in a *haudi* (interceptor chamber) rather than building an expensive waffle chamber, it has been possible to reduce the cost further. It took many months of experimentation with various designs of *haudis* and manholes before a satisfactory solution was found.

The task of extension work involved considerable time and effort. Having arrived at a successful design of *haudi* with a T-pipe connection, we found that the residents were often not following the OPP instructions. When the technical staff surveyed the lanes constructed with OPP assistance, it was found that a number of houses had been given direct connections to the main sewerage line. They had either not built the *haudis* with T-pipe connection or in some places misunderstood the instruction and made direct connection with an oversized T-pipe. This made it likely that the system would choke and fail.

Consequently OPP had to instruct all its managers and technical staff to make sure that no future direct connections were made, and those made were rectified. Our extension method — that is, how to deliver a design for successful implementation by the people — had to be improved. Plastic scale-models were made to demonstrate visually how the system works, from the commode (toilet) to the *haudi* to the main line.

People-oriented

OPP's aim is to organize the people to learn how to build a sewerage system themselves. Deviance and error of judgment is part of the process of developing local organizations and local skills and expertise, which will eventually eliminate the need to depend on the extravagantly expensive services of outside institutions and professionals. OPP is aware that it cannot build a fully integrated sewerage system immediately.

The effect of this self-help programme has been significant. When it first started in September 1981, it took three months for Dr Khan and his social

Plan (top) and elevation (below) of the OPP's standard design for sewerage house connections

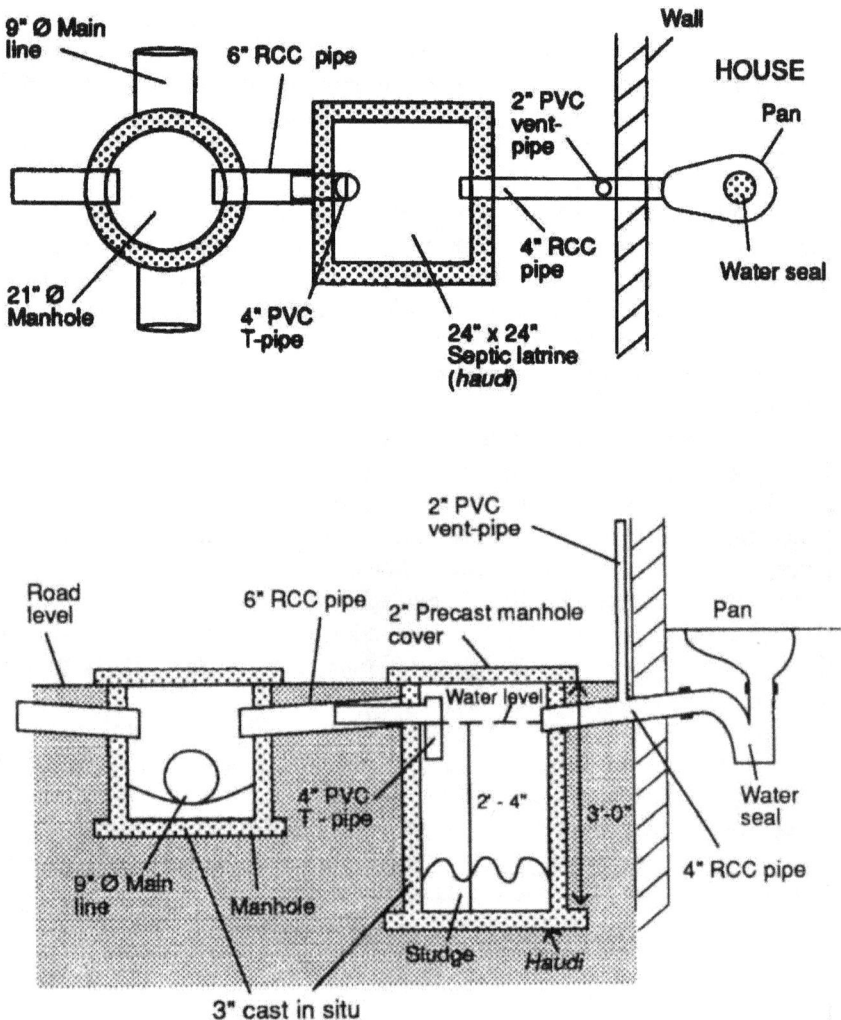

motivators to convince the residents of a single lane that the proposal was not another political gimmick and that it would work and work well. Today, applications from lane residents keep pouring in, and the OPP office is unable to keep up with the requests.

If social mobilization is the main springboard of development, then the distinct roles of social mobilization and technical expertise must be fully recognized. Otherwise one is likely to make the error of measuring an unconventional approach through narrowly 'professional' yardsticks. This is what seems to have been at the root of the conflict between the OPP and the UN Centre for Human Settlements (UNCHS or Habitat). Mr Nicholas Houghton, sent by the UNCHS to assist the OPP, felt that the approach of OPP and that of UNCHS are 'irreconcilable ... one open-ended, exploratory and evolutionary with emphasis on sociological particulars ... the other, target-oriented, systematic, with a professional and technical focus ...'

This produced a conflict which has been most unfortunate, because the UNCHS, 'uniquely equipped to provide specialized support for undertaking large-scale projects in low-income urban areas', became an adversary of a project it had come to assist. It insisted that it would assist only on its own terms or not assist at all. In fact, the project has now been split into two, one part remaining with the OPP and the other going to BCCI — the Community Development Programme of which Mr Houghton is the Chief Technical Advisor.

Conflict

As a result of this conflict with the UNCHS, OPP suddenly found itself faced with a unique challenge. Did it have to depend on foreign agenices like the UNCHS with their professionals and experts to provide an effective and viable strategy for the improvement of low-income areas, or could the work be done just as well or better by Pakistani technical and social science experts who have an interest and commitment to the people of low-income groups? This challenge has implications not only for the OPP but for low-income people in virtually every part of the Third World.

By the end of the first quarter this year, the programme had reached a stage of self-sustained growth. Requests from the majority of lanes had not needed the prompting of OPP social organizers. During this quarter, 84 lane sewerage lines and 9 secondary drains were under construction. Neither the excitement and preoccupation of elections nor the rise in the prices of pipes and other materials reduced the tempo of work.

At the same time, fairly good quality work is being maintained, and very few technical mistakes are being made by the lane managers. House-owners are inclined to consider the T-*haudi* superfluous however, because they think that as plenty of water is now available for flushing, their latrines should be connected directly to the manholes. This insistence on direct connections makes the improvement of the open *nallas*, the natural drains into which the lane sewerage lines open, very urgent.

In some places, indeed, the *nallas* are overflowing and damaging the houses and the lane sewerage lines. The OPP has therefore decided to start some research into low-cost design of large *nallas*, and persuade the lane people to take this problem on as well.

By December 1984, in OPP's area of Orangi, 1,273 of a total of 3,072 lanes had constructed sewerage lines. Of 43,424 houses, 20,470 had built sanitary latrines connected to the underground sewerage lines in the lanes.

Women's programme

Following on from low-cost sanitation, OPP has started health education, concerning personal hygiene, boiling drinking-water and profitable kitchen gardens for women in purdah, when custom requires them to stay inside their homes. Generally, such women go out only for emergencies or in exceptional circumstances. Therefore, we think that constructing Welfare Centres is ineffective, as it is quite unrealistic to expect these women to leave their homes to seek advice.

Instead, OPP is introducing a system of mobile teams, which work with women activists or contact persons in the lanes. There should be regular and continuous meetings at the activist's house, leading to the formation of small groups by each activist. Each team consists of a woman health visitor, a social organizer and a gardening expert. At present there are two teams, working under the guidance of a woman doctor. The two teams are dropped at the lane activists' houses, and brought back to the OPP office after the meetings. With this approach, it may become possible to contact and educate large numbers of families from a central office, with the help of a vehicle.

OPP is also supporting other developments which sprang from the low-cost sanitation programme. They include improving the conditions of many Orangi women, who take in stitching work, and research into low-cost house construction.

Challenging conventional approaches

The Orangi Pilot Project is by definition an experimental exercise, conceived and executed in response to the inability of official agencies to improve the lot of the low-income people. The substandard condition of any *katchi abadi* is an expression of the failure of conventional institutions and approaches, and therefore the OPP experiment has been to find viable alternatives.

It would not have been possible to make people understand the efficacy of OPP's self-help and self-financed programme had it not been for the community involvement and leadership abilities of OPP's social organizers. They are all residents of Orangi who understand the problems first-hand and feel committed to the area's improvement and well-being. Dr Akhter Hameed Khan's life-long commitment to non-elitist developmental strategy has been the guiding principle of the project. He has the vision and courage to challenge conventional approaches and has unwavering faith in the ingenuity of national expertise and local activists.

The breakthrough in the technology of low-cost sanitation has been possible largely due to the efforts and ingenuity of Mr Arif Hasan, consulting architect and a Visiting Professor at the Darwood Engineering College, Karachi, who works with the OPP as its chief technical consultant. He has been assisted by architect Parween Rahman, OPP's Joint Director (Technical).

The search for alternatives for the improvement of *katchi abadis* is a difficult task. It needs competence and patience; it needs commitment and dedication; it needs vision, ingenuity and experimentation. The end result, we hope, will be success in evolving an effective and viable strategy for improving low-income areas which have been traditionally neglected.

Further information

Much more detailed information can be found in Orangi Pilot Project, progress reports April 1980-June 1983, and the Orangi Pilot Project, 21st quarterly progress report, January-March 1985.

(Waterlines Vol. 4 No. 1, July 1985)

CHAPTER 11

Strategies for Improvement

It is imperative that projects are not only carefully monitored but also evaluated to optimize the use of resources and also to achieve objectives without adverse effects on the environment. Gunnar Schultzberg of WHO, Geneva, and Richard Feachem and Carol MacCormack of the Ross Institute, London, collaborated to produce a set of guidelines for evaluating the extent to which water supply and sanitation projects are functioning and being used. The technique is quick, allowing judgements to be made in a matter of weeks rather than months with few resources in terms of money and manpower. For this reason, it is known as the Minimum Evaluation Procedure (MEP). The first article here outlines the three consecutive steps using a set of indicators which can be observed in the community.

Chris Smith reports on the latrine acquisition curve, a simple research tool which aims to improve the planning of latrine promotion activities and to provide a basis for evaluating the effects of sanitation programmes.

The water-supply programme in Zambia's Western Province had been established for a few years before health education and community participation came to be recognized as essential elements of rural water supply. Joanne Harnmeijer reflects on the introduction of a community education and participation component into the programme.

Mathew Onduru reports on a seven-year project which aims to establish effective community-based health care in the district of Kisumu in Kenya. Evaluation of the project in 1987 showed that community participation was very strong and that the project had already improved the health status of the population served. But this progress has been achieved mainly through immunization and maternal and child health services.

Jamie Bartram and Warren Johns describe and assess the efforts of the Aguarana and the Huambisa Jungle Indian Council to integrate water supply, hygiene education and sanitation into their primary health programme. They conclude that little has been achieved, if health statistics are compared, despite some success in the control of measles and chickenpox by vaccination. But simple health statisitics may not be an adequate measure. The health programme has contributed enormously in providing a solid centre of activity. Other technologies such as the Blair latrine are being considered. They conclude that good health in the developing world can only come from the action of the people themselves. This article demonstrates that water quality surveillance (chapter 5) is a vital tool for the monitoring and assessment of drinking-water supplies (indicator W2 for the WHO Minimum Evaluation Procedure).

It is envisaged that evaluation of projects will contribute significantly to future improvements in health benefits and optimum resource use.

One step at a time: WHO's Minimum Evaluation Procedure for water-supply and sanitation projects

GUNNAR SCHULTZBERG, RICHARD FEACHAM and CAROL MACCORMACK

The WHO Minimum Evaluation Procedure looks at water-supply and sanitation projects in three consecutive steps using a set of 'indicators', which can be observed in the community.

It asks 'Is the system actually working?' (Function). If the system is not, steps must be taken to identify the reasons and remedy them before using other indicators to ask 'How widely is the system being used?' (Utilization). Again, if the indicators reveal problems, it is essential to look back into the system and put them right before expecting any improvement in people's health. This article will not deal with health impact, as the authors plan to publish a separate document on this aspect. They stress that it would be a waste of time and resources to look for improvements in the standard of health before being sure that a scheme is both capable of functioning and is actually used by the intended target population.

Water, sanitation and hygiene education schemes must be integrated with primary health care initiatives in the country concerned to maximize the possibility of improvements in the health of the people. This requires the involvement of the appropriate ministries at an early stage, a factor which has been overlooked in many studies, and has led to missed chances in many countries.

The MEP outlines some methods of collecting household information, given in Table 1 (page 288-9). It then follows a set of carefully chosen indicators to assist in evaluating firstly the functioning and then the use. There are four for the function of community water supply, three for sanitation and

Table 1. Methods of collecting information.

Method	Advantages	Disadvantages
1. *Direct observation* of a sample of households to record: 1. Types of households or neighbourhoods that do not have acess to facilities 2. Hygiene use of the facilities 3. Technical reasons for malfunctioning. 4. How much water is being collected and/or for what purposes the water is being used. 5. Use of latrines Sample question: Are the latrines kept clean or are they fouled?	Immediate, vivid understanding of problems, low cost.	Disadvantaged households and neighbourhoods may not be found and observed, especially if the evaluators are not familiar with the local area. People may object to being observed, in particular when it comes to use of latrines. The sample is small.
2. *Workshops* in project areas in which project staff, primary health care workers and representatives of the recipients (including women) work out maintenance problems in a water system. There is a problem - solving focus - and participants are chosen according to the problem.	A simple effective way to evaluate progress and develop possible modifications to design and/or implementation. Project personnel can make immediate use of the information.	Participants may not have systematically observed the functioning and utilization of facilities: quantified information may thus not be available to persuade decision makers at higher levels.
3. *Small sample household survey* using brief interview schedules and *conversational interview* technique. Enquiry is sharply focused on only a few essential topics. Sample question: Do you use this water? If the answer is 'no', questioner asks 'Why not?', sympathetically listening to all the person has to say.	Conversation, rather than direct questioning is usually perceived by rural people to be more polite, more interesting and expressing a genuine concern about them and their health. Since only a few topics are discussed in depth, the quality of information is good. Unanticipated constraints and perceptions may emerge.	There is a smaller quantity of information. Responses are not so easily coded and compared with other responses. The scope of enquiry is limited. The technique requires considerable skill of the interviewers.
4. *Stratified samples* of groups. This is not a random method of choosing, and zeroes in on groups which are most likely to be left out of water-supply and sanitation schemes, eg. the poor, lowest caste or a marginal ethnic group. Sample question: Are you receiving this service? If not, what are the reasons?	The extremes of service and/or wealth can be covered with specific samples allowing smaller total survey size than in method 5 described below. Conditions of especially disadvantaged groups in the community can be investigated and compared with the most advantaged groups.	Poor households nay not be clustered and easily identified. Methods of statistical analysis will have to be modified to deal with non-random distribution.

5. *Questionnaire survey* of households selected at random or clusters of households selected at random. Sample question: Are health education messages being understood?	The sample is both large and chosen at random. Therefore, disadvantaged households are guaranteed to be within the survey sample. Less skillful interviewers may be used.	A large sample is required to cover the whole spectrum of: (i) levels of service;(ii) social strata Questions which are needed to identify the socio-economic postion of households may be perceived as threatening. Questionnaires must be used for reasons of efficiency but may yiield superficial or evasive responses. Large surveys are costly, time-consuming and it might take a long time to process the data. Results may not be readily understood by project staff or the project beneficiaries.

four for hygiene education. On the use side, there are two for community water supply, one for sanitation and three for hygiene education, giving a total of 17. They are all described, together with data required, guidelines on how to assess findings and possible follow-up actions, for water, sanitation and hygiene education.

Function indicators: water supply

The quantity of water (Indicator W1) which designers plan to supply to each member of the population increases depending on whether the service is a standpipe, a yard connection or a house connection, and whether cattle or vegetable gardens are watered from the same source. Seasonal variation in the quantity of water available at source, and in demand, are often overlooked in planning documents. Answers to the 12 questions which make up this indicator may lead to the design criteria being revised.

Water quality (Indicator W2) targets are based on the WHO Guidelines for Drinking Water Quality[62]. 'Safe water' implies no bacteriological pollution, and with acceptable chemical properties, colour, taste and odour. Water analysis and sanitary surveillance are the important aspects of water quality control. Sanitary surveys cannot replace bacteriological analysis, but will give a good idea of factors likely to lead to bacteriological contamination. For instance, a surface water supply, eg. a river, is much more likely to be contaminated with disease-transmitting faeces, indicated by the presence of faecal coliform bacteria (mainly *E. coli*) than a protected groundwater source such as a spring. Contamination may also occur at the tap or in the home. Adult women are the best target for education in hygiene, if the latter is the case.

Reliability of water supplies (Indicator W3) is not often considered when

Flowchart of water-supply evaluation

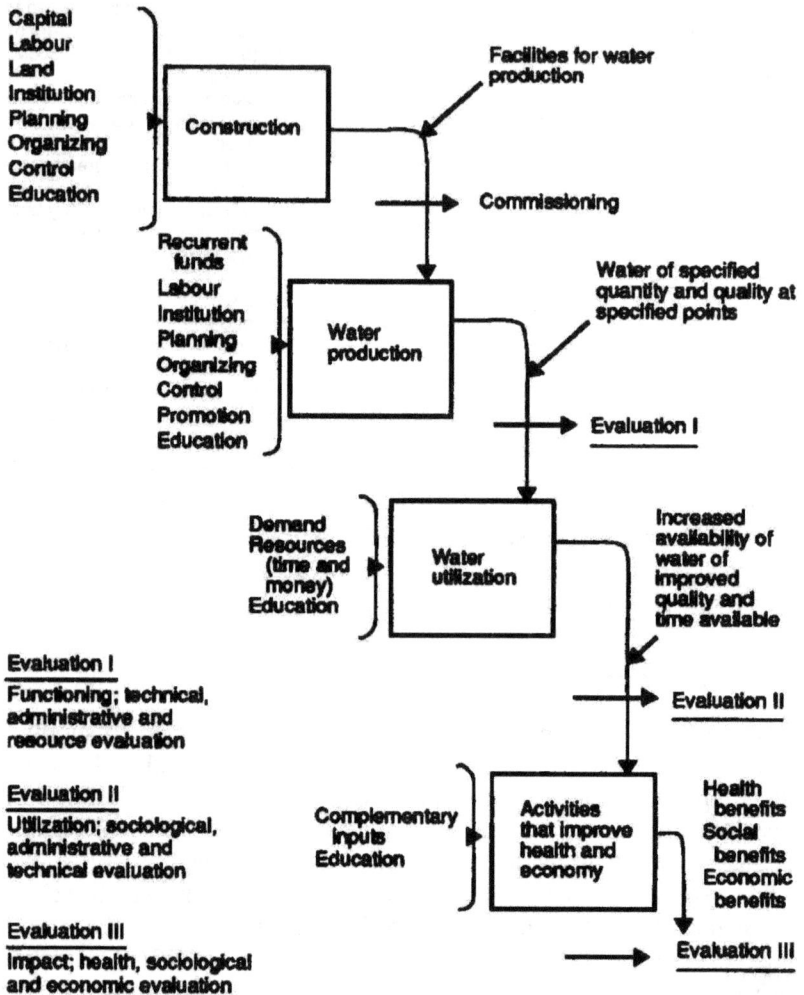

they are planned. Low reliability can be the result of poor design and construction, but is most commonly because of inadequate operation and maintenance. If maintenance is the problem, the tasks to remedy it must be clearly defined and the bodies responsible identified. Often, central government assumes that the community itself will be responsible for maintaining the supply, even though it gives the villages inadequate support, training or money.

If new clean water sources are too far from people's houses, they are more likely to use traditional polluted sources (Indicator W4, convenience of water points). Where there are marked seasonal variations in the supply, people will have to use sources further from their homes in the dry season compared with the wet season. If the proportion of households located further from a water point than planned is excessive, or if a great number of households forsake the new supply in favour of traditional sources, more water points should be constructed. A promotion programme would also help persuade people of the benefits of the new supply.

Function indicators: sanitation

Information on the proportion of households with improved latrines (Indicator S1) in the project area is collected by a house-to-house survey, followed by a special survey of households not participating in the improvements. Initially, this is to find out whether they know about the project, and, if they do, to find out whether they have chosen not to take part or whether they have been excluded (and why, and by whom). Substantial community health benefits will probably only materialize if more than 80 per cent of the population have improved latrines. The action needed to improve coverage will depend on the main reasons for people not participating in the project.

Unhygienic latrines deter people from using them, so sanitation hygiene (Indicator S2) must be evaluated, with the aim of curtailing insect-breeding, smell and fouling.

Sanitation measures need to be reliable (Indicator S3) if people are going to use them. Each type of latrine has various requirements before it can function correctly. For instance, a ventilated pit latrine must have an intact vent-pipe and mosquito screen; a pour-flush latrine must have an intact water seal, and, if emptying is required, it must be regular and sufficiently frequent. These factors can be investigated during house-to-house visits at the same time as Indicators SI and S2. If latrines are emptied by a central service, enquiries will also have to be made at headquarters and depots. Failures in reliability can often be put down to poor design and construction, operation and maintenance services such as latrine emptying.

Function indicators: health education

Each country will have to find the right mix of mass media (radio, for instance), folk media and face-to-face techniques (such as a community health worker treating diarrhoea and teaching prevention) to reach adult women. Women are the sector of the population who collect and store water, handle food, clean latrines and dispose of babies' faeces, among other things.

For health education to get through, people must be able to understand the language of the message — literally (Indicator EI). Health education messages must be in a language that the great majority of the women in the area fully understand.

The content of the health education message (Indicator E2) must be culturally suitable and built upon indigenous concepts of purity, pollution and cleanliness. Women educators will be most effective in introducing new health-promoting habits, especially where conversations about excreta may be deemed embarrassing or immoral.

Project technicians briefed in hygiene education, primary health-care workers, adult literacy teachers, political party officials and school-teachers are all in face-to-face contact with people benefiting from the project. Their role should be integrated with IDWSSD goals through national co-ordinating committees linking ministries.

Use indicators

When the evaluation team is sure the facilities are working, the next step is to evaluate how well facilities are being used.

The proportion of households using water-supply and sanitation systems in the project area is Indicator W5. A comparison between use in wet and dry seasons should be made in areas with marked seasonal differences. Users should be classified as to whether they have individual household water connections, individual or shared plot connections, communal waterpoints or wells equipped with handpumps.

Water supply should cover drinking, cooking, and washing food utensils, bodies and clothes, and Indicator W6 consists of assessing the volume of water used and for what purposes.

The proportion of people using the sanitation facilities is very difficult to assess, as people are likely to say they all use latrines even if this is not the case. Observing latrines to find out would be regarded as an invasion of privacy in many societies. A combination of subtle interviewing and observation for signs as to whether latrines are used or not is likely to give the most accurate picture of the situation. The degree to which young children use the latrines must be found out, together wih the age at which they start using them, and where they defecate before that age. Small children may require special latrine arrangements.

Effectiveness of hygiene education is measured by three indicators. The presence of a cover on the household water container is taken to represent generally hygienic behaviour in protecting stored water (Indicator E5, Water storage habits). A sample of households that have received hygiene education can be compared with a matched sample of households in an area which has not, or with a baseline survey (showing conditions or behaviours before intervention). If there has been no significant change in hygiene behaviour, it is an indication that education techniques need to be altered. This sort of comparison can also be used for hand-washing after defecation (Indicator E6). Water availability may be a constraint on hand-washing, showing that water supply and sanitation need to be linked in future projects.

Knowledge of oral rehydration therapy (Indicator E7) among mothers is taken as proxy for improvements in other health-promoting behaviour. The correctness with which it is used may be graded on a three-point scale. For instance:

(i) Does not know what oral rehydration fluid is.
(ii) Proportions of ingredients or application is grossly wrong.
(iii) Approximately correct.

Possible action to improve the situation includes linking curative and preventative services within primary health care so that workers who treat diarrhoea also teach skills to mothers.

In conclusion, this Minimum Evaluation Procedure is not exhaustive, but consists of a set of essential indicators for evaluating water and sanitation projects, within limited bounds of time and cost.

Initial work on the MEP was done at the Ross Institute, London, and commented on by a number of international bilateral agencies which have been active in the IDWSSD. It was then revised in the light of these bodies' experience and field-tested in Burma by Schultzberg and MacCormack. They were keen to use an Asian country to assess the MEP to overcome any African bias created by the fact that most of their own field experience has been gained in Africa. Dr K. Subramanyan, head of Water and Sanitation in WHO's Asian Region, advised during a further revision of the MEP in Delhi.

Further reading

Minimum evaluation procedure for water-supply and sanitation projects, WHO ETS/83.1, CDD/OPR/83.1, February 1983.

(*Waterlines* Vol. 2 No.1, July 1983)

The latrine acquisition curve: a tool for sanitation evaluation

CHRIS SMITH

In recent years, attention has been drawn to the need to understand the social aspects of rural sanitation programmes in the developing world. Methods using questionnaires asking about defecation habits have been proposed, and the importance of community consultation has been emphasized.

This article proposes an additional research tool with which to study retroactively the process of latrine acquisition in communities which already have a substantial number of latrines. The technique provides a reconstruction of the rate at which the community acquired the latrines, and gives a historical background against which to discuss the social processes involved. The tool is suggested as a way of helping those working on sanitation programmes to reach a greater understanding of the dynamics of latrine acquisition in the communities where they are hoping to conduct interventions in order to allow more rational planning and evaluation.

Method

The technique involves asking every householder two questions:
O When was your first latrine built?
O When was your house built?

In communities where a small number of houses have been abandoned or demolished over the period to be investigated, the changes in the numbers of households and latrines can be estimated using these questions.

For example, consider a village which had 100 households and 70 latrines in 1985. If 20 of the houses and 40 of the first latrines were built within the previous five years, there would have been 80 houses and 30 latrines in 1980. If 30 of the houses and 60 of the first latrines were built within the previous 10 years, then in 1975 there would have been 40 houses and 10 latrines. In this example, the percentage of households with latrines rose from 25 per cent in 1975 through 37 per cent in 1980 to 70 per cent in 1985.

Additional questions

In communities where a substantial number of houses have been abandoned or demolished during the period in question, several additional questions are required:
O When did you move into your house?
O Where did you live before?
O What happened to your house when you left it?
O If empty or demolished, when was it abandoned?

These questions allow a more precise enumeration of the changes in the number of households in the village over time.

The results can be used to plot curves of the number of households with latrines versus years, and the percentage of households with latrines versus year. The curves provide a description of the rate at which a particular community has acquired latrines, and can also be used as a basis for discussions with the community on the historical factors which affected latrine acquisition.

Examples from Palestine

The examples illustrated here are taken from studies of two West Bank Palestinian villages. The West Bank is that part of Palestine which was occupied by the Hashemite Kingdom of Jordan between 1948 and 1967, and which has been under Israeli military occupation since 1967.

Figures 1 and 2 show latrine acquisition curves (LACs) for village A, a bedouin community in the Jordan valley. Figure 2 reveals a gradual rise over a period of 20 years from 8 per cent of households with latrines in 1965 to 67 per cent in 1985. During this period, the community was making a transition from a semi-nomadic to a sedentary lifestyle.

During interviews, villagers explained that latrines had not been part of traditional bedouin life, but that two factors had encouraged their acquisition during this period: the effect of school on the children of the village and the demand for latrines from visiting guests.

United Nations' schools were available to the village from the early 1950s, and children became accustomed to using latrines while at school. Villagers explained that, when these schoolchildren grew up to be house-owners, they were more likely to build latrines for their own homes. As for the influence of guests, it was apparently a source of some embarrassment to householders without latrines when visitors to the house asked to use the toilet.

One interesting point arising from discussions with the villagers was that a campaign mounted by the UN in the 1950s to promote latrine construction had not been successful in the village. People were not persuaded to change their behaviour by argument alone; the role of education and the demands of hospitality were rated as more important factors.

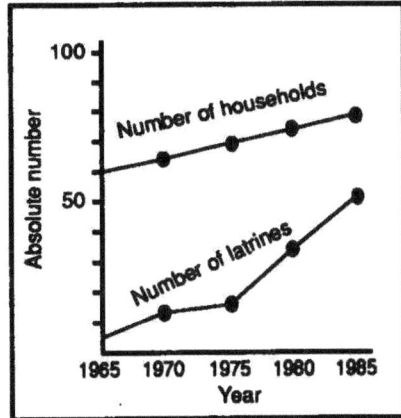

Figure 1. Latrine acquisition curve for village A (number of latrines in village vs. time).

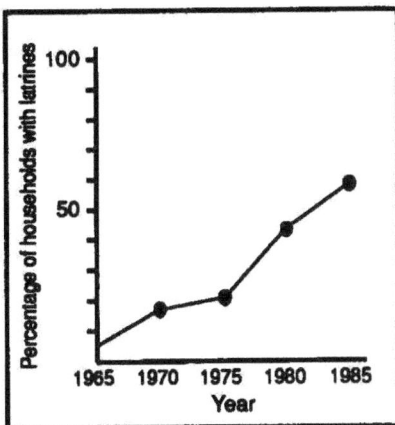

Figure 2. Latrine acquisition curve for village A (percentage of house-holds with latrines vs. time).

For the 34 per cent of households without latrines, the main reason given for not having one was the difficulty in obtaining planning permission from the Israeli authorities. Part of the village is on land which has been declared a military area, and the permission required for any kind of construction or renovation is routinely refused by the military authorities. Anyone building or renovating without a permit had their homes demolished. Villagers believe that the military are trying to encourage them to leave their homes and land, and most said they would build latrines if these restrictions were not present.

For this village, then, the process of latrine acquisition has been occurring progressively over the last 20 years. Without the construction restrictions, it is possible that almost all the houses would soon have latrines.

Figures 3 and 4 show LACs for

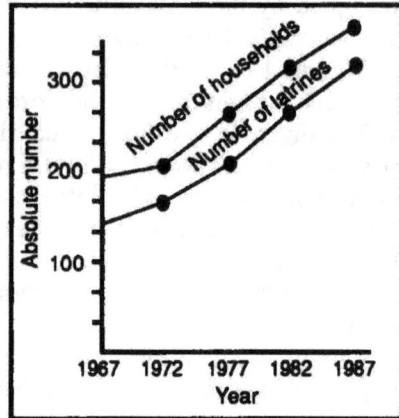

Figure 3. Latrine acquisition curve for village B (number of latrines in villages vs time).

village B in the West Bank highlands. In this village, the percentage of houses with latrines has risen from 77 per cent to 85 per cent over the last 20 years. Village B is not a bedouin village. It has been a permanent settlement for centuries.

It may have gone through a process similar to that described for village A during an earlier period in its history. For the last 20 years, B has seen a large increase in the number of households. Many of the village men had worked as labourers outside the village and had made enough money to build their own homes. These new houses built by the younger generation were mainly constructed with latrines. Most of the households which did not have latrines in 1967 still did not have them in 1987.

The sanitation problem for village B, then, is a small group of households, which have not, over the past 20 years, conformed to the sanitation norms of the village.

These examples illustrate two main points. Firstly, a single measurement

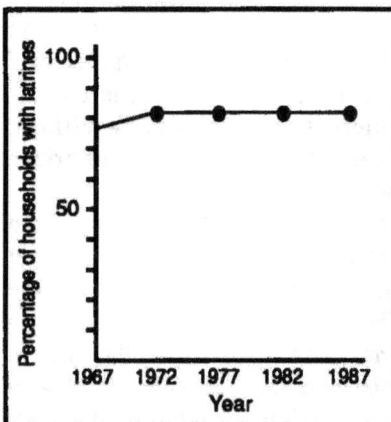

Figure 4. Latrine acquisition curve for village B (percentage of house-

of the percentage of households with latrines at a given time is less informative then the LAC. Secondly, the time-scale of the effect of a particular intervention — for example the UN school — may be several decades. Thus project evaluations which occur after only a few years may be premature.

Evaluation

The approach also raises some questions concerning the normal shapes of LACs, for which further research is needed. Figure 5 shows a possible generalized LAC. The graph is S-shaped: a slow initial period of latrine acquisition up to a point after which there is a fast increase in construction, followed by a levelling-off. The point where the 'take off' occurs could correspond to the period when latrine possession becomes a social norm (1965 to 1975 in village A). At the other end of the curve, there may be a small proportion of the community who will not, or cannot, conform to the new sanitation norms (such as 1967 to 1987 in village B).

If the reasons why people choose to build or not build latrines can be better understood, then it may be possible to design more effective promotion strategies.

In village A for example, the UN campaign, which concentrated on the message that latrines were healthy, was not successful. The latrine in the school was important, however, as was entertaining visitors. In similar situations priority might be given to latrine construction in schools, and more effective health education messages might focus, for example, on the need to make visitors feel comfortable.

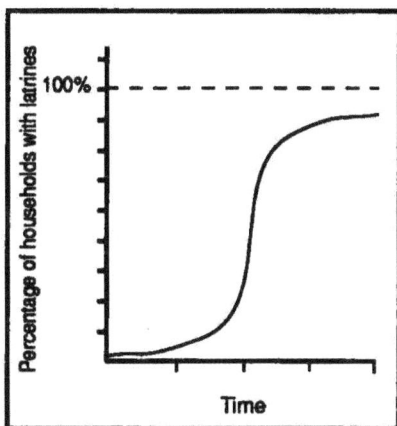

Figure 5. Hypothetical latrine acquisition curve.

In terms of project evaluation, monitoring the rates of latrine acquisition over a period of many years will provide a better understanding than a single point measurement. When a new generation learns a new technique, time is needed before that generation finds itself able to adopt the techniques and the technology. An educational intervention in school may have its effect only after 10 or 20 years have passed.

Thus it is suggested that a better understanding of the historical patterns of latrine acquisition should facilitate improved planning of latrine promotion activities and provide a basis for evaluating the effects of these activities. The latrine acquisition curve is proposed as a useful framework for studying this process.

Acknowledgments

Rita Giacaman, Muna Odeh and Sandy Cairncross made valuable comments on the first draft. Some of the information presented is from unpublished studies of the Union of Palestinian Medical Relief Committees and the Birzeit University Community Health Unit.

(*Waterlines* Vol. 7 No. 1, July 1988)

Reflections on a rural water-supply project in Zambia

JOANNE HARNMEIJER

There is a chasm between what is being written about community participation, mainly by people who have actually never done what it is they are advocating, and what is seen to be necessary, practical and affordable by those charged with managing water-supply and sanitation programmes in the developing countries.

Richard Feachem [131]

Many projects find themselves in the situation facing the Norad-funded water supply programme in Western Province, Zambia; the realization that community education and participation (CEP) must be part of any rural water supply programme is followed by the difficult task of introducing CEP into an existing project. Many questions arise. How do we introduce community participation? Where does health education come in? Who can do it? Where do we begin?

The programme in Western Province took its first steps to change in 1984 with its integration within the governmental structure of the Department of Water Affairs and the addition of a CEP component. The programme was renamed WASHE programme, an acronym for Water Supply, Sanitation and Health Education. Apart from assisting urban water schemes, the programme aimed to construct about 800 wells for rural communities. Rural water supplies consisted of hand-dug shallow wells, drilled and jetted wells.

The Health Co-ordinator

A Health Co-ordinator was employed, whose main task was to set up the CEP component of the programme. Taking up such a job amid scores of shallow-well teams, drillers and mechanics, all scratching their heads wondering what a medical doctor could contribute to water supply, makes for a humble start!

The job description of the Health Co-ordinator called for activities such as 'integrating with the Provincial Medical Officer'. One of the first steps was to listen to knowledgeable people, both inside and outside the department, to hear their ideas on what had gone wrong in the past and what should be done in the future. The basis for discussions was how to establish procedures at village level; the decision to operate through village water committees was fairly obvious since community health workers and village health committees were few and far between.

More difficult to answer was the question of how villages, once identified and approved for assistance with improved water supply, should be approached and guided through the process of site selection and choosing a village water committee. What should be the tasks of such a water committee? And on what existing structures and staff could the water programme rely?

The tasks of the village water committees were drawn up during workshops with field staff from the Ministry of Health, and included:

Preparatory stage

O Make sure all villagers are informed about the well.
O Make sure the siting of the well benefits the maximum number of people.
O Arrange the clearing of the selected site.
O Arrange for preparation of drillers'/diggers' camp (clearing, latrine, refuse pit).
O Arrange labour for well-digging and additional construction desired such as washing slabs or fencing.
O Arrange contributions for additional construction.

Continuous tasks

O Lead by example in hygienic behaviour.
O Help create responsibility in individuals to ensure proper use; instil a sense of ownership.
O Ensure contributions for spare parts.
O Report any serious repairs which are necessary.
O Maintain records such as a monitor on water quality and maintenance.

Although this list was drafted by health assistants, much of the emphasis is on non-health issues. Training, apparently, would have to focus on organizational skills and intangible issues such as co-operation. Health education was considered to have the best chance of success when taking place concurrently or immediately after construction of the well, when the enthusiasm of the community was at its height.

One important choice which had to be made at an early stage was how and where to recruit staff to carry out the CEP programme. The Department of Water Affairs itself had no staff below district level, and they were mostly plumbers and bricklayers with no training in extension work. The choices were thus fourfold: training existing technical staff of the Department of Water Affairs; employing and training school-leavers; recruiting extension staff on secondment from other departments; or relying on local extension staff from other departments in the field.

We decided on a combination of these options, with emphasis on a core-team of extension workers on secondment from various ministries at provincial level. The WASHE programme was fortunate to receive a positive response from heads of departments to the request for seconded staff; one reason for their willingness to co-operate was the level of formal and informal contact reached through the formation of the WASHE committee, an intersectoral committee at provincial level. Even so, it took more than a year to build up a CEP team of seven men and women seconded by the Ministries of Health, Agriculture and Education. Their allowances, accommodation and transport were provided by the project.

Co-operation at all levels

A water-supply project involves a chain of events in which various institutions and technical teams play a role for a finite period of time. In the WASHE project we found that although the tasks of different teams need to be defined separately, cohesion between the field staff improves when responsibility for the final product is shared. This requires a formal and informal information circuit. The informal circuit seemed to be the most important one and was based on mutual respect rather than rules and regulations. There was no point in telling the drillers that they should not start drilling if the site chosen was disputed, unless they had witnessed some of the preparatory meetings, and had come to understand the difficulties met in some communities. The CEP staff had to be skilled in communicating, but their interest in the technicalities and their willingness to use a spade proved vital to their acceptability as part of the programme.

Although the CEP team was made responsible for the software of the programme, the technical teams such as drillers and installation workers had to be convinced that CEP was part of their work as well. Workshops were organized by the Provincial Water Engineer and the Health Co-ordinator during the pay-rounds at the end of the month, when everybody was 'in town'. Discussions were easier in small groups, aided by a list of statements, which had to be rejected or supported, such as:

O A water programme will only succeed if the community is involved from the start of the planning procedures.

O Involvement of women at local level is essential for the success of rural water supply.

O A water committee supported by local leadership is necessary for rural water supply in our province.

O It is essential that villagers are able and willing to pay for the operation and maintenance of their water supply.

O Villagers will not be able to take complete responsibility for their water supply, therefore it is essential that there is support at district level in case of serious breakdowns.

O It is necessary that people recognize water-related diseases as a major concern.

The funding agency was particularly keen that the water project should be oriented towards women's needs. To make this more than just a phrase, a fairly simple and practical step was to fill vacant positions in the technical teams with women. These women were carefully selected and it was made clear to them that not only were they to learn a technical trade, they were also expected to form a link with men and women in the villages, where they would reinforce the preparatory work of the CEP teams. It was hoped that the mere presence of women talking to villagers about well-maintenance, for instance, would arouse the interest of village women in a natural way. Thus two women in each district team were recruited and trained as bricklayer or pump installer, and were made familiar with the CEP methods.

Participatory approach

The small size of the villages allowed us to address the whole community rather than train only the village water committees. The procedure chosen was to take the community through a series of four meetings during which the topics were built up from making decisions about the location of the well to the benefits of using more water and cleaner water. The technical aspects of maintenance and repair were dealt with by the installation team in the third meeting when the pump was installed: the procedure was slightly different for dug wells. The other meetings were guided by CEP staff.

Realizing that 'top-down' message delivery is ineffective and that messages should be relevant to the needs of the recipients, we decided on a participatory method in which the topics were introduced by the CEP team following a standardized approach, but the discussion was flexible and depended to a large extent on what was said by villagers during the meeting.

An example of such a participatory method dealing with diarrhoea is the 'story with a gap'. Two drawings show a child in good health and a child of the same age looking dull and skinny. People taking part in the session are asked to identify the difference and reply that the child has been ill/has had diarrhoea/is malnourished. The question is then asked: how did the child get into that condition? (This is problem analysis.) Answers by the participants cover all possible reasons known in the community. The extension worker, if necessary, will probe for other reasons. How could this child get into good shape again? (Problem solution.) Participants mention the fashionable as well as more obscure solutions. The group leader picks up points mentioned and enquires further as deemed necessary. Have any of the villagers' children been in this condition and what did they do? How else can one prevent a child from getting into such a condition? This discussion sets the scene for a practical demonstration on oral-rehydration solution.

The 'story with a gap' offers a way to start from the illness, (for example diarrhoea) and work backwards through analysis and forwards through problem-solving with the people concerned, building on what they already know and believe. The same method used for wells proves a good way to generate a discussion on the day-to-day tasks of the village water committee.

Another method which allows villagers — rather than extension workers — to talk, is the poster series 'At home' which attempts to reinforce hygienic practices in and around the home. The posters are put on a mat or table, so that everybody can see them. Participants are told that these posters depict either 'healthy living' or 'living leading to illness'. One by one, they are picked up and described by participants, after which they are assigned to either pile. Sometimes a third pile — undecided — is needed when people cannot agree. The extension worker may decide to emphasize some of the points raised by asking questions, but normally villagers give quite convincing explanations without being probed. Sometimes people must talk about the benefits of having things they don't usually think about.

Materials for education

Since there was no suitable education material available, one of the Health Co-ordinator's first tasks was to employ a local artist. There are a few rules for making visual aids, which are aptly described in the book *Making the Links*[132]. For the participatory approach to be successful, it is essential that the material can be handled by the participants. We chose A4-size black-and-white posters covered in transparent plastic; these could be copied. The materials were carried around by extension staff arranged by topic in a big file. Apart from posters, numerous songs, dramas and stories were developed which mostly dealt with organizational aspects.

All this took 12 months, during which time the expanding CEP team gradually established its procedures, the materials were continuously adapted and new ideas were tried out in response to the situations faced. Thus, the development of the approach and of the education materials was a learning process for everyone, not least the Health Co-ordinator. Eventually, the materials and ideas were all put together in a 90-page file, which was made available to extension staff of other departments and to other departments and water-supply projects in the country.

It was an interesting and enjoyable experience to build up the CEP component of the WASHE programme, in a joint effort relying on the inspired assistance of a local artist and motivated staff. Health education was treated as part of community education and efforts were made wherever possible to work through the local extension staff of other departments.

The lack of a blueprint enhanced the creativity and self-confidence of the CEP team, which slowly overcame scepticism among other staff. It proved important that the technical teams were committed to CEP as well and showed this commitment in their day-to-day work with the communities. The introduction of female skilled labour in the technical teams was particularly helpful.

(Waterlines Vol. 7 No. 1, July 1988)

The Kisumu Primary Health Care Project

MATHEW ONDURU

The Kisumu Primary Health Care Project was launched as a result of the 1981 Aga Khan Foundation/World Health Organization Conference on the Role of Hospitals in Primary Health Care. In July 1982, the Aga Khan Health Services, Kisumu, and the Aga Khan Foundation co-sponsored the Kisumu Primary Health Care Planning Seminar, which was attended by delegates from local government health services, the central Ministry of Health, UNICEF, WHO, Aga Khan Foundation, the Ford Foundation and the African Medical & Research Foundation (AMREF).

The participants concluded that the projects should cover two locations in the Kisumu District of Nyanza Province: North and Central Nyakach and Kajulu. The estimated population of Nyakach is 40,000, and growing at 3.8 per cent per year, while in Kajulu the population is around 20,000, rising at a rate of 6 per cent per year. Communities in both areas shared similar health problems: a high infant mortality rate; malaria; intestinal parasites; cholera and other diarrhoeal diseases; respiratory infections; various communicable and infectious diseases and poor sanitation and unsafe water supplies.

Before the project could be set up, it was important to carry out a detailed baseline community health survey. (See table for some of these results.)

Deaths in the past year: results of baseline survey

The survey revealed very high mortality rates: it was reported that there had been 102 deaths in the past 12 months. All the mortality rates are higher than the national averages also shown below:

	National per 1,000	Nyakach per 1,000	Kajulu per 1,000
Crude birth rate (CBR)	55	59	70
Crude death rate (CDR)	14	16.3	19.7
Infant mortality rate (IMR)	80	194	236
Child mortality rate (CMR)	13	22.1	25.3

Objectives

Following an analysis of the baseline survey, a broad objective was drawn for the project, namely to improve the health and nutritional status of people in the project areas, particularly children under five and women of child-bearing age. Five more specific objectives were also recommended:

O To increase the community's awareness of their health problems and to motivate them to undertake disease prevention and health promotion activities at the individual, family and community levels.

O To increase the availability, accessibility and acceptability of health services, principally by employing a community-based health care approach and by training community health workers (CHWs).

O To improve environmental health conditions by providing a clean water supply and waste disposal system through community participation and self-help efforts.

O To reduce infant and child mortality.

O To reduce malnutrition among children and women by promoting growth monitoring, improving weaning practices, better food selection and preparation, and increasing local production of nutritious foods.

One of the recommendations of the planning seminar had been that the project should be run in close collaboration with the Ministry of Health and the Municipal Council of Kisumu in order to carry out certain activities more effectively. These included community mobilization, training of CHWs, maternal and child health care and family planning (MCH/FP), water and sanitation improvements, and a participatory school health programme.

Training

Training is essential to enable participants in primary or community-based health care to fulfil their roles effectively. The project carries out training at community level for CHWs, traditional birth attendants (TBAs), women's groups, schools and community leaders, and at the central level for trainers and facilitators.

Community health workers are trained for a period of 60 days at the village level, in a school, church or community hall. The curriculum is based on health problems common to the area and training is geared to action, that is the development of practical skills, rather than simply acquiring knowledge. CHWs are required to practise what they learn before they begin to advise other members of the community.

When training has been completed, each CHW covers an average of 30 to 50 households, depending on distance between the houses, where they carry out a number of activities:

O Encouraging communities to dig pit latrines within their homesteads and to keep the area tidy.
O Encouraging households to use dish-racks.
O Advising mothers to take their children to be immunized.
O Educating families on good nutrition for their children.
O Teaching parents how to control diarrhoea.
O Weighing children.
O Giving health talks at community gatherings, for example at churches.
O Carrying out home visits to assess hygiene conditions there and give advice accordingly.
O Advising pregnant women on feeding, and encouraging them to attend antenatal clinics.
O Treating minor ailments and referring cases too difficult to handle to health facilities.
O Supplying essential drugs and organizing growth monitoring sessions.

Apart from normal training of 60 days, refresher courses are also organized for CHWs.

Maternal and Child Health/Family Planning

The project provides MCH/FP services to mothers and children under five years of age. These services are run at health centres and at mobile sites, always emphasizing community participation. Immunization sites are organized by the community through their leaders. CHWs are then provided with a record of all the children under the age of five; it is their job to make sure that the children complete immunization. The TBAs, after delivering a baby at home, also advise mothers to take their children to be immunized. CHWs assist at the clinics by helping project staff weigh children and advise mothers on nutrition.

Water is a major concern to the people in the project areas, in terms of both quality and quantity. The major sources of water — rivers, streams and ponds — are used to fulfil all the requirements of the human and domestic animal population. Most of the rivers and streams are seasonal, and the women may have to walk over five kilometres in search of water during the dry season. At these times, water is precious to them, yet it may contain cholera vibrio, which can be a killer.

Water and sanitation

The government and non-governmental organizations have protected water sources for communities in Kenya in the past. However, most of these sources have not been used for a long time, because when they break down, no one is responsible for their repair. The water source may be used by the community, but it is called 'the Ministry's well', piped water-line or spring, and is considered to be the responsibility of the government.

This lack of identification, ownership and responsibility has led to the failure of many otherwise successful programmes. Yet the concept of CBHC calls for reciprocal responsibility and self-reliance. It was with this in mind that the project drew up the criteria for helping communities to acquire safe water and proper sanitation. The communities have to fulfil these criteria before the project staff begin to work with them on water source protection:

O Raise an adequate sum of money for well protection, spring protection and 10 per cent of the total cost for piped water. This money is kept at the project office as long as the project exists, but will be given back to the community for future maintenance when they take over the responsibility for the water supply.
O Bring to the site a sufficient amount of locally available materials, mostly sand and stone.
O Agree on a site where the well is to be dug.
O Accommodate and provide for the diggers and masons, who are supplied by the project.
O Provide ample unskilled labour.
O Agree to undertake maintenance and repair once the source is completed and handed over to the community.

Before work is started, a meeting must be held between the community and project staff to plan the progress of the work and delegate tasks. After the meeting, the project undertakes to assist the community with technical support, materials which are available within the community such as cement and iron rods, payment for skilled labour which includes masons and skilled diggers, and the provision of handpumps.

The community response has been almost too good. After a slow start because some communities did not believe they could undertake such big projects by themselves, the demand for water services has now exceeded what the project staff alone can do. Most of the project's water activities are with rural communities and are initiated by women or clan groups, which are stronger and more organized.

With community participation, it has been very easy for the project's Public Health Officer to carry out supervision as the community handles most of the problems and if there is anything they cannot solve themselves, they usually organize a meeting with project staff. It has been found that the community contributes almost half the total cost of protecting a water source.

Participatory school health programme

The children of today will be the leaders and parents of tomorrow, and to be good leaders and parents, they need information and skills. Thus the Kisumu Primary Health Care Project has joined hands with parents and children to work towards a healthier present and future through the participatory school health programme.

There are many reasons why this programme is so important. Through schools a large number of children can be reached; over 70 per cent of school-age children in the country attend primary schools. At a young age, children are better able to learn, accept, remember and practice what they are taught, and the practices learnt and used during the early years become part of everyday life. Older children look after and teach their younger brothers and sisters many of their first lessons in life, so the quality of knowledge they have will enable them to do a better job. Thus, from an early age, children join their parents and community in improving and maintaining a clean, healthy environment.

Before the programme was adopted, meetings were held so that teachers and parents could share their thoughts and make plans. As both teachers and parents were involved from the outset, there has been no conflict.

Because it was important for the teachers to understand the concept of PHC/CBHC, a workshop was organized to define self-reliance and the roles of teachers and pupils in CBHC.

Each school is involved in four or five activities, activities which pupils can carry out both in the school and at home:

O Tree planting.
O Making dish-racks.

O Making a pit-latrine cover.
O Diarrhoea management by using sugar and salt solution.
O Destruction of mosquito breeding sites.
O Cleaning compounds at school and at home.
O Giving information about health.
O Composing songs and poems about health.
O Growth monitoring.
O Immunization monitoring.
O Personal hygiene.
O Reducing scabies.

Project staff assist in training when requested to do so by the schools, otherwise everything is done by pupils, teachers and parents, and the activities are assessed by pupils and teachers.

Evaluation

Evaluation of the project was carried out in May 1987, and several outstanding achievements were highlighted. Community participation is very strong in activities such as the training of community members, construction of latrines, protection of water sources and environmental improvement. Awareness of PHC/CBHC is evident among women's groups, teachers and other members of the community. The project has already improved the health status of the population served. In Kajulu, the infant mortality rate has dropped from 236 in 1984 to 171 in 1987. In Central Nyakach, it fell from 194 to 110, and in North Nyakach to 147. This progress has been achieved mainly through immunization and maternal and child health services.

The process of establishing community-based health care has been quite effective, particularly in terms of co-ordination and collaboration between other NGOs operating in the area and government health institutions. Some 325 CHWs have been trained and of these, 71 per cent are considered fully active; 149 TBAs have also undergone training.

Other activities to improve health have focused on water supply. So far, 10 wells, six springs and six piped water-lines have been connected to various communities through community participation.

In the future, there are plans to develop the Kisumu Primary Health Care Project into a regional resource centre in PHC/CBHC for Western Kenya, with a small but highly capable staff, technical materials and an up-to-date library. The centre will further develop the methods and support mechanisms for establishing, managing and maintaining community-based health care.

(*Waterlines* Vol. 7 No. 1, July 1988)

Water supply in primary health care: experiences of Amazon Indian communities

JAMIE BARTRAM and WARREN JOHNS

The Aguaruna & Huambisa Jungle Indian Council has developed what is, in many ways, a model primary health care programme; yet, over the course of 11 years, it has failed to make any real change in the pattern and incidence of diseases suffered by the population. Recent improvements in the health programme revealed the fundamental problem to be the lack of emphasis on preventive measures. As a result, an improvement strategy integrating water supply, hygiene education and sanitation is being developed.

Area, lifestyles and changes

The 35,000 Aguaruna and Huambisa Indians living in Peru occupy an area of 22,000 km² in the northern jungle. The area has always been isolated, protected by a combination of impassable rapids, mountains and dense jungle; only relatively recently have Western influences penetrated significantly. The main communication and transport routes are the rivers. The few roads, restricted to a small area in the south, are often impassbale after rain. Telephone, telegram and mail services are non-existent for most people.

The soil of the area is poor so, paradoxically, the luxuriant forest is a potential desert. It survives by an intense recycling of nutrients in a delicate ecological balancing act. Although, to outsiders, the upland rain forest often appears under-used, a large amount of land is needed to maintain the traditional lifestyle. The forest-dwelling Indians have evolved ways of life which respect this delicate equilibrium: their own survival depends on the rational management of the forest and its resources.

The traditional way of life of the Aguaruna and Huambisa is largely subsistence, based on slash-and-burn agriculture, hunting, fishing and the collection of jungle fruits. The tribes lived in semi-dispersed extended family groups, each maintaining a number of clearings, cut by the men, but maintained by the women for growing cassava and plantain, the food staples. The clearings were cropped for about seven years, after which they were no longer considered viable, and fresh clearings cut. Hunting was a male preserve, as was fishing except barbasco fishing, when a large number of people would work together to dam and poison a stretch of river and then collect the affected fish. Families would move on when suitable land was exhausted or local game depleted. During the 1950s and 1960s, however, the tribes were attracted by the schools and new trading opportunities and began to form larger, more fixed communities, migrating towards the banks of the five principal rivers.

Other changes affected the lifestyle of the Aguaruna and Huambisa at this time. The jungle began to be viewed by outsiders as an under-exploited resource. There was a frontier war with Ecuador and reports of land seizures by outside colonists: these factors led many of the communities to form the Aguaruna & Huambisa Jungle Indian Council (CAH) in 1977. The CAH has over 100 affiliated communities and has developed five principal programmes — including one on health.

The health programme

The new, larger and more stable communities created greater competition for the limited resources available. Nearby cultivable land gradually became exhausted, the rivers depleted of fish, and over-hunting demanded ever longer journeys to find game. Greater population density and increased community contact both within the tribes and with outsiders have also brought new diseases to a population previously isolated from them: there have been epidemics of measles and whooping cough, and the transmission rate of the faecal-oral diseases has intensified.

With the increasing scarcity of traditional nutritional sources and increasing competition for land to cultivate around the communities, malnutrition is a serious problem. At the same time, diarrhoea is the most common disease, and the parasite carrier rate is 54 per cent. Children are quickly drawn into the cycle of diarrhoea-malnutrition, and the nutritional losses are difficult to regain; consequently 53 per cent of children under five are anaemic. The health programme obviously has an important role to play in helping these communities to reduce the incidence of disease.

The health programme is based around a network of about 100 health promoters; communities select their own promoters and build a health post. Using a community fund to purchase medicine, promoters can obtain about 30 essential drugs from the central pharmacy. The health programme also has an impressive support network of five health centres, one on each of the principal rivers. Each river has its own elected supervisor while the promoters themselves attend yearly re-training courses; courses are also arranged for newly appointed promoters.

The health programme has, based at the health centres, five laboratory technicians, who carry out basic tests: haemoglobin, blood smears for malaria, stools for parasites, urine for infection and sputum for tuberculosis to help diagnosis and treatment.

Health centre laboratories are traditionally viewed as small-scale hospital laboratories with a diagnostic role affecting treatment. The CAH's experience has shown that this alone is not viable; what is also needed is a 'community diagnostic', not just individual treatment but also the determination of fundamental community health problems, which would allow long-term preventive planning, including water monitoring. The laboratories now work at three levels: water monitoring, patient diagnosis and survey work. The latter includes examining haemoglobin to assess the general occurrence of anaemia and surveying parasite carriage to see what preventive and community treatment measures are needed. Both diagnostic and survey work are now carried out from portable laboratory kits, while water surveillance centres around sanitary inspection and a portable batttery-powered water-testing kit.

Water surveillance and community diagnosis

Carrying out water-supply surveillance in the northern jungle required first a 'diagnosis' of the existing problems, resulting in improved programmes, and continuing surveillance thereafter, where it was considered to be worthwhile.

The first results from the diagnosis were surprising. It had always been assumed that the *pozos* (shallow springs) provided good water unless they were directly contaminated. When they were actually tested, however, they showed a variable, but high level of contamination, as did the principal rivers (Table 1). On the other hand, the *quebaradas* (shallow streams) that ran through the communities, which had been assumed to be inferior sources, generally provided better water.

In retrospect, this should have been foreseen. The *pozos* are shallow depressions in the impermeable layer into which water slowly filters, rather

Table 1. Drinking-water quality by source type in communities affiliated to the Aguaruna & Huambisa Council

Source type	A (%)	B (%)	C (%)	D (%)
Pozo (shallow spring)	36	17	27	20
Quebrada (shallow stream)	57	28	0	14
River	-	-	-	100

Note: Water quality defined by faecal coliform count by membrane filtration and cultivation on membrane lauryl sulphate broth at 44°C.

A = 0/100ml   B = 1-10/100ml   C = 11-50/100ml   D = >50/100ml

Source: Archive of the Health Programme, Aguaruna and Huambisa Council; quoted in Jamie Bartram, *Saneamiento Ambiental en las Comunidades Afriliades al Consejo Aguaruna y Huambisa; Problematica, Prioridades y Objectivos*, 1987.

than fast-flowing springs, and for convenience they are often dug near the dwellings. Although they were probably adequate when the tribes lived in small dispersed extended family units, which moved regularly, as they grouped together — and especially as they started to build latrines — these springs became increasingly contaminated and contributed more and more to the exposure of community members to water-related diseases.

The *quebradas*, however, are surface waters, so it should be assumed that they would carry higher levels of contamination, yet in practice their faecal contamination was generally lower. The reason for this was that communities are generally at the end of a *quebrada* where it joins the princiapal river; there is no tradition of keeping domestic animals except within the confines of the community itself, nor are there other communities above them on the same watercourse, so the water is relatively clean. Although *quebradas* may become contaminated as they pass through the community itself, any contamination introduced by stepping into the water or from dirty collection vessels is quickly carried away by the fast-moving current.

The community diagnostic did not end with the water collection sites: the household storage of food and water and the use of latrines were also considered by the laboratory workers (Table 2).

Household water is generally stored in an open bucket or pot on the floor, making it open to contamination by both the children and animals. In contrast, the cassava beer is carefully tended in lidded pots, often raised off the ground. Whether this should be used as a model for household water storage, or whether drinking beer should replace water drinking was the subject of considerable discussion.

At first, food storage appears to be a problem, since fruit and vegetables are stored at ground level, but whether there is a real health risk is not clear, as most food is eaten hot and freshly cooked.

Like many jungle groups, the Aguaruna and Huambisa Indians have

Table 2. Household hygiene in the communities affiliated to the Aguaruna & Huambisa Council

Household practice	%
Domestic animals kept within the dwelling	83
Raw fruit and vegetables stored above ground level	62
Cooked food stored under a lid	62
Drinking-water container stored above ground level	32
Drinking-water container kept under a lid	43

Source: Archive of the Health Programme, Aguaruna and Huambisa Council; quoted in Jamie Bartram, *Saneamiento Ambiental en las Comunidades Afriliades al Consejo Aguruna y Huambisa; Problematica, Prioridades y Objectivos*, 1987.

scrupulous personal hygiene, but this may not always have direct health benefits. Hand-washing, for example, is invariably practised after eating, but rarely before.

Although there are many latrines in the area, their contribution to health is doubtful as they are simple pit latrines, built close to the home and often inundated with water because of the high water-table. Their dampness gives them an unpleasant and unacceptable smell and also causes a fly nuisance near dwellings, with the accompanying health risks.

Achievements and prospects

The persistently high level of intestinal parasites and anaemia as demonstrated by the laboratory survey has shown that over the years no fundamental improvement has occurred in real health status (Table 3). The prestige of curative work has overshadowed the less glamorous work of greater longterm importance: that of prevention. Without approaching the fundamental cause — the hygiene habits that promote the diseases — patterns will not change.

So, after 11 years of developing a model primary health care programme, the CAH appears to have achieved little, if simple health statistics are compared, although some successes can be seen, notably in the control of measles and chicken-pox by vaccination. But simple health statistics may not be an adequate measure. Forty years ago, the communities of the Aguaruna and Huambisa tribes were scattered, lacked co-ordination and

Table 3. Community Health Diagnosis Results

	Adults (%)	Age Group 6 to 11 (%)	0 to 5 (%)	Total (%)
With intestinal parasites	56	67	53	54
Anaemic (HB< 10g/dl)	23	38	53	34
Hookworm carriers	34	38	27	-
Healthy (non-anaemic with no intestinal parasites)	36	28	25	-

Source: *Informe do una encuesta de las frecuencia de anemia y parasitosis intestinál en 17 communidades nativas del Alto Maranon relaizada por el Programa de Salud del Consejo Aguaruna y Huambisa.* Asesores del Programa de Salud, CAH, 1988.

were under pressure from both the state and colonizers, whom they were in no position to resist, and who were likely to destroy their way of life along with much of the environment in which they lived.

The CAH has provided a solid centre of activity for cohesion and autonomy, to which the health programme has contributed enormously. The work of these years has built a solid infrastructure on which to build further, and disease prevention by vaccination has had some success. Individual treatment is under way and after a recent evaluation, new strategies for preventive medicine are being developed. Some communities have started to experiment with rain-water catchment; the latrine problem is also seen as important, but the population has lost faith in traditional latrines, and Blair latrines are being considered as a more promising alternative.

It seems that the achievement of good health in the developing world can only come by the actions of the people themselves — it will never come from outside.

(Waterlines Vol. 7 No. 1, July 1988)

References and further reading

1 United Nations Economic and Social Council, 'UNICEF/WHO joint study on water and sanitation components of primary health care'. *UNICEF Document E/ICEF/L 1386*, December 15, 1978.

2 *The International Drinking-Water Supply and Sanitation Decade: review of national progress (as at December 1983)*, (WHO, Geneva, 1986).

3 *Technology for water supply and sanitation in developing countries*, WHO Technical Report Series, 742, (WHO, Geneva, 1987).

4 N. Imboden, 'Induced change in health behaviour: a study of a pilot environmental sanitation project in Uttar Pradesh', *Publication No. 356*, Planning Research and Action Institute, (Lucknow, India, 1968).

5. R.G. Feachem et al, *Water health and development: an inter-disciplinary evaluation*, (Tri-Med Books, London, 1978).

6. M.L. Elmendorf, 'Field notes from Sri Lanka', excerpts in *Decade plan for water supply and sanitation*, (American Public Health Association, Washington DC, USA, 1980).

7. G. Eoff, *Las Catanas: a case study of a traditional subsistence-oriented peasant community (mimeo)*, (USAID, Honduras, 1977).

8. R.I. Rodriguez, C. Pineo and M.L. Elmendorf, 'Nicaragua: Country report', in 'Seven case studies of rural and urban fringe areas in Latin America', ed. Elmendorf, *Appropriate technology for water supply and sanitation*, Volume 8, (The World Bank, Washington DC, USA, 1982).

9. B.L. Hall, 'Mtuni Afya: Tanzania's health campaign', *Clearing-house on Development Communication Publication 9*, (Washington DC, USA, 1978).

10. J.D. Skoda, J. Medis, J. Bertrand, and M. Chia, *A survey in rural Bangladesh on diarrhoeal morbidity, water usage and related factors*, (UNICEF/WHO, Geneva, Switzerland, 1978).

11. M.L. Elmendorf and P.K. Buckles, *Sociocultural aspects of water supply and excreta disposal*, (World Bank, Washington DC, USA, 1980).

12. M.G. McGarry and M.L. Elmendorf, 'What is appropriate technology? A Maya village asks', in *Appropriate technology for water supply and sanitation* Vol. 8, (The World Bank, Washington, DC, USA, 1982).

13. R.G. Feachem, 'Rural water and sanitation', *Proceedings of the Royal Society Series of London*, B Volume 209, (UK, 1980).

14. A.U. Kirkby, 'The development of a user-choice approach in rural water supply', *Rural water supply and sanitation working paper 7*, (International Development Research Centre, Lausanne, Switzerland, 1973).

15. A. Whyte, and I. Burton, in R.G. Feachem, M. McGarry and D. Mara, (eds) *Water, waste and health in hot climates*, (Wiley, London, UK, 1977).

16. A. Whyte, *Draft guidelines for the design of a national support programme for community education and participation in water supply and sanitation*, (WHO/IRC, The Hague, Netherlands, 1980).

17. M.L. Elmendorf, 'Community participation: a human dimension with promise and problems', *Safe water and waste disposal for health: a reference manual*, (National Demonstration Water Project, Washington, DC, 1981).

18. A. White, *Community participation and education in community water and sanitation programmes: Methods and strategies*, (WHO/IRC, Rijswijk, Netherlands, 1981).

19. A. Iwanska, *Purgatory and Utopia*, (Schenkman Press, Cambridge, Massachusetts, USA, 1971).

20. F.C. Miller and C.A. Cone, 'Latrines in Valuc: a twenty-year perspective', *Appropriate Technology for water supply and sanitation*, Volume 8, (The World Bank, Washington DC, USA, 1982).

21. P.K. Buckles, 'The introduction of potable water and latrines: a case study of two rural communities in Guatamala', ed. Elmendorf, 1982.

22. K. Jorgenson, *Water supply problems in rural Africa: the implications for women*, (Centre for Development Research, Copenhagen, Denmark, 1980).

23. J. Briscoe, R.G. Feachem, and M.M. Rahaman, *Evaluating Health Impact: Water Supply, Sanitation, Hygiene Education*, (IDRC, Ottawa, 1986).

24. P. Bifani, K. Adagala and P. Kariuki, *The impact of development on women in Kenya*, (UNICEF, Nairobi, 1982).

25. J.E. Rohde, 'To drink or not to drink', *Diarrhoea Dialogue* 2: 4-5, (London 1980).

26. 'BRAC's oral rehydration programme', *Glimpse* 2 (1): 1-2 1980.

27. S.P. Erasmus et al, 'Composition of oral solutions prepared by Jamaican mothers for treatment of diarrhoea', *The Lancet* March 14: 1981. pp 600-601

28. R.G. Feachem, 'Oral rehydration with dirty water?' *Diarrhoea Dialogue* 4:7 1981.

29. M.U. Khan, 'Interruption of shigellosis by handwashing', Transactions of the Royal Society of Tropical Medicine and Hygiene, Vol 76 (2): 164-168, 1982.

30. G. Davidson, 'Who doesn't want to eradicate malaria?' *New Scientist* 96 (1336), 731-736, (London, 1982).
31. P.F. Russel, L.S. West and R.D. Maundwell, *Practical Malariology*, (W. B. Saunders Co, London 1946).
32. *Manual on environmental management for mosquito control*, Offset publication No. 66, (WHO, Geneva 1982).
33. S.A. Hossain, 'Low cost on housing in Bangladesh', *Proceedings of conference on low cost housing*, (Bangkok, 1977).
34. *Indian Census Returns* Series 19, Part 4; 1971.
35. S. Denyer, 'African traditional architecture', (Heinemann, London, 1978).
36. C.A. Gollmer, 'Journals', (un-published, 1859).
37. N.L. Hall, 'Has thatch a future?' *Appropriate Technology*, Vol 8, No 3, (London 1981).
38. J.J.A. Janssen, Personal communication, 1982.
39. 'Specification', (Architectural Press, London, 1982).
40. W.J. van Zijil, N. Blioumel and D.G. Schliessmann, Report of studies on diarrhoeal diseases, (The WHO Diarrhoeal Advisory Team in co-operation with the Ministry of Health, Khartoum, 1961).
41. Samia Al Azharia Jahn, 'Attempts to improve the traditional clay jars for water storage by insertion of plastic taps', *Progr. Water Techn. II*, 1979.
42. Zohour H. Hammad and A Dihar Hamid, 'Microbiological examination of sebeel water', *Applied and Environmental Microbiology 43*, 1982, pp 1238-1243.
43. Samia Al Azharia Jahn, *Traditional water purification in tropical developing countries - Existing methods and potential applications*, Manual, ed. (GTZ (Deutsche Gesellschaft für Technische Zusammenarbeit), Ser. No. 117 , Eschborn, 1981).
44. S.B. Watt, 'Water jars from cement mortar', *Appropriate Technology*, Vol 2, No 2, pp 10-11, (London, 1975).
45. S.B. Watt, *Ferrocement Tanks and their Construction*, (Intermediate Technology Publications, London, 1978).
46. E. Green, *A knowledge, attitudes and practices survey of water and sanitation in Swaziland*, (Academy for Educational Development, Inc., 1982).
47. T.A. Dillaha and W.J. Zolan, *An investigation of the water quality of roof-top rainwater catchment systems in Micronesia*, (University of Guam, 1983).
48. H.W. deKoning, K.R. Smith and J.M. Last, 'Biomass fuel combustion and health', *Bulletin of WHO*, 63(1), 11-26, 1985.
49. A.E. Khairy, 'Water supply and nutritional status in rural drinking-water in a Nile Delta village', *Journal of Hygiene*, Cambridge, 88, 57, 1982.

312 COMMUNITY HEALTH AND SANITATION

50. F.D. Miller, 'Problems of water storage in the rural village home: the Egyptian zir', *Journal of Tropical Medicine and Hygiene*, 87, 53-59, 1984.

51. Sathian Lim Phongpand, 'Bacterial contamination in home-made electrolyte solution', *Ramathibodi Medical Journal*, 2:208, 1979.

52. W.J. Lewis, S.S.D. Foster, B. Drasar, *Report 1: Groundwater pollution from unsewered santitation: a critical review in relation to site evaluation and risk assessment*, (IRCWD, Zurich, Switzerland, 1982).

53. Rajagopalan and Shiffman, *Guide to simple measures for the control of enteric disease*, (WHO, Geneva, 1974).

54. S.B. Watt and W.E. Wood, Hand-dug wells and their construction, (Intermediate Technology Publications, 1976).

55 J.T. Visscher, R. Paramasivan and M. Santacruz, 'IRC's Slow Sand Filtration Project', *Waterlines* Vol. 4, No. 3, 1986.

56. S. el Basit and D. Brown, 'Slow Sand Filter for the Blue Nile Health Project', Waterlines, Vol. 5, No. 1, 1986.

57. M. Wegelin, *Horizontal-flow Roughing Filtration: a design, construction and operational manual*, (IRCWD Report No. 6, 1986).

58. M. Wegelin, 'Horizontal-flow Roughing Filtration: An appropriate Pretreatment for Slow Sand Filters in Developing Countries', *IRCWD News*, No. 20, 1984.

59. N.C. Thanh and E.A.R. Ouani, 'Horizontal-flow Coarse Material Prefiltration', (AIT, Research Report No. 70, 1977).

60. M. Wegelin and T.S.A. Mbwette, *Slow Sand Filter Research Report Nos 1-3*, (University of Dar es Salaam, 1980-81).

61. M. Wegelin, M. Boller and R. Schertenleib, 'Particle Removal by Horizontal-flow Roughing Filtration', *AQUA*, No. 3, 1986.

62. *Guidelines for Drinking-Water Quality, Vol. I, Recommendations; Vol. II Health Criteria and Other Supporting Information; Vol III Drinking-Water Quality Control in Small Community Supplies*, (WHO, Geneva, 1984-5).

63. *Surveillance of Drinking-Water*, (WHO, Geneva, 1976).

64. Peter Morgan and Ephraim Chimbunde, *Appropriate Technology*, Vol. 9 No. 2, London.

65. Peter Morgan and Duncan Mara, *Ventilated improved pit latrines: recent developments in Zimbabwe*, World Bank Technical Paper No. 3, (World Bank, Washington).

66. R. Feachem and S. Cairncross, 'Small excreta disposal systems', *Ross Bulletin No. 8*, (Ross Institute, London, 1978).

67. E.G. Wagner and J.N. Lanoix, 'Excreta disposal for rural areas and small communities', (WHO, 1985).

68. 'The latrine project, Mozambique', *IDRC Report MR58e*, (IDRC, Ottawa, Canada).

. J.M. Kalbermatten, D.S. Julius and C.G. Gunnerson, *Appropriate Technology for water supply and sanitation: Vol. II. A Sanitation field manual*, (World Bank, Washington, DC, 1980).
. E.G. Wagner and J.N. Lanoix, 'Excreta disposal for rural areas and small communities', (WHO Monograph Series 39, 1958).
. K.D. Iwugo, 'Sanitation technology for developing countries (with special reference to Africa)', *Public Health* London 95:1891-206, 1981.
. G.B. Williams, *Sewage disposal in India and the Far East*, (Thacker, Spink & Co., India, 1924).
. C. Sebastian and I.C. Buchanan, 'Feasibility of concrete septic privies for sewage disposal in Anguilla, British West Indies', *Public Health Reports*, 80(12):1113-1118, 1965.
. M. Assar, Guide to sanitation and natural disasters, (WHO, Geneva, 1971).
. R.J. Biellik, *The evaluation of public health components of international disaster relief operations: Indochinese refugees in Thailand, 1979-82*, (Doctor of Public Health Dissertation, University of Texas School of Public Health, Houston, Texas, 1983).
. K. Kiljunen, 'The tragedy of Kampuchea'. *Disasters* 7(2):129-141, 1983.
. E.F. Gloyna, *Waste stabilization ponds. Monograph Series No. 60*, (WHO, Geneva, 1971).
. J.P. Lumbers, 'Waste stabilization ponds: design considerations and methods', *Journal of the Institute of Public Health Engineers*, Vol 7, No 2, April, 1979.
. E.J. Middlebrooks, C.H. Middlebrooks, J.H. Reynolds, G.Z. Walters and D.B. George, *Waste water stabilization lagoon design performance and upgrading*, (First edition, Macmillan Publishing Co. Inc, 1982).
. 'Evaluation of facultative waste stabilization ponds', *US Environmental Protection Agency Reports* 600/2-77-085, 086, 109 and 167, (EPA, Washington, 1977).
. M.G. McGarry and M.B. Pescod, 'Waste stabilization pond criteria for tropical Asia', *Proceedings of the second international symposium on waste treatment lagoons*, p114, (Kansas City, USA, 1970).
. D.D. Mara and S.A. Silva, 'Sewage treatment in waste stabilization ponds: recent research in north-east Brazil', *Progress in Water Technology* Vol II No 2 p340, 1982.
. J.P. Arthur, 'The development of design equations for facultative waste stabilization ponds in semi-arid areas', *Proceedings of the Institution of Civil Engineers* Vol 71 (2) p197, 1981.
. Hideo Kawai, 'Waste stabilization pond design in Brazil',

Companhaide Technologia de Saneamento Ambiental, (Sao Paolo, Brazil, 1982).

85. R.M. Bradley, 'BOD removal efficiencies in two stabilization lagoons in series in Malaysia', *Journal of Water Pollution Control* Vol 82 No 1, 1983.

86. J.P. Lumbers, 'Discussion: the development of design equations for facultative waste stabilization ponds in semi-arid areas, by J.P. Arthur, *Proceedings of the Institution of Civil Engineers Part 2*, Vol 73 p225, 1982.

87. D.D. Mara, *Sewage treatment in hot climates*, (Wiley, London, 1976)

88. P.J. Meynell, *A feasibility study for a sanitaiton scheme to produce biogas from human waste in Kiriiapone Shany, Colombo, Sri Lanka*, (Report for Save the Children Federation, Intermediate Technology Consultants Ltd, London, 1979).

89. P.J. Meynell, *Methane, planning a digester*, Second edition, (Prism Press, Dorchester, UK, 1982).

90. Bioenergy systems report, (USAID, March 1982).

91. P.J. Meynell and C. McKone, *A proposal for an FAO programme for energy use and conservation in agricultural co-operatives and other rural groups*, (Plunkett Foundation, Oxford, UK, 1981).

92. ESCAP *Guidebook on biogas development*, Energy Resources Development Series No 21, (United Nations, New York, USA, 1980).

93. S. Subramian, with A. Barnett and L. Pyle, *Biogas technology in the Third World: a multidisciplinary review*, (IRDC, Ottawa, Canada, 1978).

94. M. McGarry and J. Stainforth, *Compost, fertiliser and biogas production from human and farm wastes in the People's Republic of China*, (IDRC, Ottawa, 1978).

95. R. Feachem et al, *Health aspects of exreta and wastewater management*, Energy, Water and Telecommunications Department, (The World Bank, Washington DC, USA, 1978).

96. *Manual of septic tank practice*, Publication No 526, (US Department of Health, Education and Welfare, Public Health Service, Washington DC, USA, August 1959).

97. *Participation of women in water supply and sanitation, roles and realities*, (IRC, The Hague, Netherlands).

98. United Republic of Tanzania, 'Water master plans for Iringa, Ruvuma and Mbeya Regions', *Socio-Economic Studies*, Vol 13, 1983.

99. D.J. Bradley, 'Water supplies: the consequences of change', in *Human rights in health*, ed. K. Elliott, Ciba Foundation Symposium 23, (Associated Scientific Publishers, Amsterdam, 1974, pp. 81-98).

100. R.G. Feachem, D.J. Bradley, H. Garelick and D.D. Mara, *Appropriate Technology for Water Supply and Sanitation*, Vol 3 'Health aspects of

excreta and sullage management', p.62, (World Bank, Washington DC, 1981).

11. T. McKeown, *The role of medicine*, (Blackwell, Oxford, 1979); also T. McKeown and C.R. Lowe, *An introduction to social medicine*, (Blackwell, Oxford, 2nd edition, 1974, page 15).

2. C. Dyhouse, 'Good wives and little mothers: social anxieties and the school-girl's curriculum, 1890-1920', *Oxford Review of Education*, Vol 3 (1977), pp 21-35.

3. Everett M. Rogers, *Modernization among peasants*, (Holt, Rinehart and Winston, New York, 1969, p.71).

. Two factors that have contributed to high literacy in Kerala are (a) the educational traditions of the long-established Christian community, and (b) a high level of political awareness leading to wide newspaper circulation in the local language: the latter is connected with a long history of trade union activity and the rivalry between two communist parties. Reading habits are discussed by Aiyappan, *Social revolution in a Kerala village*, pp 92-5, Asia Publishing House, London, 1965.

05. The ultimate source for the statistics quoted here is usually the Office of the Registrar General, New Delhi, which publishes *Sample Registration Bulletin* (twice yearly) and *Provisional population totals; census of India 1981* (editor P. Padmanabha). But due to the many problems of interpretation of the data, more useful sources are R.H. Cassen, *India: population, economy, society*, (Macmillan, London and Basingstoke, 1978); and T. P. Dyson, 'Preliminary Demography of 1981 Census', *Economic and Political Weekly* (Bombay), vol. 16, No 33, August 15, 1981, pp. 1349-54. I have also benefitted from more informal contact with T. P. Dyson and Professor K.N. Udupa.

06. A. Aiyappan, *Social revolution in a Kerala village*, (Asia Publishing House, London, 1965, pages 102-4).

07. Consortium on Rural Technology, *Rural sanitation: technology options*, Delhi, Institute of Social Studies Trust, 1981, pages 32, 49-68.

08. In 1973, for example, per capita expenditure on public health was 2.92 Rupees in Kerala compared with an average of 3.76 Rupees in all-India. Spending on clinics and other aspects of medicine, by contrast, was higher than average.

09. C. Goyder, 'Voluntary and government sanitation programmes', in *Sanitation in developing countries*, ed. Arnold Pacey, (Wiley, Chichester and New York, pages 162-167).

10. R. Chambers, R. Longhurst and A. Pacey, *Seasonal dimensions to rural poverty*, (Frances Pinter, London, 1981, page 231).

11. R.H. Cassen, *India: population, economy, society*, Macmillan, London and Basingstoke, 1978; also, P.M. Blaikie, *Family planning in India*, (Edward Arnold, London, 1975).

112. Rogers, op. cit. (see ref 103 above), page 68.
113. Aiyappan, op. cit. (see ref 106 above), pp. 92-101.
114. N.T. Mathew and W. Scott, *A development monitoring service at the local level*, Vol 1, 'Socio-economic observation areas in Kerala', (Geneva, UNRISD, 1980).
115. W.A. Smith, 'Do visual instructions make a difference?', *Appropriate technology for health*, a WHO Newsletter, No 10, 1981, pages 14-15.
116. S.M.L. Laver, *Designing instructional support media for sanitation development projects at community level in Zimbabwe. An interim report on the development of media strategies*, (Mimeograph, Department of Community Medicine, University of Zimbabwe, September, 1985).
117. R.A. Boydell, *An evaluation of a number of Blair VIP latrines, drilled boreholes, hand-dug wells and hand-augered boreholes recently constructed in Masvingo Province*, (Mimeograph, Ministry of Health/GTZ, Zimbabwe, September 1984.
118. R.G. Feachem, 'Interventions for the control of diarrhoeal diseases among young children: promotion of personal and domestic hygiene', *Bulletin of the World Health Organization* 62(3), 467-476, 1984.
119. T.M. Boot, *Making the links: Guidelines for hygiene education in community water supply and sanitation*, (IRC, The Hague, 1984).
120. H. Perret, *Social feasibility analysis in low-cost sanitation projects*, TAG No. 5, (World Bank, Washington DC, 1983).
121. M. Herbert-Simpson, *Methods for gathering socio-cultural data for water supply and sanitation projects*, TAG Tech. Note No. 1, (World Bank, Washington, 1983).
122. A. Acra et al., *Solar disinfection of drinking water and oral rehydration solutions*, (UNICEF, Jordan, 1986).
123. J.H. Hubley, 'Principles of health education', *British Medical Journal*, 289, 1054-1056, 1984.
124. H. Perret, *Planning of communication support (information motivation and education) in sanitation projects and programmes*, TAG Tech. Note No. 2, (World Bank, Washington, 1983).
125. D. Hilton, *Health teaching for West Africa - stories, drama and song*, (MAP International, Illinois, 1980).
126. J. Jenkins, *Mass media for health education*, IEC Broadsheets on Distance Learning No. 18, (International Extension College, Cambridge, 1983).
127. E.M. Rogers, L.Shoemaker, *Communications of innovations - a cross-cultural approach*, (Free Press, New York, 1971).
128. *Diarrhoeal disease control - examples of health education materials*, (WHO Diarrhoeal Diseases Control Programme, Geneva, 1982).
129. B. Karlin, R.B. Isely, *Developing and using audio-visual materials in*

water supply and sanitation programs, Wash Technical Report No. 30, (Water and Sanitation Health Project (WASH/USAID), Washington, DC, 1984).

0. A. White, *Community participation in water and sanitation. Concepts, strategies and methods*, Tech. Paper Series No. 17, (IRC, 1981).

1. R. Feachem, 'Community participation in appropriate water supply and sanitation technologies', *Proc. R. Soc. Lond*, B 209, 1980.

2. M. Boot, *Making the Links*, Occasional Paper, (IRC, Rijswijk, The Netherlands, 1984).

www.ingramcontent.com/pod-product-compliance
Lightning Source LLC
Chambersburg PA
CBHW070906030426
42336CB00014BA/2316